Monitoring
Critical Functions

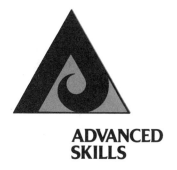

**ADVANCED
SKILLS**

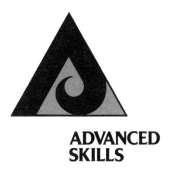

ADVANCED SKILLS

Monitoring Critical Functions

Springhouse Corporation
Springhouse, Pennsylvania

Staff

Executive Director, Editorial
Stanley Loeb

Senior Publisher
Matthew Cahill

Art Director
John Hubbard

Senior Editor
Stephen Daly

Clinical Project Director
Patricia Dwyer Schull, RN, MSN

Editors
Elizabeth Weinstein, Neal Fandek, Kathy Goldberg, Elizabeth Mauro

Clinical Editors
Tina R. Dietrich, RN, BSN, CCRN; Mary Jane McDevitt, RN, BS

Copy Editors
Cynthia C. Breuninger *(supervisor)*, Doris Weinstock, Priscilla DeWitt, Nancy Papsin

Designers
Stephanie Peters *(associate art director)*, Matie Patterson *(senior designer)*, Linda Franklin, Joseph Laufer

Illustrators
Michael Adams, Jackie Facciolo, Jean Gardner, John Gallagher, Linda Gist, Frank Grobelny, Bob Jackson, Robert Neumann, Judy Newhouse, Gary Phillips, George Retseck, Larry Ward

Art Production
Anet Oakes, Ann Raphun, Robert Wieder

Typography
David Kosten *(director)*, Diane Paluba *(manager)*, Elizabeth Bergman, Joyce Rossi Biletz, Phyllis Marron, Robin Mayer, Valerie Rosenberger

Manufacturing
Deborah Meiris *(manager)*, Anna Brindisi, T.A. Landis

Production Coordination
Patricia W. McCloskey

Editorial Assistants
Maree DeRosa, Beverly Lane, Mary Madden

AS5-010693

Library of Congress Cataloging-in-Publication Data
Monitoring critical functions.
    p.   cm. — (Advanced Skills)
    Includes bibliographical references and index.
    1. Intensive care nursing.
    2. Patient monitoring.
    I. Springhouse Corporation. II. Series.
    [DNLM: 1. Monitoring, Physiologic — methods. WB 142 M744 1993]
RT120.I5M65 1993
610.73'61 — dc20
DNLM/DLC   93-3447
ISBN 0-87434-555-3   CIP

Contents

Advisory board

At the time of publication, the advisors
held the following positions.

Cecelia Gatson Grindel, RN, PhD
Nurse Researcher
Lehigh Valley Hospital
Allentown, Pa.

Judith Ski Lower, RN, MSN, CCRN, CNRN
Nurse Manager, Neurology Critical Care Unit
Johns Hopkins Hospital
Baltimore

Kathleen M. Malloch, RN, BSN, MBA, CNA
Vice President, Patient Care Services
Del Webb Memorial Hospital
Sun City West, Ariz.

Marguerite K. Schlag, RN, MSN, EdD
Director, Nursing Education and Development
Robert Wood Johnson University Hospital
New Brunswick, N.J.

Karen L. Then, RN, MN
Assistant Professor, Faculty of Nursing
University of Calgary, Alberta

Contributors

At the time of publication, the contributors held the following positions.

Marcy L. Diethorn, RN, MSN
Director, Professional Education Services
Baxter Healthcare Corp.
Edwards Critical-Care Division
Irvine, Calif.

Tina R. Dietrich, RN, BSN, CCRN
Staff Nurse, Coronary Care
St. Luke's Hospital
Bethlehem, Pa.

Ellie Z. Franges, RN, MSN, CCRN
Patient Care Manager
Lehigh Valley Hospital
Allentown, Pa.

Paula Harrison Gillman, RN, MSN, CCRN
Clinical Affairs Specialist
Baxter Healthcare Corp.
Edwards Critical-Care Division
Irvine, Calif.

Jan M. Headley, RN, BS
Senior Education Consultant
Baxter Healthcare Corp.
Edwards Critical-Care Division
Irvine, Calif.

Pamela Kasold, RN, BSN, CCRN
Clinical Education Manager
St. Jude Medical, Inc.
Cardiac Assist Division
Chelmsford, Mass.

Dianne M. Lameier, RN, MSN
Electrophysiology Clinical Nurse Specialist
University of Cincinnati Medical Center

Barbara Leeper, RN, MN, CCRN
Cardiovascular Clinical Nurse Specialist
Baylor University Medical Center
Dallas

Patricia A. McGaffigan, RN,C, MS
Clinical Education Manager
Nellcor, Inc.
Hayward, Calif.

Suzanne D. Skinner, RN, MS
Nursing Education Consultant
Severna Park, Md.

Gloria Sonnesso, RN, MSN, CCRN
Pulmonary Clinical Specialist
Philadelphia

Eileen Suida, RN
Staff Nurse, Labor and Delivery
Abington (Pa.) Hospital

FOREWORD

More than ever before, your responsibilities are likely to include the use of sophisticated monitoring devices. And working with monitors can challenge even the most seasoned nurse: You must first carry out complex procedures to initiate monitoring and then be ready to respond if something goes wrong. You must also constantly update your knowledge to stay abreast of equipment advances, new procedures, and revised techniques.

To meet these responsibilities effectively, you need more than just a passing familiarity with monitoring techniques. You need complete, up-to-date information. Until now, to keep up with technological changes and to learn the required skills, you had to search through journals, manuals, and reference books. Fortunately, *Monitoring Critical Functions* puts an end to your search. The latest book in the Advanced Skills series, it presents both background information and the specific skills you need to monitor your patient effectively.

This book will guide both the nurse who is new to monitoring and the experienced nurse who needs a quick, up-to-date reference. What's more, it emphasizes patient-centered care to help you avoid a common pitfall—becoming so involved in the technical details of monitoring that you inadvertently overlook some aspect of your patient's care.

The book consists of 10 chapters. The first chapter covers cardiac monitoring, including continuous electrocardiographic (ECG) monitoring and ST-segment monitoring. Chapter 2 helps you understand the whys and hows of hemodynamic monitoring. Reading this chapter will prepare you for the two chapters that follow, which cover arterial pressure monitoring (Chapter 3) and pulmonary artery pressure and central venous pressure monitoring (Chapter 4).

Chapter 5 explains how to monitor cardiac output, a key index of cardiac function. Chapter 6 describes how to monitor your patient's neurologic status, including intracranial pressure (ICP) monitoring and cerebral blood flow monitoring. Chapter 7 presents the latest techniques in monitoring gas exchange, such as pulse oximetry, transcutaneous oxygen and carbon dioxide monitoring, and end-tidal carbon dioxide monitoring.

Chapter 8 makes the complicated procedures of fetal monitoring easy to understand. In this chapter, you'll learn how to initiate both external and internal electronic fetal monitoring. Chapter 9 explains how to monitor your patient's fluid and electrolyte status — essential for safeguarding his renal and metabolic functions. Chapter 10 covers important monitoring techniques outside the scope of the other chapters. The topics here include intra-aortic balloon counterpulsation, automated vital signs monitoring, and pulse amplitude monitoring.

For your convenience, most chapters follow the same format. After a brief introduction, the chapter reviews essential physiology. Next come separate entries, each covering a different monitoring method or technique. Each entry includes a section that describes the equipment you'll work with, explains how to prepare the patient and equipment, presents the procedure you'll use to initiate monitoring and obtain values, explains how to interpret findings, and discusses nursing considerations that will help you ensure high-quality care.

In a departure from the standard format, Chapter 2 focuses on the physiologic and technical factors that affect pressure monitoring, the chief components and setup procedure for any pressure monitoring system, and ways to verify the accuracy of the values you obtain.

As you use this book, you'll come upon logos — graphic devices that focus your attention on key pieces of information. The *Advanced equipment* logo signals a detailed look at sophisticated and sometimes new equipment you'll be working with. *Troubleshooting* highlights information that will help you detect and correct monitoring problems. *Complications* alerts you to patient problems that may arise during monitoring. *Physiology* accents the basic body functions associated with a particular type of monitoring. *Clinical preview* presents a case study of a hospitalized patient, showing how a particular monitoring technique was used corrrectly or incorrectly by the health care team.

You'll also find many helpful monitor strips, photographs, illustrations, and charts throughout the book. For example, Chapter 1 includes ECG strips that indicate various arrhythmias,

and Chapter 8 presents a wide range of fetal monitor strips. In Chapter 7, a photographic guide shows how to set up a mixed venous oxygen saturation monitoring system. Chapter 6 includes a chart that compares four types of ICP monitoring systems.

Following the last chapter is a listing of other books and articles on monitoring recommended by the authors. Next, you'll find the *Advanced skilltest,* a multiple-choice self-test that lets you assess what you've learned and detect which areas of monitoring you need to review. The answers, along with complete rationales, immediately follow the test.

I recommend *Monitoring Critical Functions* for all nurses. You'll appreciate the many useful features and the straightforward writing. As you monitor your patients, you'll turn to this comprehensive, easy-to-use guide again and again. Whether you're maintaining a sophisticated monitoring system for a gravely ill patient or analyzing your patient's serial laboratory values for dangerous trends, this book will enhance your skills and boost your confidence. By drawing on its wealth of knowledge, you can monitor your patients in the safest, most effective way.

Gloria Sonnesso, RN, MSN, CCRN

Pulmonary Clinical Specialist
Philadelphia

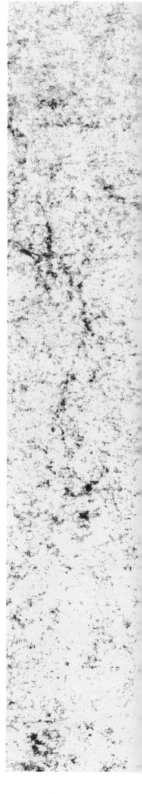

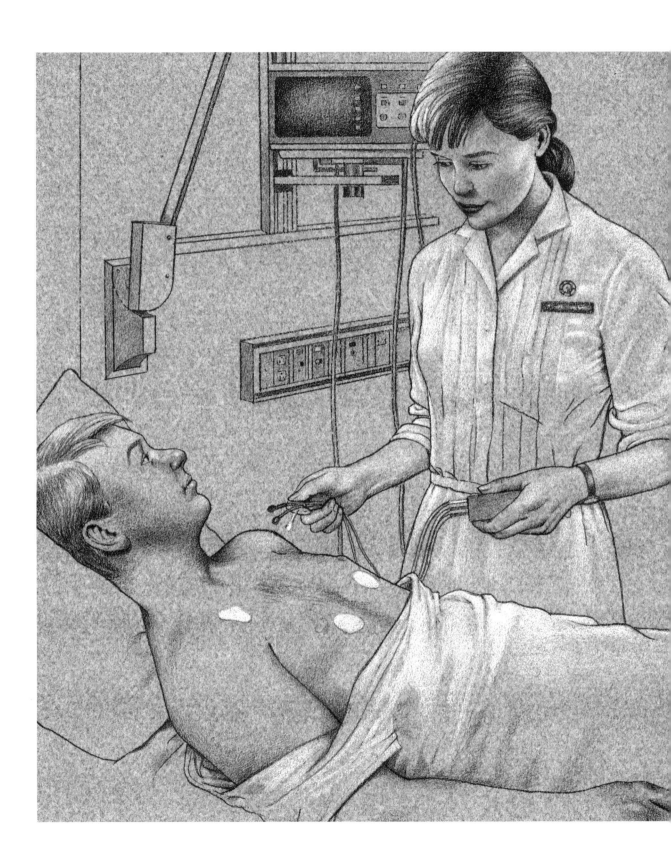

CHAPTER

Performing cardiac monitoring

Cardiac monitoring has gained extensive use since the first coronary care unit opened in the United States in 1962. Nurses now rely on this technique to monitor the patient's heart rate and rhythm, detect arrhythmias, and help evaluate a patient's response to drug therapy. In fact, the technology for cardiac monitoring systems now exists to store recorded arrhythmias electronically for several hours, to record multiple leads on the strip chart, and to monitor ST segments for displacement during myocardial ischemia or other events.

During the past 30 years, clinicians have developed more reliable criteria for diagnosing arrhythmias and conduction disturbances through cardiac monitoring. They've also identified precursors to such life-threatening arrhythmias as ventricular tachycardia, ventricular fibrillation, and asystole.

Using cardiac monitoring, you can recognize these disturbances quickly and intervene immediately to save the patient's life. In fact, over

PHYSIOLOGY

The heart's conduction system

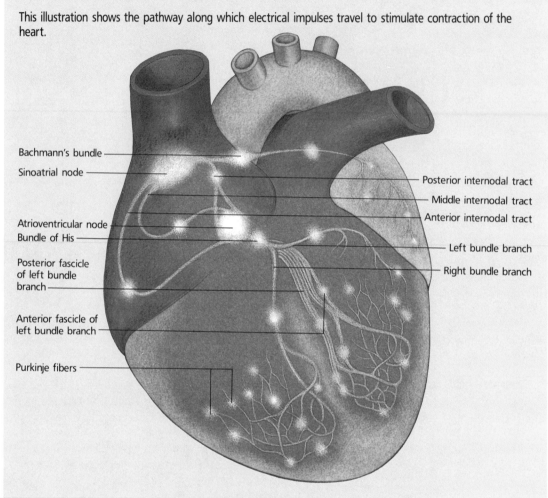

This illustration shows the pathway along which electrical impulses travel to stimulate contraction of the heart.

Bachmann's bundle

Sinoatrial node

Atrioventricular node

Bundle of His

Posterior fascicle of left bundle branch

Anterior fascicle of left bundle branch

Purkinje fibers

Posterior internodal tract

Middle internodal tract

Anterior internodal tract

Left bundle branch

Right bundle branch

the past three decades, cardiac monitoring and early nursing intervention have reduced in-hospital mortality associated with myocardial infarction (MI) from roughly 50% to about 15%.

Previously, patients undergoing cardiac monitoring had to remain directly connected to a bedside monitor via hardwire cables. Now, with telemetry as an option, patients can be monitored from a remote location. Telemetry is widely used in intensive care units, step-down or intermediate care units, recovery rooms, emergency departments, and labor and delivery departments. Some patients even use it at home.

In this chapter, you'll find a review of the principles underlying cardiac monitoring. The chapter also discusses the equipment required for continuous electrocardiogram (ECG) and ST-segment monitoring and tells how to prepare the patient and the equipment for each procedure. After describing the steps you'll take to initiate monitoring, the chapter explains how to interpret findings and presents important nursing considerations.

Cardiac conduction

The heart's conduction system consists of a specialized group of tissues that generates, receives, and transmits electrical impulses. These impulses travel through the myocardium, causing the myocardial cells to depolarize and then mechanically contract. Afterward, they repolarize, becoming electrically recharged until they reach a resting, or polarized, state.

Normally, an electrical impulse begins in the sinoatrial (SA) node, located near the right atrium where the superior vena cava joins the right atrium. The SA node acts as the heart's primary pacemaker because its automatic firing rate exceeds that of the heart's other pacemaker tissues.

From the SA node, the impulse travels through the right atrium along internodal tracts to the atrioventricular (AV) node. Situated in the right atrium between the coronary sinus and the septal cusp of the tricuspid valve, the AV node briefly delays the impulse to give the atria time to contract.

From the AV node, the impulse travels through the bundle of His and the right and left bundle branches to the Purkinje fibers, where it triggers ventricular depolarization. (See *The heart's conduction system.*)

Continuous ECG monitoring

Electrical impulses moving through the heart's conduction system create electrical currents, or vectors, that can be monitored on the body's surface. Electrodes placed on the patient's extremities and chest wall detect the vectors and transmit them to the ECG machine. This device measures and averages the differences between the electrical potential of each electrode site for each lead and graphs them over time. This creates the ECG complex, or waveform.

The various components of the ECG waveform represent the phases of the depolarization-repolarization cycle. The P wave represents

ECG waveform components

The three basic components of an electrocardiogram (ECG) waveform are the P wave, the QRS complex, and the T wave. These components can be further broken down into a PR interval, QT interval, ST segment, and U wave.

The *P wave* represents atrial depolarization. The *QRS complex,* a series of deflections, represents ventricular depolarization. Its normal duration is 0.10 second or less. The *PR interval,* representing atrioventricular conduction, measures from the beginning of the P wave to the beginning of the QRS complex. Normally, it has a duration of 0.12 to 0.20 second but remains constant in each individual.

The *ST segment,* representing part of ventricular repolarization, measures from the end of the QRS complex to the beginning of the T wave. It's usually an isoelectric line. The *T wave* represents ventricular repolarization. The *U wave* sometimes follows the T wave.

The *QT interval* shows the time the ventricle takes to depolarize and repolarize. It extends from the beginning of the Q wave to the end of the T wave.

Normal ECG waveform

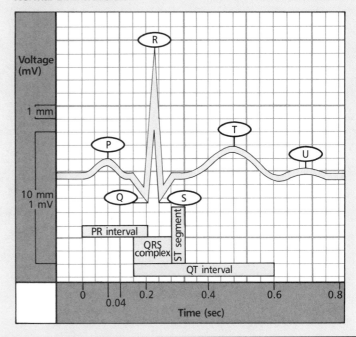

atrial depolarization; the PR interval, impulse conduction through the AV node and bundle branches; and the QRS complex, ventricular depolarization. (See *ECG waveform components.*)

(Text continues on page 6.)

Creating monitoring leads

This chart shows the correct electrode positions for some of the monitoring leads you'll use most often. For each lead, you'll see electrode placement for a five-leadwire system, a three-leadwire system, and a telemetry system.

In the two hardwire systems, the electrode positions for one lead may be identical to the electrode positions for another lead. In this case, you simply change the lead selector switch to the setting that corresponds to the lead you want. In some cases, you'll need to reposition the electrodes.

In the telemetry system, you can create the same lead with two electrodes that you do with three, simply by eliminating the ground electrode.

The chart uses these abbreviations: RA, right arm; LA, left arm; RL, right leg; LL, left leg; C, chest; and G, ground.

FIVE-LEADWIRE SYSTEM	THREE-LEADWIRE SYSTEM	TELEMETRY SYSTEM
Lead I		

| **Lead II** | | |

| **Lead III** | | |

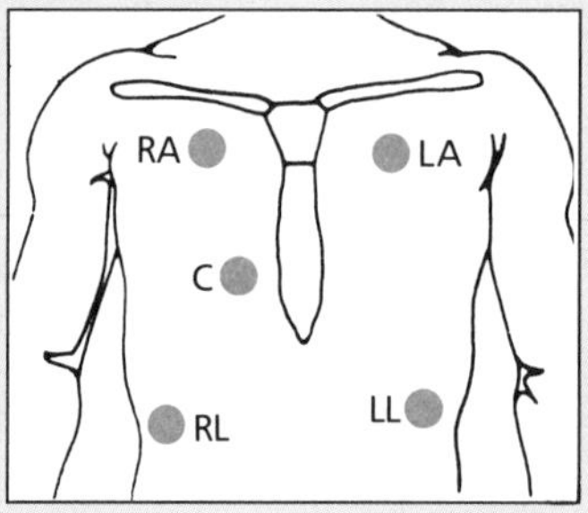

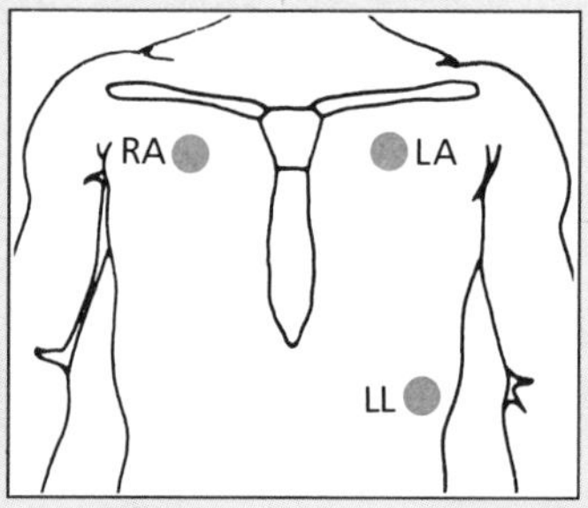

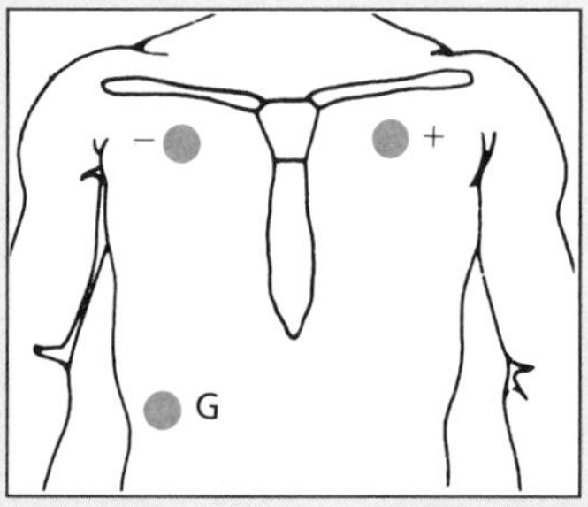

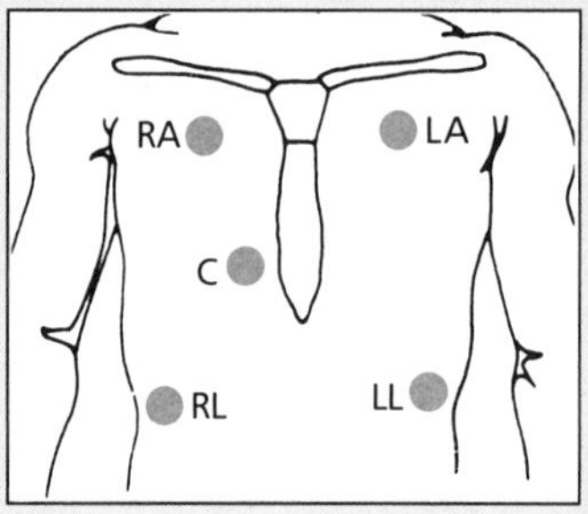

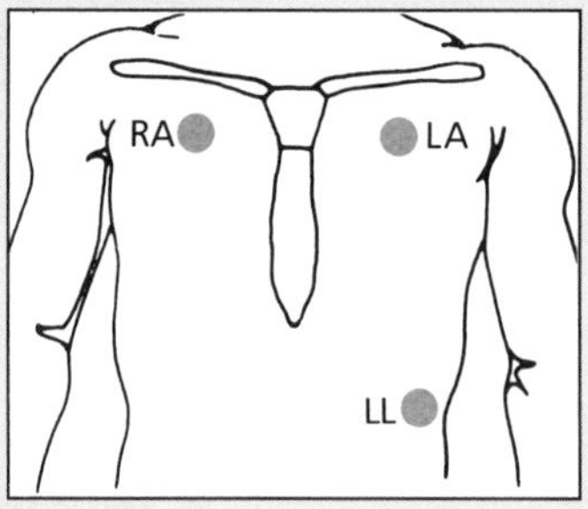

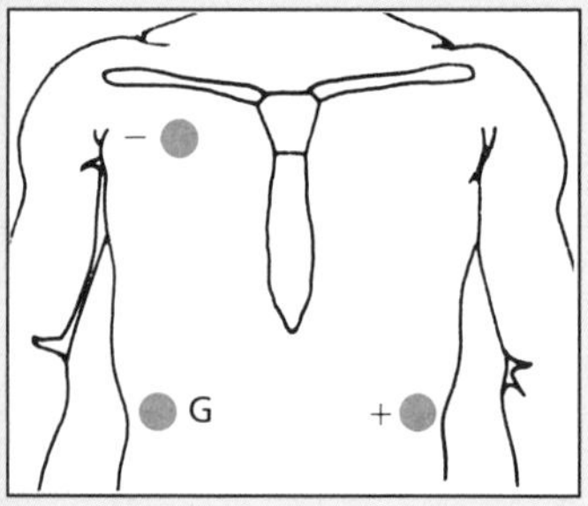

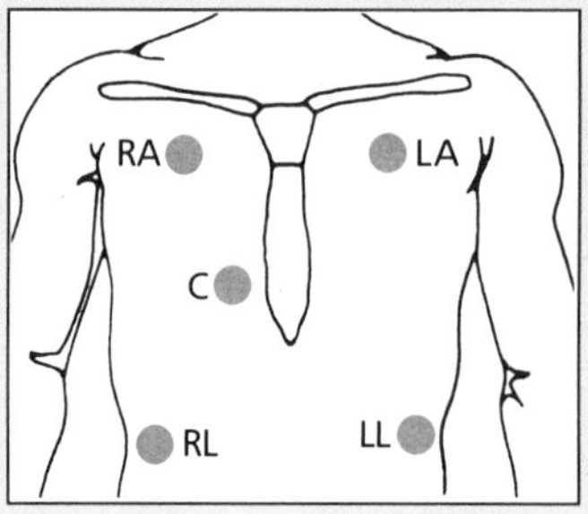

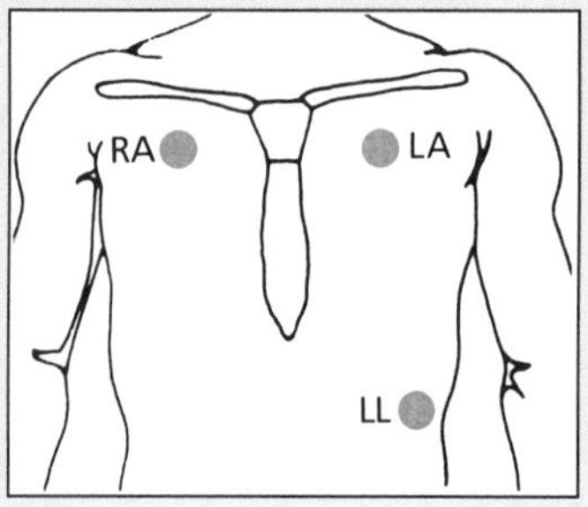

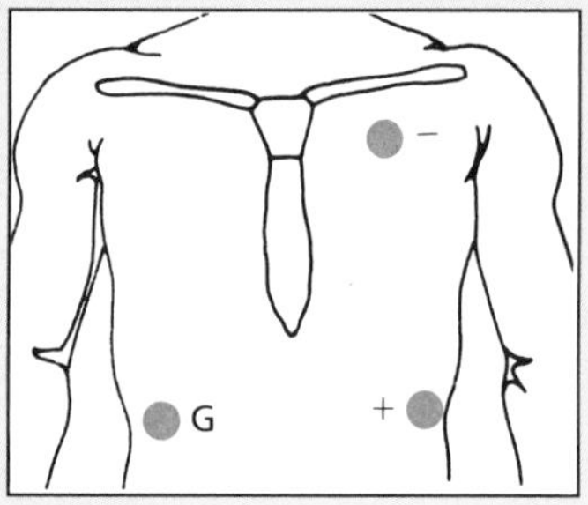

FIVE-LEADWIRE SYSTEM	THREE-LEADWIRE SYSTEM	TELEMETRY SYSTEM

Lead MCL₁

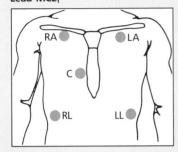 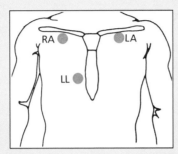 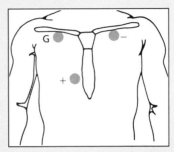

Lead MCL₆

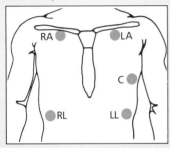 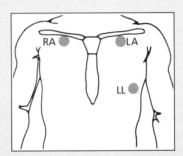 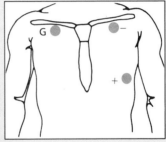

Sternal lead

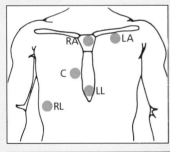 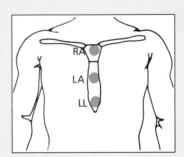 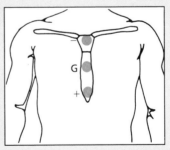

Lewis lead

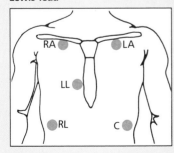 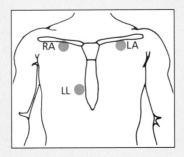 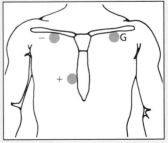

Monitoring leads

ECG waveform configuration depends on electrode position relative to the heart's electrical field. ECG monitoring leads may be bipolar or unipolar. A bipolar lead consists of two electrodes (one positive and one negative), placed at opposite poles of the heart's electrical field. A unipolar lead consists of a positive electrode placed on the skin and a central terminal within the ECG machine.

The positive electrode serves as the recording electrode. When electrical current travels *toward* this electrode, the ECG machine records a positive complex (one that's deflected above the baseline). When the current travels *away* from the positive electrode, the ECG machine records a negative complex (deflected below the baseline). If the current travels perpendicular to the positive electrode, the ECG records an isoelectric complex (equal deflections above and below the baseline).

In a standard 12-lead ECG, the first six leads show the heart's electrical activity from the frontal plane. These leads include three standard bipolar limb leads (I, II, and III) and three augmented unipolar limb leads (aV_R, aV_L, and aV_F).

Bipolar limb leads measure the difference in electrical potential between two electrodes. Placement of the negative and positive electrodes varies with each lead. For lead I, the negative electrode is placed on the patient's right arm and the positive electrode on the left arm. For lead II, the negative electrode goes on the right arm, the positive electrode on the left leg. For lead III, the negative electrode goes on the left arm, the positive electrode on the left leg. These three leads form an equilateral triangle around the heart.

With unipolar limb leads, the positive electrode is placed on the right arm for aV_R, on the left arm for aV_L, and on the left leg for aV_F. The axis of each unipolar limb lead lies perpendicular to the axis of one of the bipolar leads. Leads I and aV_L face the lateral wall of the left ventricle, whereas leads II, III, and aV_F face the inferior surface, and lead aV_R faces the posterior surface of the heart.

The other six leads in a 12-lead ECG, called chest or V leads, are unipolar and record the heart's activity on the horizontal plane. The positive electrode for these leads is placed at specific points across the anterior chest wall. Leads V_2, V_3, and V_4 face the anterior wall of the left ventricle, whereas leads V_5 and V_6 face its lateral wall. V_1 is the only routinely recorded chest lead that faces the right side of the heart. (See *Creating monitoring leads,* pages 4 and 5.)

Normally, electrical impulses travel through the heart in a leftward, inferior direction, toward the left iliac crest. As a result, leads I, II, and aV_F largely display an upward deflection, whereas lead aV_R displays a downward deflection. Leads III and aV_L vary. Lead V_1 displays mostly a downward deflection. The rest of the leads show a gradual increase in R-wave amplitude and a gradual decrease in S-wave depth. Thus, leads V_5 and V_6 display a largely upward deflection.

Two other leads, the Lewis lead and the sternal lead, may also be used. The varying P waves associated with atrial arrhythmias are particularly visible when you monitor in the Lewis lead. With the sternal lead, electrode placement on the sternum helps stabilize the ECG pattern.

Modified chest lead

Initially, lead II was the standard lead used for continuous, single-lead ECG monitoring. However, the modified chest lead (MCL), a bipolar lead, now is sometimes used instead. MCL shows the heart from the horizontal plane, producing a view similar to the one shown by the six chest leads. Place the negative electrode on the patient's left shoulder, just below the middle of the clavicle; place the positive electrode at any of the six positions used for chest leads. This lead is further labeled according to where you place the positive electrode—for instance, MCL_1 if you place it in the fourth intercostal space along the right sternal border, or MCL_6 if you place it in the fifth intercostal space along the left midaxillary line.

Equipment

Most monitoring systems display a single lead on the monitor and simultaneously record one or two leads. However, some models display

Simultaneous monitoring

Monitoring in two leads provides a more complete picture than monitoring in one lead. With simultaneous dual monitoring, you'll generally review the first lead—usually designated as the primary lead—for arrhythmias. A two-lead view also helps detect episodic beats or rhythms. Leads II and V₁ are the two leads most often monitored simultaneously.

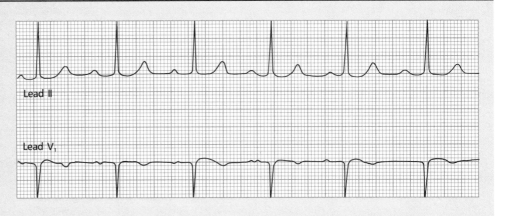

Lead II

Lead V₁

---

multiple leads and graphically record two or more leads. (See *Simultaneous monitoring.*)

You'll probably use a three- or five-electrode system. A three-electrode system permits monitoring of one or two leads. With a five-electrode system, you can monitor seven leads (I, II, III, aV_R, aV_L, aV_F, and one chest lead).

Preparation
Preparing the patient
Explain the purpose of ECG monitoring to the patient and his family to help reduce their anxiety. Explain how the rate alarms work. If your unit or department has a central station with a telemetry technician, reassure the patient that a staff member will observe the monitor at all times. Emphasize that the monitor will *not* alert caregivers to symptoms, such as pain or shortness of breath.

Remove all nongrounded electrical equipment from the patient's room. These items may interfere with the waveform and thus give false readings. To prepare the patient's skin for electrode placement, first shave any excess hair at the site you wish to place the electrode. Then remove all dirt, moisture, surface hair, and old skin, using alcohol sponges if desired to clean the skin. To promote better skin-electrode contact and ensure good tracing quality, rub the skin until it's red.

Various electrode patches are available. Some consist of a foam pad with a small sponge in the center; the sponge is permeated with a conduction gel that promotes impulse transmission. Other electrode patches consist of paper tape with a sponge center.

For best results, attach the electrode to the monitoring wire before applying it to the patient. To attach the electrode, simply snap it onto the monitoring wire.

Preparing the equipment
Turn the bedside monitor on and set the upper and lower limits of the heart rate alarm. If the patient has a pacemaker, activate the pacemaker channel to avoid double sensing of pacemaker artifacts and QRS complexes. For telemetry monitoring, make sure to use the appropriate transmitter. Some transmitter models are designed for a specific channel on the central display station. With others, a transmitter can be assigned to a channel when the patient is admitted; should the unit malfunction, another transmitter is assigned to that channel.

Procedure
• Correct electrode placement is crucial for obtaining clear, accurate information. For a five-electrode system, place each of the four limb

electrodes as follows. Place the *white* (right arm) electrode below the right clavicle, the *black* (left arm) electrode below the left clavicle, the *green* (right leg) electrode on the right lower anterior rib cage, the *red* (left leg) electrode on the left lower anterior rib cage, and the *brown* (chest) electrode in any one of the chest lead positions (V_1 through V_6).

Be especially careful when placing the electrodes for leads II and V_1 or MCL_1. Some caregivers mistakenly place the positive electrode for lead II too high on the patient's chest. To ensure accurate results, make sure to place it below heart level (lower than the sixth intercostal space). Be sure to place the positive electrode for V_1 or MCL_1 on the fourth intercostal space rather than over the rib, on the sternum, or on any other intercostal space.
• Once you've properly positioned the electrodes and attached the leadwires, move the cable to one side of the patient's gown to allow movement.
• For telemetry monitoring, place the transmitter on one side of the patient's body. Or you may place it in a special disposable holder, if available. (For instance, some holders can be tied around the patient's neck.) Some hospitals supply special patient gowns with a front pocket designed to hold the transmitter.

Interpretation of findings

An arrhythmia is classified as a sinus, atrial, junctional, or ventricular arrhythmia or an AV block.

Sinus arrhythmias result from functional disturbances in the SA node, the heart's primary pacemaker. Normally, the SA node has the least negative charge during the resting phase of the depolarization-repolarization cycle. Also, depolarization normally begins during the resting phase. A sinus arrhythmia may occur if other conduction tissue has a more negative charge or if depolarization doesn't begin during the resting phase. Sinus arrhythmias include sinus bradycardia, sinus tachycardia, sinus arrhythmia, and sinus arrest.

Reentry of an impulse or enhanced automaticity of atrial tissue may cause *atrial arrhythmias*. The most common arrhythmias, atrial arrhythmias may shorten diastole, reduc-

ing ventricular filling and coronary artery perfusion. They also may diminish atrial kick. When reentry triggers an atrial arrhythmia, the underlying cause may be ischemia, electrolyte abnormalities, or drugs that lead to slow, one-way impulse conduction through atrial tissue. When enhanced automaticity triggers an atrial arrhythmia, the underlying cause may be digitalis toxicity, elevated catecholamine levels, hypoxia, or electrolyte abnormalities. Atrial arrhythmias include premature atrial contraction, atrial tachycardia, atrial flutter, and atrial fibrillation.

Junctional arrhythmias originate in the AV junction—the area around the AV node and the bundle of His. These arrhythmias usually result from suppression of a higher pacemaker or impulse blockage at the AV node. Junctional arrhythmias include junctional rhythm, premature junctional contraction, and junctional tachycardia.

Ventricular arrhythmias arise in ventricular tissue below the bifurcation of the bundle of His. They may result from reentry, enhanced automaticity, or afterdepolarization. Ventricular arrhythmias include premature ventricular contraction, ventricular tachycardia, and ventricular fibrillation.

AV blocks are caused by an abnormal interruption or delay in conduction of atrial impulses to the ventricle. Such blocks may be partial or total and may occur in the AV node, bundle of His, or Purkinje system. Studies show that AV block can occur in patients with normal hearts when atrial rates reach 125 to 150 beats/minute.

Each arrhythmia causes distinctive changes in the ECG waveform. (For the characteristics of common arrhythmias, see *Recognizing common arrhythmias*.)

Nursing considerations

• Be sure to check the expiration dates on the electrodes before placing them on the patient.
• Observe the ECG monitor for changes that suggest arrhythmias and other problems at least every 15 to 30 minutes.
• Regularly assess the patient's skin for redness

(Text continues on page 13.)

Recognizing common arrhythmias

If your patient is undergoing cardiac monitoring, you can use the descriptions and waveforms below to help identify some common arrhythmias.

Sinus arrhythmia

Distinguishing characteristics
◆ *Atrial rhythm:* irregular; difference between longest and shortest P-P interval exceeds 0.12 second
◆ *Ventricular rhythm:* irregular; difference between longest and shortest R-R interval exceeds 0.12 second
▲ *P wave:* normal size and configuration; P wave precedes each QRS complex

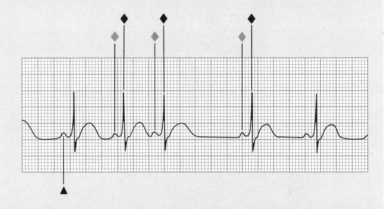

Wandering pacemaker

Distinguishing characteristics
◆ *Atrial rhythm:* varies slightly, irregular P-P interval
◆ *Ventricular rhythm:* varies slightly, irregular R-R interval
▲ *P wave:* changing size and configuration because of changing pacemaker; the P wave may also be absent or inverted, or it may appear after the QRS complex; a combination of these P-wave variations may appear on the waveform

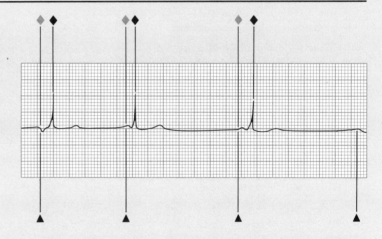

Premature atrial contractions

Distinguishing characteristics
▲ *P wave:* premature and abnormally shaped; possibly lost in previous T wave

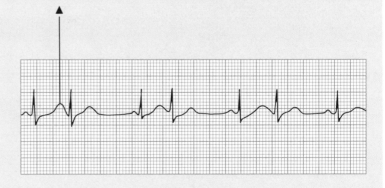

(continued)

Recognizing common arrhythmias *(continued)*

Paroxysmal atrial tachycardia

Distinguishing characteristics
- ◆ *Atrial rhythm:* regular
- ◆ *Ventricular rhythm:* regular
- ● *Atrial rate:* 160 to 250 beats/minute
- ● *Ventricular rate:* 160 to 250 beats/minute
- ▲ *P wave:* configuration abnormal
- ▲ *Other:* one P wave for each QRS complex

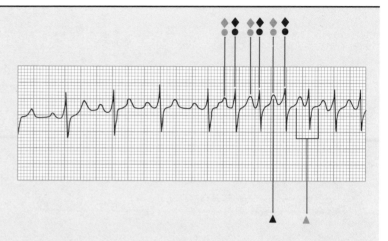

Fine atrial fibrillation

Distinguishing characteristics
- ◆ *Atrial rhythm:* grossly irregular
- ◆ *Ventricular rhythm:* grossly irregular
- ● *Atrial rate:* almost indiscernible; usually above 400 beats/minute
- ▲ *P wave:* absent; F waves with an erratic baseline (fibrillatory waves) appear in their place. Arrhythmia is termed *coarse atrial fibrillation* when F waves are pronounced, *fine atrial fibrillation* when they're not pronounced.
- ■ *QRS complex:* duration usually within normal limits

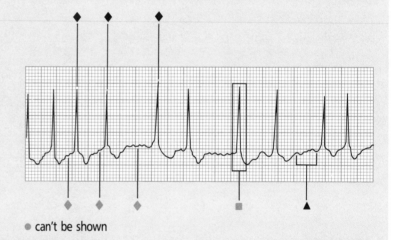

● can't be shown

Junctional tachycardia

Distinguishing characteristics
- ● *Atrial rate:* exceeds 100 beats/minute (usually from 100 to 180 beats/minute); however, rate may be impossible to determine if P wave is absent or hidden in QRS complex or preceding T wave
- ● *Ventricular rate:* exceeds 100 beats/minute (usually from 100 to 180 beats/minute)
- ▲ *P wave:* usually inverted; may appear before or after QRS complex or be hidden in QRS complex; may be absent
- ■ *PR interval:* if P wave occurs before QRS complex, PR interval is shortened (less than 0.12 second); otherwise, it can't be measured.
- ■ *QRS complex:* duration usually within normal limits; configuration usually normal

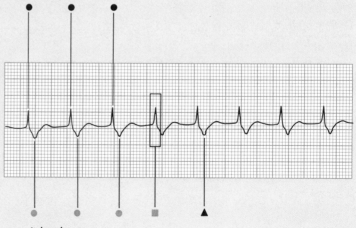

■ can't be shown

Recognizing common arrhythmias *(continued)*

Wolff-Parkinson-White (WPW) syndrome

Distinguishing characteristics
- *PR interval:* less than 0.1 second
- *QRS complex:* duration greater than 0.1 second; beginning may be slurred, producing a delta wave. In Type A WPW syndrome, delta wave and QRS complex are upright in precordial leads, as shown on this ECG strip. In Type B WPW syndrome, delta wave and QRS complex are inverted in V_1 and upright in V_5 and V_6.

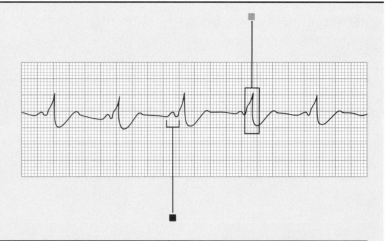

Type II second-degree atrioventricular (AV) block

Distinguishing characteristics
- *Atrial rhythm:* regular
- *Ventricular rhythm:* regular or irregular; pauses correspond to dropped beat
- *P wave:* normal size and configuration, but some P waves aren't followed by QRS complex; P-P interval containing nonconducted P wave equals two normal P-P intervals.
- *QRS complex:* periodically absent

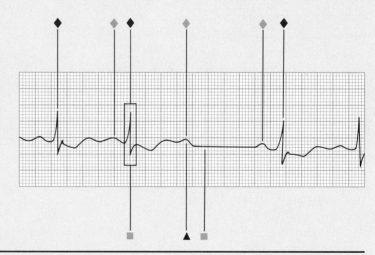

Complete AV dissociation

Distinguishing characteristics
- *Atrial rhythm:* regular, no relationship between atrial and ventricular rhythms
- *Ventricular rhythm:* regular
- *Atrial rate:* usually equal to ventricular rate
- *Ventricular rate:* usually equal to atrial rate, depending on underlying cause
- *QRS complex:* may be wide and bizarre, depending on location of ventricular pacemaker
- *T wave:* abnormal; may be altered or inverted, depending on the underlying cause

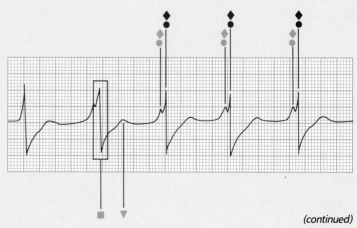

(continued)

Recognizing common arrhythmias *(continued)*

Premature ventricular contractions

Distinguishing characteristics

▲ *P wave:* absent

■ *PR interval:* not measurable

▨ *QRS complex:* occurs earlier than expected; duration exceeds 0.12 second; bizarre configuration

▼ *T wave:* occurs in direction opposite QRS complex

▲ *Other:* horizontal baseline, called compensatory pause, may follow the T wave.

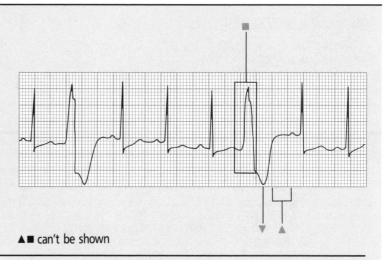

▲■ can't be shown

Ventricular tachycardia

Distinguishing characteristics

◆ *Atrial rhythm:* can't be determined

◆ *Ventricular rhythm:* usually regular but may be slightly irregular

● *Atrial rate:* can't be determined

● *Ventricular rate:* usually rapid (100 to 200 beats/minute)

▲ *P wave:* usually absent; may be obscured by QRS complex; retrograde P waves may be present

■ *PR interval:* not measurable

▨ *QRS complex:* duration exceeds 0.12 second; bizarre appearance, usually with increased amplitude

▼ *T wave:* occurs in opposite direction of QRS complex

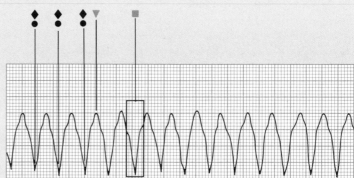

◆●▲■ can't be shown

Ventricular fibrillation

Distinguishing characteristics

◆ *Atrial rhythm:* can't be determined

◆ *Ventricular rhythm:* no pattern or regularity

● *Atrial rate:* can't be determined

● *Ventricular rate:* can't be determined

▲ *P wave:* indiscernible

▨ *QRS complex:* duration indiscernible

▲ *Other:* waveform is a wavy line; when the waves are large, the rhythm is coarse fibrillation; when the waves are small, the rhythm is fine fibrillation.

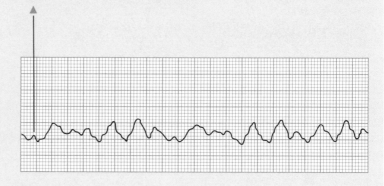

◆◆●●▲■ can't be shown

and blisters and note any complaints of itching at the electrode skin sites. These signs and symptoms may indicate an allergy to the electrode patch or conduction gel. Remove the electrode and try another type of electrode or gel.

• If recommended by the manufacturer, change the electrode patches daily. (Some electrodes remain effective for 3 days and are waterproof, allowing bathing.)

• If your patient is being monitored for tachycardia, use lead V_1 (or MCL_1) or V_6 (or MCL_6) to differentiate tachycardias with wide QRS complexes. *Don't* use lead II for this purpose because it doesn't provide enough information.

• To detect a new bundle-branch block in a patient who's had an MI, use lead V_1 (or MCL_1) or V_6 (or MCL_6). Don't depend on lead II to provide adequate information to differentiate right and left bundle-branch blocks.

• If your patient is being monitored to detect ischemia and muscle injury after an MI, thrombolytic therapy, or percutaneous transluminal coronary angioplasty (PTCA), the choice of ECG lead depends on which vessel or muscle mass region was affected. If it was the inferior wall of the left ventricle or the right coronary artery, use lead II to detect changes. If it was the anterior wall of the left ventricle, use anterior chest leads V_2, V_3, and V_4 (or MCL_2, MCL_3, and MCL_4). To monitor for changes in the lateral wall of the left ventricle, use lateral leads I, aV_L, V_5 (or MCL_5), and V_6 (or MCL_6).

• Many ECG monitoring systems can analyze heart rhythm trends. For instance, some can determine the number of premature beats, detect the length of tachycardic episodes, and count the number of pauses that may occur if an AV conduction abnormality is present. You may be able to program the bedside monitor according to the patient's needs, specifying which information to analyze for trends. The device may display the resulting data on a time line or provide a printout and a description of each cardiac event.

• If the monitor's display and graphic printout are poor, check for patient movement or other potential causes. (See *Identifying cardiac monitor problems,* page 14.)

• Follow your hospital's policy regarding post-

ing and interpreting rhythm strips in the patient's medical record. The Joint Commission on Accreditation of Healthcare Organizations requires that each rhythm strip include the patient's name and the date and time the strip was recorded. Also, the measured intervals and interpretation must appear next to the strip or in the nurses' notes.

• Document the patient's rhythm strip at least every 8 to 12 hours. Be sure to document a strip recorded after each change in the patient's condition and the ensuing intervention, as well as one recorded after the intervention to document whether it was effective.

• If the patient will be monitored by telephone at home after discharge, provide appropriate teaching. (See *Transtelephonic cardiac monitoring,* page 15.)

Discontinuing ECG monitoring

• When the doctor decides to discontinue ECG monitoring, remove the electrode patches and clean the sites.

• If telemetry monitoring was used, be sure to retrieve the transmitter and return it to the central station or other designated area. (The transmitter is expensive, but it may be so small that staff members may accidentally remove it with the bed linens, or the patient may take it home.) After retrieving the transmitter, clean it with a mild cleaning solution, according to the manufacturer's recommendations.

• Document that monitoring has been discontinued.

ST-segment monitoring

A relatively new technique, ST-segment monitoring helps detect myocardial ischemia, electrolyte imbalances, coronary artery spasm, and hypoxic events. The ST segment represents early ventricular repolarization, and any changes in this waveform component reflect alterations in myocardial oxygenation. Any monitoring lead that views an ischemic heart region will reveal ST-segment changes. A devia-

(Text continues on page 16.)

Identifying cardiac monitor problems

PROBLEM	POSSIBLE CAUSES	INTERVENTIONS
False-high-rate alarm	• Monitor interpreting large T waves as QRS complexes, which doubles the rate • Skeletal muscle activity	• Reposition electrodes to lead where QRS complexes are taller than T waves. • Place electrodes away from major muscle masses.
False-low-rate alarm	• Shift in electrical axis from patient movement, making QRS complexes too small to register • Low amplitude of QRS complex • Poor contact between electrodes and skin	• Reapply electrodes. Set gain so height of QRS complex exceeds 1 millivolt. • Increase gain. • Reapply electrodes.
Low amplitude	• Gain dial set too low • Poor contact between skin and electrodes; dried gel; broken or loose leadwires; poor connection between patient and monitor; malfunctioning monitor	• Increase gain. • Check connections on all leadwires and monitoring cable. Replace electrodes as necessary. Reapply electrodes, if required.
Wandering baseline	• Poor position or contact between electrodes and skin • Thoracic movement with respirations	• Reposition or replace electrodes. • Reposition electrodes.
Artifact (waveform interference)	• Patient having seizures, chills, or anxiety • Patient movement • Electrodes applied improperly • Static electricity • Electrical short circuit in leadwires or cable • Interference from decreased room humidity	• Notify doctor and intervene as ordered. Reassure patient and keep him warm. • Help patient relax. • Check electrodes and reapply them, if necessary. • Make sure cable doesn't have exposed connectors. Change static-causing bedclothes. • Replace broken equipment. Use stress loops when applying leadwires. • Regulate room humidity to 40%.
Broken leadwires or cable	• Stress loops not used on leadwires • Cable and leadwires cleaned with alcohol or acetone, causing brittleness	• Replace leadwires and retape them, using stress loops. • Clean cable and leadwires with soapy water. *Do not allow cable ends to become wet.* Replace cable as necessary.
60-cycle interference (fuzzy baseline)	• Electrical interference from other equipment in room • Patient's bed grounded improperly	• Attach all electrical equipment to common ground. Check plugs to make sure prongs aren't loose. • Attach bed ground to the room's common ground.
Skin excoriation under electrode	• Patient allergic to electrode adhesive • Electrode on skin too long	• Remove electrodes and apply nonallergenic electrodes and nonallergenic tape. • Remove electrode, clean site, and reapply electrode at new site.

Transtelephonic cardiac monitoring

Using a special recorder-transmitter, patients at home can transmit electrocardiograms (ECGs) to a central monitoring center by telephone for immediate interpretation. This new technique, called transtelephonic cardiac monitoring (TTM), helps reduce health care costs and has gained widespread use. Nurses play an important role in TTM. Besides performing extensive patient and family teaching, they may run the central monitoring center and help interpret the ECGs sent by patients.

TTM helps caregivers assess transient conditions that can cause symptoms such as palpitations, dizziness, syncope, confusion, paroxysmal dyspnea, and chest pain. Such conditions can make diagnosis difficult and costly. TTM lets the patient transmit an ECG recording from his home when the symptom appears, avoiding the need to go to the hospital for diagnosis. The patient may keep the equipment for an extended time to aid diagnosis.

TTM home care

TTM can also be used by patients undergoing cardiac rehabilitation at home. As the patient performs the prescribed activities, the nurse calls him periodically to receive transmissions and assess his progress. Thus, TTM helps reduce the anxiety felt by many patients and their families after discharge, especially if the patient suffered a myocardial infarction.

TTM is especially valuable for assessing the effects of drugs and for diagnosing and managing paroxysmal arrhythmias. In both cases, it can eliminate the need to admit the patient to the hospital for evaluation and a potentially lengthy stay.

Understanding TTM equipment

TTM requires three main pieces of equipment. An ECG recorder-transmitter converts electrical activity from the patient's heart to acoustic waves. (Some models have a built-in memory, which stores the cardiac event so the patient can transmit it later.) A standard telephone line is used to transmit information. A receiver converts the acoustic waves into ECG activity, which is recorded on ECG paper for interpretation and documentation in the patient's chart.

The recorder-transmitter has two types of elec-

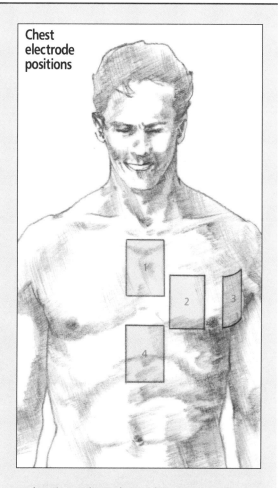

Chest electrode positions

trodes. Finger electrodes produce ECG tracings similar to those produced by leads I and II. Chest electrodes produce tracings resembling those of the precordial leads of a 12-lead ECG, depending on where they're placed on the chest. When placed on area 1 in the above illustration, they produce tracings similar to those of leads V_1, V_2, and V_3 (showing the septal and anterior heart portions). When placed on area 2, they view the lateral ventricular wall, as shown by lead V_5. When placed on area 3, they produce tracings similar to those of leads V_5 and V_6, which show the lateral and posterior ventricle walls. Electrodes placed in area 4 view the inferior ventricular wall, as shown by leads II, III, and aV_F.

When to use ST-segment monitoring

Monitoring ST-segment changes as they occur proves especially useful for patients at risk for silent ischemia. Consider, for instance, that you're caring for Frank Chung, age 50.

Initial care
Mr. Chung was admitted to the emergency department (ED) complaining of mild, nonradiating, substernal chest pain. His medical history revealed hypertension and an inferior-wall myocardial infarction. An electrocardiogram (ECG) taken in the ED showed mild ST-segment depression in leads II, III, and aV$_F$ and a 1-mm elevation of the ST segment in lead V$_1$. Mr. Chung then received two sublingual nitroglycerin tablets. A short time later, he reported that his pain had subsided. His doctor then admitted him to your unit for close observation.

Care on your unit
After greeting Mr. Chung, you repeat an ECG and find that his ST segments have returned to normal. You then connect him to a bedside ECG monitor with ST-segment monitoring capabilities. Your subsequent assessments reveal normal findings until 2 hours later when Mr. Chung, pale and short of breath, complains of severe substernal chest pain that radiates down his left arm. You quickly check his ST segments and find a 5-mm elevation in leads V$_1$ to V$_4$. A 12-lead ECG confirms this finding.

You report your findings immediately to the doctor, who orders oxygen (3 liters/minute) via a nasal cannula, morphine sulfate I.V. for pain, and tissue plasminogen activator (tPA).

Within 60 minutes of symptom onset, as Mr. Chung receives the tPA infusion, you note that his ST segments are less elevated. Thirty minutes later, you see that his ST segments have returned to baseline and his vital signs have stabilized. Mr. Chung tells you that he feels much better and that his pain is gone.

Subsequently, Mr. Chung shows no further ST-segment changes and remains free from pain. The next morning, with a cardiac crisis averted, he'll be able to undergo the doctor's prescribed treatment: percutaneous transluminal coronary angioplasty.

tion of more than 1 mm from the original baseline is considered significant and may indicate myocardial ischemia.

The monitor depicts ST-segment changes as they occur. This makes ST-segment monitoring especially useful for patients at risk for silent ischemia, allowing prompt assessment and immediate treatment that can prevent myocardial necrosis. The technique also helps caregivers evaluate the effectiveness of specific treatments in returning the ST segment to baseline. (See *When to use ST-segment monitoring*.)

Candidates for continuous ST-segment monitoring include patients with coronary artery disease, those who've undergone PTCA, intraoperative and postoperative patients at high risk for myocardial injury, and those who've received thrombolytic therapy. ST-segment monitoring also may be indicated for patients with head injury, chest trauma, major vascular trauma, bundle-branch block, pacemaker rhythms, electrolyte imbalances, pericarditis, hypothermia, or pulmonary infarction. Patients who are undergoing suctioning or receiving drugs such as vasopressors, potassium supplements, and digitalis glycosides also may benefit from ST-segment monitoring.

Equipment
Current equipment used for ST-segment monitoring can analyze two, three, or four leads chosen from any of the standard 12 ECG leads, as well as the right-sided chest leads V$_3$R, V$_4$R, and V$_5$R. Depending on how the monitor has been programmed, it may display one or more leads. (Monitors that display up to 12 leads will be available soon.)

The monitor software establishes a template of the patient's normal QRST pattern from the selected leads, and then displays ST-segment changes. Some monitors display such changes continuously, others only on command. With some models, the changes appear over the original template; with other models, the template and ST-segment changes appear side by side.

Placing leads for ST-segment monitoring

To ensure accuracy, you must place leads precisely for ST-segment monitoring. The first illustration shows where to place the four limb leads. The second illustration shows where to place the chest or V leads. You may place the positive electrode at any precordial (V lead) position.

Limb leads

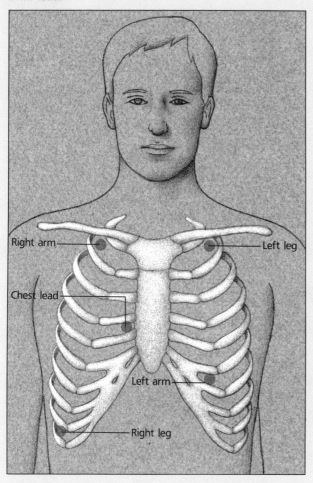

V leads

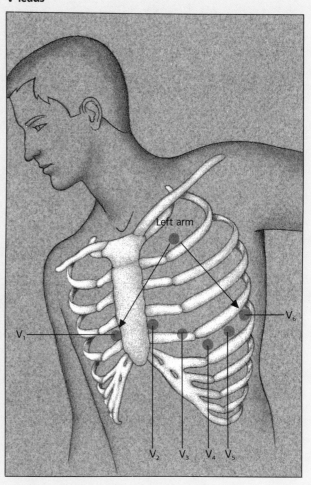

Preparation

Preparing the patient

If necessary, explain the purpose of ST-segment monitoring to the patient and his family. Emphasize why such monitoring is important to the patient's treatment regimen.

Prepare the patient's skin by shaving any excess hair and thoroughly cleaning the sites where the electrodes will be placed. Dry the skin completely before placing the electrodes. To promote better contact between the skin and electrodes, rub the skin briskly.

ST-segment recording

This waveform, produced by ST-segment monitoring, displays ST-segment changes as an overlay on the patient's normal pattern. The numbers beneath the waveform denote millimeters of ST depression or elevation.

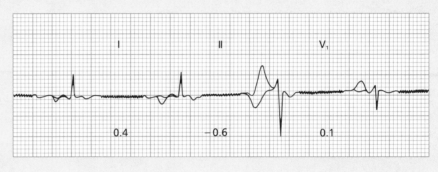

Preparing the equipment

Follow the manufacturer's recommendations for ST-segment monitoring. The specific leads you'll use depend on the patient's needs and clinical status. The primary channel may be the best lead to use when monitoring for specific arrhythmias or blocks to which the patient is predisposed.

The second channel should be used to detect ischemic changes. Research shows that leads V_2 and V_3 can best detect ST-segment elevation during occlusion of the left anterior descending coronary artery. Lead III is recommended for detecting occlusion of the left circumflex coronary artery; lead II or aV_F, for detecting right coronary artery occlusion. Use lead V_4R or lead V_6R to monitor for right ventricular ischemia.

Procedure

Apply the electrodes to the patient as appropriate for the selected leads. Be sure to position the electrodes precisely to allow accurate detection of ST-segment changes. (See *Placing leads for ST-segment monitoring,* page 17.)

Interpretation of findings

The monitoring system analyzes each ST segment for changes. Some systems analyze a block of ECG complexes, whereas others analyze individual complexes. Most systems compare ST segments with baseline data. Be sure to find out how the system you're using analyzes ST segments. Also find out how often it updates baseline data, how it's affected by artifact, and how you can adjust it to get the most accurate analysis.

Monitoring systems that analyze *trends* in ST-segment changes can be especially valuable in coordinating nursing and patient self-care activities. You can determine, for example, how long the patient can be active before the ST segment changes. Be sure you understand how the software performs trend analysis so you can interpret findings accurately. (See *ST-segment recording.*)

Nursing considerations

• Be sure to watch the monitoring system closely. Subtle changes in the patient's ST segment may be precursors to major changes in his condition.

• Assess electrode skin sites regularly for signs of an allergic reaction to the conduction gel or electrode patch (such as redness and blisters), and switch to different types of gel or electrode patches if necessary. You should also note if the patient complains of any itching or irritation.

• Change the electrode patches according to the manufacturer's recommendations or your hospital's policy.

• Obtain rhythm strips at least every 8 to 12 hours, and place them in the patient's chart. You should also obtain rhythm strips whenever you note ST-segment changes, during interventions, and after each intervention to document its result.

• The doctor will tell you when to discontinue ST-segment monitoring, but make sure you note it in the nurses' notes.

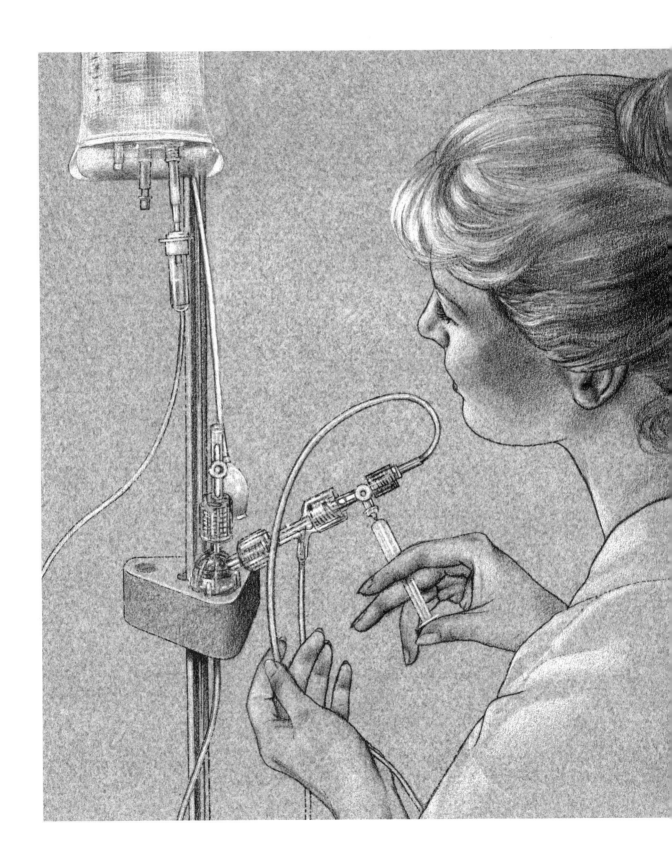

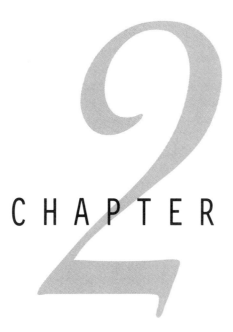

CHAPTER 2

Understanding hemodynamic monitoring

Scientists have made enormous strides in recording and monitoring physiologic pressures since Stephen Hales recorded the first vascular pressure in 1734. In the 1970s, doctors began using the pulmonary artery catheter to record pressures at the bedside, avoiding the need to transport patients to a catheterization laboratory for assessment.

Since then, technologic advances in invasive pressure monitoring have made simple blood pressure measurement nearly obsolete. Bedside monitoring provides hemodynamic information that helps caregivers assess the patient's status and choose appropriate interventions. Such routine monitoring has revolutionized nursing practice.

Today's nurse must possess expert skills in using sophisticated pressure monitoring systems—skills once reserved for the biomedical engineering staff. To set up a pressure monitoring system, identify adequate dynamic response, and verify the accuracy of pressure values, you'll need to understand the technical and physiologic aspects of pressure monitoring.

All systems used to monitor vascular pressure possess the same underlying principles and share certain essential components. This chapter provides the knowledge base you'll need to use any type of pressure monitoring system. It also prepares you to troubleshoot the system — a skill that's crucial to ensuring accurate pressure values and waveforms.

The chapter begins by discussing the factors that affect pressure monitoring, such as flow dynamics and signal transmission. Then it describes the basic components of a pressure monitoring system, explains how to set up the system, and tells how to verify the accuracy of the pressure values.

Flow dynamics

Reviewing flow dynamics within the vessels will help you understand the components of pressure waveforms and the requirements for pressure monitors. Within the circulatory system, pressure results from the contractile force of the heart's left ventricle and the arteries. Because vessels constrict and dilate and ventricular contractions vary, vascular pressures are dynamic.

Vascular pressure measurement is based on Pascal's law, which holds that a pressure change at any given point in a confined fluid results in a similar pressure change throughout the entire fluid volume. Pascal's law also states that in a fluid-filled tube, pressure at both ends of the tube is equal.

Hydrostatic pressure
The ends of the tube must rest on the same level to avoid the influence of *hydrostatic pressure* — the force or weight of a fluid pushing against a surface. When using a pressure monitoring system, you apply this principle by making sure both ends of the pressure tubing are at the same level. This eliminates the influence of hydrostatic pressure, ensuring that pressures recorded at both ends of the system are the same.

An important factor in intracardiac and arterial pressure measurement, the hydrostatic pressure of fluid in a given column increases with the vertical height and density of the fluid. For example, pressure in a column of water 5' (152 cm) tall exceeds pressure in a column only 2' (61 cm) tall. Also, pressure in a mercury column exceeds pressure in a water column of the same height because mercury is denser than water.

Dynamic flow changes
Within vessels and heart chambers, dynamic flow changes occur. As blood is propelled through the vessels or chambers, the velocity of the flow causes turbulence. Called the *dynamic pressure component,* turbulence can be misleading if the lumen of the catheter points toward the flow of blood or if flow rates are extremely high.

The residual or static pressure used to assess systolic and diastolic blood pressures is even more relevant to caregivers. (Although systolic and diastolic pressures change, they're considered static because we record a single high and low rather than the changing pressures that result from turbulent flow.) For example, if a central aortic pressure line is placed near a stenotic aortic valve, the pressure monitoring system may record multiple systolic waveforms that are very high and multiple diastolic waveforms that are very low.

Pressure monitoring systems are designed to accurately reproduce only the changes in systolic and diastolic pressures. The accuracy of the values obtained depends on the fidelity with which the monitoring system transmits the residual pressure (which varies with the cardiac cycle).

Pressure signal transmission

Accurate reproduction and transmission of pressure signals detected by the monitor depend on many factors. Transmitting a pressure signal from a vessel or a heart chamber requires that you insert a catheter and attach fluid-filled tubing to a transducer. (Fluid acts as a conductor for flow and pressure changes.) Flow and pressure changes are converted to an electrical signal that's displayed on an oscilloscope as a numerical value, a waveform, or both. Although numerical values are important, observing waveforms will indicate trends in your patient's blood pressure and enhance assessment.

Damping

Damping refers to the diminishing of the system's vibrations, which in turn causes a reduction in amplitude of the pressure tracing. Ideally, a system should be critically, or optimally, damped for accurate reproduction of the tracing and accurate pressure values. (See *Terms used in pressure monitoring.*)

With *overdamping,* the pressure tracing has an overly diminished amplitude and an unclear dicrotic notch, with false-low systolic pressure. Causes of overdamping include compliant pressure tubing, use of additional stopcocks, and large air bubbles near the transducer. Compliant pressure tubing may lead to overdamping because it doesn't carry vibrations as well as stiffer tubing. Stopcocks, used to change the direction of the flow of fluid or pressure, may diminish vibrations by interrupting the fluid-filled path. Air bubbles may cause overdamping because air is compressible and acts as a shock absorber to vibrations within the tubing.

With *underdamping,* the natural frequencies of the system and the patient are too similar. This causes false-high systolic pressure and false-low diastolic pressure. This tracing shows overshoot or whipping. Common causes of underdamping include pressure tubing that's too long, use of additional stopcocks, and small air bubbles near the catheter insertion site.

Determining the dynamic response helps evaluate whether the system is optimally damped. One method of determining this is to calculate the frequency response and damping coefficient.

Terms used in pressure monitoring

Damping: decrease in the amplitude of signals produced, caused by drainage of energy from the oscillating system to overcome frictional or other resistive forces. A critically, or optimally, damped system reproduces physiologic signals accurately. In an overdamped or underdamped system, signals are distorted.

Damping coefficient: speed with which a pressure system's vibrations come to rest after being displaced; the ratio of successive amplitudes of oscillating waves divided by the natural frequency. Plotting this value on a dynamic response graph helps determine if the system is optimally damped.

Dynamic response: ability of a system to accurately record physiologic (patient) pressures; is affected by such factors as the type of catheter and pressure tubing used, tubing length, number of stopcocks, and air bubbles in the line.

Frequency response: ability of a system to accurately display the frequencies or vibrations applied to it. To reproduce an accurate signal, the system must respond faster than the fastest occurring physiologic signal.

Harmonic: multiple of the natural frequency. For instance, if the natural occurring vibration is 3 hertz (Hz) or 3 cycles/second, the monitoring system should be 10 harmonics higher (30 Hz) to accurately reproduce the pressure waveform.

Hertz (Hz): unit of frequency equal to 1 cycle/second; an index of how fast the system vibrates. Each type of catheter and pressure monitoring system has its own hertz. Such factors as type of tubing, type of catheter, and number of stopcocks in the line affect the hertz and frequency response of the system. The catheter should have a hertz above 20.

Natural frequency: vibration that occurs when a system is momentarily displaced from the resting state; also called resonant frequency.

Components of pressure monitoring systems

Regardless of the type of pressure you'll be monitoring, all systems share certain components: a catheter, stopcocks, pressure tubing, flush device, transducer, monitor, and amplifier.

Catheter

A catheter provides access to the patient's vessels for monitoring intravascular pressure. Common catheter insertion sites include the radial, brachial, femoral, subclavian, and jugular arteries.

The ideal catheter for pressure monitoring is short, with a large internal diameter. For adults, an 18G or #7 French catheter provides the most reproducible signals.

Stopcock

Attached to the tubing at multiple points along the monitoring system, stopcocks perform various functions. A one-way stopcock can be turned on or off. A three-way stopcock, the most common type, allows fluid to flow with the stopcock port turned upright; turning the handle redirects the fluid path. A four-way stopcock can be directed so that three lumens are open at the same time.

Most systems include a stopcock located on or near the transducer. Typically, this stopcock serves as the zeroing port or vent port when zeroing the transducer to atmospheric pressure.

Some stopcocks can be used for blood sampling. They are attached directly to the catheter or to extension pressure tubing. By turning the stopcock handle, you can isolate the fluid from the tubing and withdraw blood through a syringe.

To attach a stopcock, you push or twist it on. Using a luer-lock stopcock helps prevent inadvertent disconnection.

Pressure tubing

The ideal pressure tubing is short and noncompliant—stiffer than normal I.V. tubing. Compliant tubing will dissipate the physiologic signals from the patient and cause over-damped tracings. Long tubing lengths may distort pressure signals. Ideally, the system should include no more than 4' (122 cm) of pressure tubing from the catheter to the transducer.

Flush device

A flush device provides a continuous flow of solution through the line when under pressure to help keep the system patent. (However, a flush device is *not* used in intracranial pressure monitoring systems.) For adults, the normal flow rate is 1 to 5 ml/hour. A small capillary restrictor inside the flush device limits the flow continuously. However, the restrictor can be bypassed by activating the actuator, allowing infusion of more fluid. This feature is useful during initial filling, when priming the line, and when a fast flush is needed (such as when performing the square wave test).

When monitoring a pediatric or neonatal patient, you'll use a faster flow rate for the flush device—about 30 ml/hour. Using an I.V. controller with the flush device lets you administer less fluid on a continuous basis while preventing flow rates above 30 ml/hour.

Transducer

The transducer converts physiologic signals to the electrical signals displayed on the monitor. A transducer may be reusable or disposable. Reusable transducers must be attached to a dome. Filled with solution, the dome isolates the nonsterile transducer from the patient. Adding a few drops of sterile water to the transducer promotes easier coupling of the dome. Disposable transducers come with an integrated dome.

Transducers work mainly by displacement of the sensing diaphragm in the dome. When pressure from within the patient's vessel is exerted on fluid in the line, the fluid depresses the dome's diaphragm. The transducer converts the pressure on the diaphragm into electrical energy, and then transmits it to the monitor. The monitor displays the pressure reading.

Conventional transducers use a resistive device—typically a Wheatstone bridge—to convert fluid movement from the sensing diaphragm to an electrical signal. Newer disposable transducers convert the signal via a microchip. The signals generated are quite small—about 3 millivolts. These signals are amplified and processed by the bedside monitor and amplifier.

Monitor and amplifier

The amplifier, incorporated into the bedside monitor, enhances transducer-generated signals about 250 to 1,000 times. Many amplifiers include filters that eliminate unwanted "noise," or extraneous high-frequency signals. The amplifier must have a frequency response that's high enough to respond to and reproduce physiologic signals. However, an excessively high frequency response would cause the amplifier to detect very small or rapid oscillations from the catheter to the screen. To prevent this, amplifiers provide some form of damping.

The bedside monitor displays the amplifier-enhanced signals on an oscilloscope or strip chart recorder. It also displays other parameters, depending on the model and which type of pressure is being monitored. Typically, the monitor displays digital readouts of systolic, diastolic, and mean pressures.

The oscilloscope shows the pressure tracing. The vertical axis has a scale for pressure readings; the horizontal axis moves with time. Tracings move across the screen at a standard speed of 25 mm/second. With most systems, however, you can change this speed to allow waveform analysis.

The monitor prints out a hard paper copy of pressures and tracings, either at the bedside or the central station. The strip printout is essential for waveform analysis and documentation in the patient's chart.

Zeroing the transducer

Because physiologic pressures are relative to atmospheric pressure, you must zero the transducer to atmospheric pressure to obtain accurate readings. By zeroing, you're establishing atmospheric pressure as the baseline, thus preventing it from affecting pressure readings. Zeroing is performed to offset other influences from within the system, such as hydrostatic

pressure from the pressure tubing or pressure within the transducer.

To ensure proper zeroing, let the transducer warm up beforehand. A disposable transducer usually takes about 5 minutes to warm up sufficiently. Typically, you'll use the stopcock located at the transducer to zero the system. The zeroing point is the point at which you open the stopcock to air—not to the transducer. Be sure to position the patient and transducer on the same level each time you zero the transducer.

First, remove the nonvented cap from the stopcock. Then, turn the handle so it's off to the transducer and open to air. Next, position this air-fluid interface port level with the reference point. Typically, the reference point is the phlebostatic axis, located midway between the patient's anteroposterior chest wall and the fourth intercostal space. (See *Identifying the phlebostatic axis*, page 26.) After zeroing, failing to keep the zero port level with the phlebostatic axis can cause inaccurate pressure readings. Every centimeter difference between the level of the port and the level of the phlebostatic axis will cause an inverse 0.74 mm Hg pressure difference. As a rule of thumb, expect a 2 mm Hg error in the pressure reading for every 1" (2.5 cm) off the proper level. For example, if the zeroing port is 1" too high, the recorded value will be falsely low by 2 mm Hg. If it's 1" too low, the value will be falsely high by 2 mm Hg.

Next, press the ZERO or BALANCE button on the monitor. The tracing on the monitor should move to the 0, and the digital readout should show 0. If the monitor has zero offset (doesn't show zero), you can use another knob to adjust it so it shows zero.

Depending on which system you're using, you can either place the transducer on a pole or mount it on the patient's arm or chest. Keep in mind that you're using the air-fluid interface of the stopcock—not the transducer diaphragm—as the zeroing point. This means you can use a stopcock other than the one at the transducer to zero the system.

Also remember that you must rezero and relevel the transducer after patient transport. Otherwise, the pressure values and tracings

Identifying the phlebostatic axis

When zeroing a pressure transducer, use the phlebostatic axis, which bisects two thoracic planes. Using this intersected point allows the head of the bed to be raised or lowered.

To identify the phlebostatic axis, locate the patient's fourth intercostal space; then draw an imaginary line that extends down the lateral thoracic area. Next, identify a second point at the midpoint between the anterior and posterior chest walls. The site at which these two reference points bisects is the phlebostatic axis.

Some nurses use the midaxillary line rather than the midpoint between the anterior and posterior chest walls as the lateral plane. However, this line doesn't always coincide with the midheart level. Also, one caregiver may identify the midaxillary line differently than another. For reproducibility and accuracy, regard the midpoint as more accurate.

Keep in mind that the key to ensuring accurate pressure values isn't just locating the phlebostatic axis precisely but identifying it consistently for all readings. Therefore, be sure to mark the reference spot on the patient's torso to ensure a consistent leveling point.

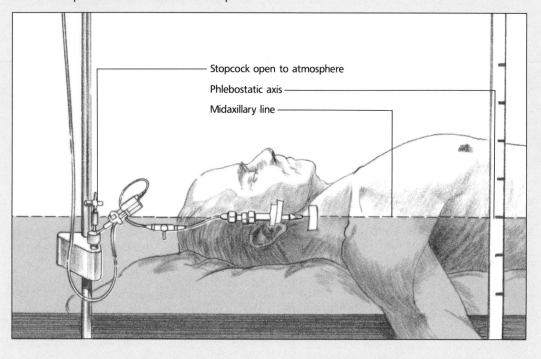

Stopcock open to atmosphere

Phlebostatic axis

Midaxillary line

you obtain will be inaccurate. (See *A transducer problem?*)

Calibrating the system

With prolonged use, transducers lose some sensitivity and become less accurate. Calibrating the system helps ensure accurate readings by verifying the electronic calibration of the monitor and the sensitivity of the transducer.

With most monitors, you calibrate by pressing the AUTO-CAL feature or a self-calibrating button. Typical calibration values are 100 mm Hg or 200 mm Hg.

Reusable transducers lose calibration more easily than disposable ones. With these trans-

A transducer problem?

How do you know whether a sudden drop in hemodynamic values results from a physiologic complication or a monitoring problem? To help you decide, consider the case of Samuel Williamson, a 66-year-old garment worker who underwent surgery for an abdominal aortic aneurysm.

Before surgery, the doctor inserted an arterial line and a pulmonary artery catheter. Mr. Williamson's surgery went well. Afterward, in the postanesthesia recovery unit, his nurse starts a nitroprusside drip at 6 mcg/kg/minute. She measures a heart rate of 80 beats/minute, a blood pressure of 148/78 mm Hg, a pulmonary artery pressure (PAP) of 35/14 mm Hg, a mean arterial pressure (MAP) of 21 mm Hg, a pulmonary artery wedge pressure (PAWP) of 12 mm Hg, and a cardiac output (CO) of 3.8 liters/minute.

Once Mr. Williamson's condition becomes stable, he's transferred to the surgical intensive care unit (ICU). On admission, his nurse, Sarah Jenkins, records a heart rate of 92 beats/minute, a blood pressure of 92/48 mm Hg, a PAP of 25/10 mm Hg, a MAP of 15 mm Hg, a PAWP of 8 mm Hg, and a CO of 3.4 liters/minute. Ms. Jenkins immediately reports these findings to the doctor, who orders a decrease in the nitroprusside infusion and administration of 500 ml of albumin to boost Mr. Williamson's blood pressure.

After implementing these orders, Ms. Jenkins realizes that the pressure transducer hadn't been releveled or rezeroed since Mr. Williamson's admission to the ICU. She promptly relevels and rezeroes the transducer, then records these values: a heart rate of 95 beats/minute, a blood pressure of 140/80 mm Hg, a PAP of 42/23 mm Hg, a MAP of 29 mm Hg, a PAWP of 22 mm Hg, and a CO of 3.2 liters/minute.

Reviewing the care

Obviously, Ms. Jenkins leapt to an erroneous conclusion about Mr. Williamson's condition. Based on the values she reported, the doctor ordered treatment that led to undesirable changes in the patient's hemodynamic status.

This situation also points out the need to question the accuracy of the monitoring system when both blood pressure and PAP drop to the level of Mr. Williamson's values. PAP rarely drops this low during hypotension. Also, the lack of a dramatic change in CO should have alerted Ms. Jenkins to potential transducer misplacement.

To check the dynamic response of the pressure monitoring system, Ms. Jenkins could have performed a square wave test. However, she would have obtained low values because the problem was lack of releveling and rezeroing, not the system itself.

---

ducers, you should verify calibration routinely or whenever you question the pressure values you've obtained. If the calibration is inaccurate, you may make another adjustment to the monitor or note the difference on the transducer. The biomedical department is a good resource for calibration.

With newer disposable transducers, the manufacturer typically verifies and checks calibration. These transducers incorporate a fixed sensitivity that's standard for all monitors. Calibration should remain intact during the short time the system is used for bedside monitoring.

Setting up the pressure monitoring system

First, make sure the bedside monitor is turned on and has the appropriate pressure module (or modules for multiple pressure monitoring). Let the monitor warm up for 15 to 30 minutes (longer for older models).

Next, gather appropriate supplies (including a catheter) for the type of monitoring to be performed. Remove the pressure monitoring kit from the sterile wrapping, and tighten all connections. (They may loosen during transport.)

Position all stopcocks so the flush solution will flow through the entire system, as shown below.

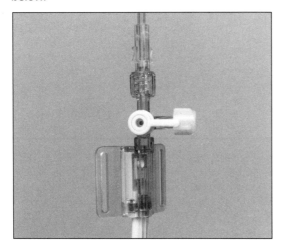

Use clear plastic stopcocks so you'll be able to see any air bubbles that become trapped. To help prevent disconnection after the system has been attached, use luer-lock stopcocks.

When filling the system, make sure all inner openings and ports are cleared of air to prevent air contamination and overdamped waveforms.

Replace the vented caps on the stopcocks with sterile nonvented caps as shown.

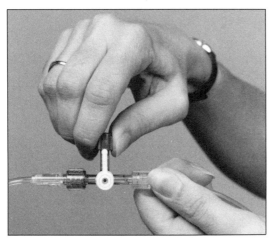

Make sure a drop of fluid shows to verify that no air is trapped. Use aseptic technique so you don't touch the end of the nonvented cap or vent port opening, possibly causing contamination.

Connect the pressure tubing to the transducer. Be sure to use rigid tubing in this segment. However, you may use standard I.V. tubing from the drip chamber of the flush solution to the transducer because this segment doesn't transmit pressure waveforms from the patient.

Use a pressure bag to apply a continuous pressure to the system. Typically, you'll use 300 mm Hg of pressure to help keep the line patent through the flush device restrictor. During initial flushing of the system, however, *don't* apply pressure on the bag. Instead, simply hang the bag on an I.V. pole about 2 feet above the end of the tubing. This will apply 45 mm Hg of hydrostatic pressure—enough to fill the system without causing turbulence and bubbling.

Flushing the system

When flushing the system, squeeze the continuous flush device slowly (as shown below) and turn the stopcocks so each stopcock port is filled in turn. Cap each stopcock after a drop of fluid shows to verify lack of air contamination.

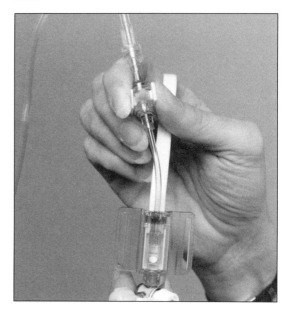

When fluid reaches the transducer, hold the transducer at a 45-degree angle (as shown in the following photograph) so air will rise up and out of the vented stopcock.

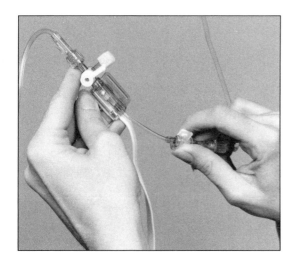

After flushing the tubing and stopcocks and replacing the nonvented stopcock caps, pressurize the pressure bag to 300 mm Hg.

Attach the transducer cable to the patient cable. Keep the patient cable connection dry. Moisture can cause corrosion of the reusable cable portion and may lead to erroneous values. If the values change rapidly after initial zeroing, give the transducer more time to warm up, and then rezero it.

Next, level the zeroing port to the phlebostatic axis. You can use a leveling tool, such as a carpenter's level or a *bubble level* on a string, to do this. Place one end of the leveling tool at the port you used to zero the transducer, and place the other end at the phlebostatic axis. Make sure the port and the phlebostatic axis are at the same level to eliminate the influence of hydrostatic pressure.

Alternatively, you may use a penlight to verify a straight line from the vent port to the phlebostatic axis. Shine the light from the vent port toward the patient's lateral chest wall. This creates a straight line, and you can then assume the port and phlebostatic axis are level.

Now the system is ready to be connected to the patient's catheter. (For a photograph of how the pressure monitoring system should look when fully assembled, see *Pressure monitoring setup,* page 30.)

Verifying the dynamic response

If you suspect that the values displayed on the bedside monitor are inaccurate or if the tracings aren't clear, you can quickly verify the dynamic response (accuracy) of the pressure system by performing the square wave test. However, this test can be done only if the flush device has a restrictor that opens and closes rapidly, as do most flush devices with a pull or snap tab. (See *Assessing the dynamic response,* page 31.)

First, squeeze the actuator on the flush device by rapidly activating the pull or snap tab. Then quickly release the actuator. The monitor should show a waveform that rises suddenly and sharply, tops off, then declines sharply. As you release, several oscillations should appear on the screen, indicating an optimal dynamic response. (See *When to perform the square wave test,* page 32.) *Note:* Although flicking the pressure line can cause enough oscillation for a square wave test, this method isn't as accurate.

The square wave test also helps you assess the patency of the system. If the system is occluded (such as from a clot or fibrin buildup in the catheter tip), the waveform will appear overdamped. (See *Pinpointing a monitoring problem,* page 33.) Be aware that heparin is typically mixed with the flush solution (1 to 2 units of heparin per milliliter of solution) to prevent clotting. However, some patients may develop heparin-induced thrombocytopenia if heparin is added to the flush solution. A nationwide study is currently evaluating the need for heparin.

Verifying transducer accuracy

If the manufacturer has supplied a calibration device, you can verify transducer accuracy by simply attaching the device to the back of the transducer and applying a negative pressure.

ADVANCED EQUIPMENT

Pressure monitoring setup

This photograph shows how a pressure monitoring system should look after you complete the setup.

Regardless of the type of pressure you'll be monitoring, all systems share certain components: a catheter, stopcocks, pressure tubing, flush device, transducer, monitor, and amplifier (monitor and amplifier not shown).

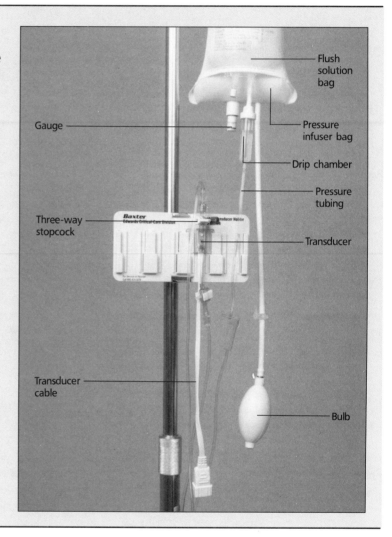

Negative pressure is automatically converted to a positive pressure on the monitor.

If the manufacturer hasn't supplied a calibration device, you must apply a known value to the transducer to verify its accuracy. To do this, you may use one of two methods. In the first, you remove the cuff from a mercury sphygmomanometer and attach the end of it to a separate sterile, fluid-filled extension pres-sure tubing, which you attach to the stopcock's zero port. Turn off the stopcock to the patient. Then squeeze the hand bulb on the sphygmomanometer until 200 mm Hg shows, indicating that 200 mm Hg of pressure has been applied to the transducer diaphragm. Now look at the monitor's digital readout. An accurate transducer should show 200 mm Hg.

To verify linear accuracy of the transducer,

Assessing the dynamic response

The square wave test helps you assess the dynamic response of the pressure monitoring system. To perform it, pull the snap tab or pull tab on the flush device, and then release it quickly. As you do this, watch the monitor screen.

Critically damped tracing
With critical damping (indicating an optimal dynamic response), you'll see the tracing rise sharply, top off after you pull the tab, then decline sharply after you release it. One or two oscillations appear above and below the baseline after release. The tracing at right shows a clear dicrotic notch.

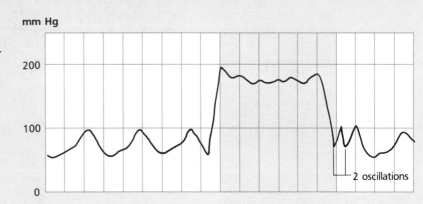

Overdamped tracing
If the system is overdamped, the tracing will have fewer than 1½ oscillations below the baseline, as in the tracing at right. In an arterial or pulmonary artery pressure tracing, the dicrotic notch won't be clear or sharp. Overdamping results in false-low systolic pressures but usually accurate diastolic pressures.

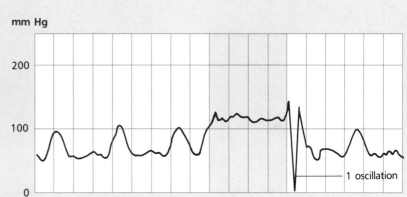

Underdamped tracing
In an underdamped tracing, you'll see "ringing" or oscillations below and above the baseline, as in the tracing at right. Underdamping leads to false-high systolic pressures and false-low diastolic pressures. Peak systolic tracings may show more than one sharp upstroke, and diastolic points are hard to differentiate.

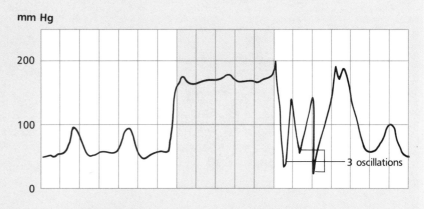

When to perform the square wave test

Performing the square wave test can help you distinguish hemodynamic complications from equipment problems. To understand how, consider that you're caring for Hannah Beaton, age 86, who was admitted to your unit with pulmonary hypertension. The admitting doctor had diagnosed her condition as acute respiratory distress and then inserted a pulmonary artery catheter to measure her pulmonary artery pressure (PAP) and monitor her fluid volume and respiratory status.

On initial assessment, you note a PAP of 98/46 mm Hg.

Conducting the test
To determine if the PAP value and tracing are accurate, you then perform the square wave test and obtain the tracing below.

Reviewing the results
This square wave test shows optimal damping. As a result, you can assume that the PAP values and tracings produced by Mrs. Beaton's monitoring system are accurate. The apparent whipping and "ringing" of the waveform (which suggest underdamping) result from pulmonary hypertension. Underdamping may result from noncompliant vessels (as in pulmonary or systemic hypertension) or vasoconstriction from excessive cooling (a possible result of coronary bypass surgery).

By performing the square wave test, you could determine that the whipping and ringing were caused by Mrs. Beaton's condition rather than the system. By wedging the catheter, you can eliminate whipping and ringing and monitor pulmonary artery wedge pressure intermittently. Keep in mind that elderly patients with pulmonary hypertension are at risk for pulmonary artery rupture. So use caution when performing a wedge tracing in these patients.

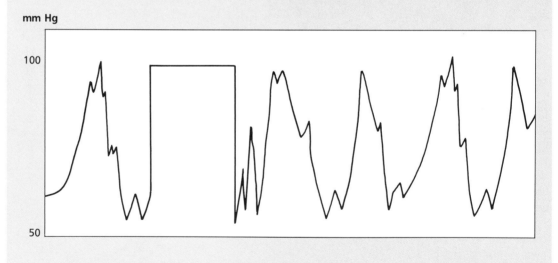

slowly release the pressure on the sphygmomanometer. As the pressure drops, check whether the reading on the sphygomanometer correlates with the monitor reading. If the two values are within 2 mm Hg, good linearity exists.

Important: This method may introduce air and bacteria into the system. For extra safety, add a micropore filter to the extension tubing.

In the second method for verifying transducer accuracy, you apply a water column to

TROUBLESHOOTING

Pinpointing a monitoring problem

If a problem occurs when your patient has a pressure monitoring system in place, ask yourself the following questions to help pinpoint the cause.

Monitor-related problems
• Is the monitor plugged into the wall outlet and turned on?
• Is the pressure module plugged in?
• Does the monitor show the right scale?
• Are all cable connections dry and tight?
• Is the viewing contrast knob turned up?

Transducer-related problems
• Is the zeroing port at the correct level?
• Has the zeroing port been turned off to the patient and opened to air?
• Has the transducer been rezeroed?
• Are all stopcock connections tight?
• Are there any air bubbles in the system, including the tubing and stopcocks?

Patient-related problems
• Is the catheter kinked?
• Has a clot formed at the tip of the catheter?
• Has the patient's clinical status changed?

---

the transducer. This method is less likely to cause contamination and is easier to perform with a disposable transducer. After setting up and priming the system, take the end of the pressure tubing that attaches to the patient, and hold it vertically 12″ (30.5 cm) above the transducer level. This applies a known hydrostatic pressure of approximately 22 mm Hg. The bedside monitor should read between 20 and 24 mm Hg.

If the monitoring system is already attached to the patient, you may attach 12″-long extension tubing to the zero port of the transducer. Turn off the stopcock to the patient; then activate the flush device so that fluid fills the extension tubing. Hold the tubing vertically from the transducer. The water column applies the pressure to the transducer.

Next, convert inches of tubing length to centimeters of H_2O, and then convert centimeters of H_2O to millimeters of mercury to obtain pressure. Keep in mind that 2.54 cm = 1″ and 1.36 cm H_2O = 1 mm Hg. For example:

$$12″ \ H_2O \times 2.54 \ cm = 30.48 \ cm \ H_2O.$$
$$30.48 \ cm \ H_2O \div 1.36 \ cm \ H_2O = 22.41 \ mm \ Hg.$$

Your calculations should yield the same value shown on the monitor.

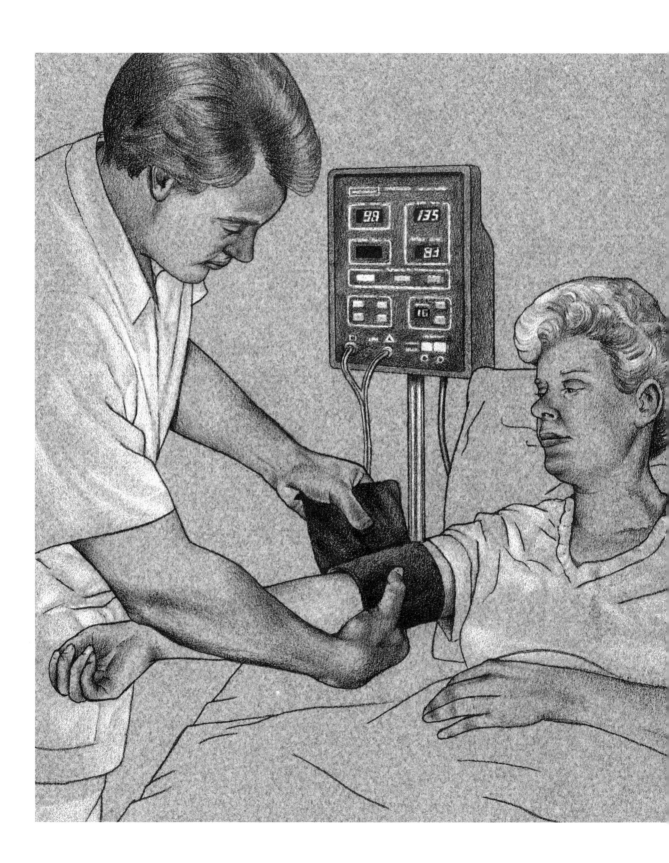

CHAPTER 3

Monitoring arterial pressure

Among the most frequently monitored physiologic indices, arterial pressure serves as an important guide to your patient's cardiovascular status — one that both aids diagnosis and guides therapy. It can be measured directly by an arterial line or indirectly by noninvasive means.

Direct monitoring is invaluable for critically ill patients. In this method, an indwelling arterial catheter is attached to a fluid-filled pressure transducer system. A flush system continuously infuses a heparinized saline solution under pressure to reduce the risk of clot formation. The transducer senses arterial pressure and converts the pressure signal to a waveform on the bedside monitor. The waveform reflects pressure generated by the left ventricle during systole (not the pressure of ejected blood, which travels more slowly). The monitor also displays numerical pressure values.

Physiology

Arterial pressure – the lateral force exerted by blood on the arterial walls – depends on the force of ventricular contraction, arterial wall elasticity, peripheral vascular resistance, and blood volume and viscosity. Systolic (maximum) pressure reflects the greatest force caused by left ventricular contraction. Diastolic (minimum) pressure occurs during left ventricular relaxation; it reflects both peripheral vascular resistance and arterial wall elasticity.

Pulse pressure – the difference between systolic and diastolic pressure – varies inversely with arterial wall elasticity. In patients with hypovolemic shock, narrowing of pulse pressure commonly precedes a drop in diastolic pressure.

Mean arterial pressure (MAP) is the average pressure during a complete cardiac cycle – the period from the beginning of ventricular systole to the end of ventricular diastole. This pressure can be used with other measurements to help evaluate afterload and myocardial contractility.

With direct pressure monitoring, you may obtain the MAP value from the readout on the monitor. Although technologies vary, MAP is calculated by dividing the area under the pressure curve by the base length – the portion extending from the upstroke of systolic pressure to the end of diastolic pressure. To calculate MAP from indirectly obtained pressure measurements, you may use an equation. (See *Calculating MAP.*)

Arterial pressure monitoring

Direct arterial pressure monitoring permits continuous measurement of systolic, diastolic, and mean pressures and allows arterial blood sampling. Because direct measurement reflects systemic vascular resistance as well as blood flow, it's generally more accurate than indirect methods (such as palpation and auscultation of

Korotkoff, or audible pulse, sounds), which are based on blood flow.

Direct monitoring is indicated when highly accurate or frequent blood pressure measurements are required – for example, in patients with low cardiac output and high systemic vascular resistance. It also may be used for hospitalized patients who are obese or have severe edema, if these conditions make indirect measurement hard to perform. What's more, it may be used for patients who are receiving titrated doses of vasoactive drugs or who need frequent blood sampling. The procedure, however, does have risks. Direct monitoring, for instance, can cause such complications as arterial bleeding, infection, air embolism, arterial spasm, or thrombosis.

Indirect monitoring carries few associated risks. A common method, applying pressure to an artery (such as by inflating a blood pressure cuff around the arm) decreases blood flow. As pressure is released, flow resumes and can be palpated or auscultated. Korotkoff sounds presumably result from a combination of blood flow and arterial wall vibrations; with reduced flow, these vibrations may be less pronounced. (See *Auscultating blood pressure,* page 38.)

To measure blood pressure indirectly, you may palpate or auscultate blood flow or use a special noninvasive device. (See *Alternative methods for auscultating blood pressure,* page 39.)

Equipment
For catheter insertion and system setup
Equipment may vary with the doctor's preference and with hospital policy and procedure. Typically, you'll gather gloves, gown, mask, and protective eyewear (for universal precautions); sterile gloves; 16G to 20G catheter (type and length depend on the insertion site, patient's size, and other anticipated uses of the line); preassembled preparation kit (if available); sterile drapes; sheet protector; sterile towel; ordered local anesthetic; sutures; pressure bag; preassembled arterial pressure tubing with flush device and disposable pressure transducer (in some units, a reusable transducer may be used; refer to manufacturer's policy for setup);

Calculating MAP

To obtain mean arterial pressure (MAP) from indirect measurements of your patient's systolic and diastolic blood pressures, you may use either equation shown here. In equation 2, you can obtain the pulse pressure by subtracting the diastolic pressure from the systolic pressure.

Equation 1

$$MAP = \frac{(2 \times diastolic) + systolic}{3}$$

Equation 2

$$MAP = diastolic + \frac{1}{3}\ pulse\ pressure$$

For example, if your patient's blood pressure is 115/85 mm Hg, the MAP would be calculated as follows using equation 1.

$$MAP = \frac{(2 \times 85) + 115}{3}$$

$$= \frac{170 + 115}{3}$$

$$= \frac{285}{3}$$

$$MAP = 95$$

To the right you'll see the locations of the systolic, diastolic, and mean pressures on an arterial waveform.

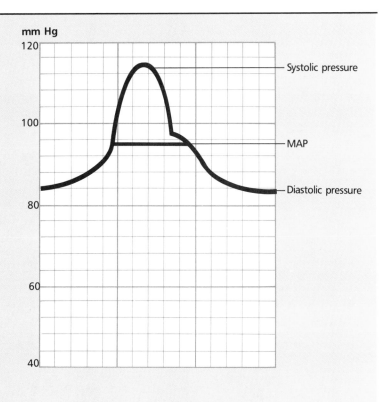

---

bedside monitor; cable (to connect the transducer to the bedside monitor); 500-ml I.V. bag; I.V. flush solution (such as dextrose 5% in water [D_5W] or 0.9% sodium chloride solution); heparin, 500 or 1,000 units (in some hospitals, premixed heparin flush solutions may be available); syringe and needle (21G to 25G, 1"); I.V. pole; tubing and medication labels; site care kit (containing sterile dressing, antimicrobial ointment, and nonallergenic tape); and arm board and soft wrist restraint (for a femoral site, an ankle restraint). For femoral artery insertion, also gather a shaving kit.

For blood sample collection

If an *open system* is in place, gather gloves; gown; mask; protective eyewear; sterile 4" × 4" gauze pads; sheet protector; 500-ml I.V. bag; 5- to 10-ml syringe for discard sample; syringes of appropriate size and number for ordered laboratory tests; laboratory request forms and labels; 16G or 18G needles (depending on hospital policy); and Vacutainers.

If a *closed system* is in place, gather gloves; gown; mask; protective eyewear; syringes of appropriate size and number for ordered laboratory tests; laboratory request forms and labels; alcohol swab; blood transfer unit; and Vacutainers.

For arterial line tubing changes

Gather gloves; gown; mask; protective eyewear; sheet protector; preassembled arterial pressure tubing with flush device and dispos-

Auscultating blood pressure

Before auscultating your patient's blood pressure, be sure to wait at least 30 minutes after the patient eats, smokes, or exercises and 5 minutes after he changes position. Make sure the patient is relaxed. He may sit, stand, or lie down during measurement.

Initially, take blood pressure measurements in both arms. (However, check the patient's history first. Taking blood pressure in a particular arm may be contraindicated by a history of a mastectomy, arteriovenous fistula used for dialysis, or other circulatory abnormalities.) A significant bilateral pressure variance may indicate occlusive disease of the subclavian artery, coarctation of the aorta, dissecting aortic aneurysm, or traumatic injury.

Applying the pressure cuff and stethoscope

Choose a pressure cuff of appropriate size for the patient's arm. Bladder width should be 40% of arm circumference at midpoint; bladder length should be 80% of arm circumference. A cuff that's too narrow will cause a false-high reading; a cuff that's too wide will cause a false-low reading.

Wrap the cuff snugly around the upper arm above the antecubital area (inner aspect of the elbow). Position it ¾" to 1¼" (2 to 3 cm) above the brachial artery.

Place the mercury manometer at eye level. When using a sphygmomanometer, place the aneroid gauge level with the patient's arm. (The indicator needle should point to the zero mark.) Keep the patient's arm at heart level by resting it on a table or chair arm or by supporting it with your hand. (Errors of up to 10% may occur if the arm is too high or too low.) Do not let the patient hold up the arm by using his muscle strength; the muscle tension can elevate systolic pressure.

After positioning the cuff, palpate the brachial pulse just below and slightly medial to the antecubital area. While observing the manometer or gauge, pump the bulb until the pulse disappears; then observe the pressure reading.

Obtaining the reading

With the stethoscope earpieces in your ears, place the head of the stethoscope over the brachial artery, just distal to the cuff or slightly beneath it. Apply the stethoscope firmly, but with as little pressure as possible to prevent distortion of Korotkoff sounds (pulse sounds). Typically, you'll use the flat diaphragm to auscultate the pulse. However, you may use the bell of the stethoscope if the patient's pulse is diminished or hard to find; the bell more effectively detects the low-pitched sound of arterial blood flow.

Watching the manometer or gauge, pump the bulb until the pressure level is about 30 mm Hg above the point at which the pulse disappeared. Slowly open the air valve and watch the mercury drop or the gauge needle descend. Release the pressure at a rate of about 2 to 3 mm Hg per second, and listen for Korotkoff sounds.

Produced by blood movement and vessel vibration, Korotkoff sounds occur in five phases. During phase I, you'll hear clear, faint tapping sounds of increasing intensity. During phase II, you'll hear a soft, swishing sound or murmur. Phase III is characterized by return of clear, crisp tapping of increasing intensity. During phase IV (the first diastolic phase), sounds become abruptly muffled and take on a blowing quality. During phase V (the second diastolic phase), pulse sounds disappear.

Recording the readings

As soon as you hear blood start to pulse through the brachial artery, note the reading on the manometer or gauge. Record this reading as systolic pressure. When you hear pulse sounds disappear (phase V), record this reading as diastolic pressure. (For children and highly active adults, phase IV [muffling] may more accurately reflect diastolic pressure.)

The American Heart Association and World Health Organization recommend documenting pressures from phases I, IV, and V. However, phase IV pressure is not commonly documented in clinical practice. To avoid confusion and aid interpretation of blood pressure changes, record pressures as *systolic/muffling/disappearance*; for example, "120/80/76 mm Hg." Also document the extremity used and the patient's position during measurement. (*Note:* If you measured blood pressure in the leg, expect pressure to be 5 to 10 mm Hg higher than brachial pressure.)

able pressure transducer; sterile gloves; 500-ml bag of I.V. flush solution (such as D_5W or 0.9% sodium chloride solution); 500 or 1,000 units of heparin; syringe and needle (21G to 25G, 1"); alcohol swabs; medication label; pressure bag; site care kit; and tubing labels.

For arterial catheter removal
Gather gloves; mask; gown; protective eyewear; two sterile 4" × 4" gauze pads; 500-ml I.V. bag; sheet protector; sterile suture removal set; dressing; alcohol swabs; and nonallergenic tape. For *femoral line* removal, gather additional sterile 4" × 4" gauze pads, a small sandbag (which you may wrap in a towel or place in a pillowcase), and an adhesive bandage. If the doctor has ordered a *catheter tip culture,* also gather sterile scissors and a sterile container.

Preparation
Preparing the patient
Explain the procedure to the patient and his family, including the purpose of arterial pressure monitoring and the anticipated duration of catheter placement. Make sure the patient signs a consent form. If he's unable to sign, ask a responsible family member to give written consent.

Position the patient for easy access to the catheter insertion site. Place a sheet protector under the site. (See *Arterial catheter insertion sites,* page 40.)

If the catheter will be inserted into the radial artery, perform Allen's test to assess collateral circulation in the hand. To perform this test, press the radial and ulnar arteries while holding the patient's arm above heart level. Exercise the patient's hand, or have him clench his fist, until you see blanching. Then lower the hand and release the ulnar artery. If blanching disappears within 6 seconds (indicating blood filling the vessels), radial catheterization can proceed safely.

Preparing the equipment
Before setting up and priming the monitoring system, wash your hands thoroughly. Maintain

---

Alternative methods for auscultating blood pressure

If your patient isn't undergoing direct blood pressure monitoring, you must assess his blood pressure indirectly. Besides auscultation, alternative methods include palpation; return-to-flow, oscillatory, and Doppler methods; and automated systems. You must use reliable equipment and proper technique to ensure accurate, reproducible findings.

Palpation
To palpate the arterial pulse using a blood pressure cuff, first inflate the cuff, and then deflate it slowly. When you detect the pulse, record the reading as systolic pressure.

Return-to-flow method
Inflate a blood pressure cuff to a measurement above the patient's anticipated or previously recorded systolic pressure. Then slowly deflate the cuff until you establish return of blood flow, such as by palpating the pulse or checking the manometer. The manometer reading at return to flow corresponds to approximate systolic blood pressure. You may also verify return to flow by using a Doppler device or, if an arterial line is in place, watching for a waveform on the bedside monitor.

Oscillatory method
Inflate the blood pressure cuff and then deflate it slowly. Record systolic pressure when you observe oscillation of the mercury column or needle gauge. Record mean arterial pressure when maximum oscillation occurs. (This method does not determine diastolic pressure.)

Doppler method
Inflate the blood pressure cuff and then deflate it slowly. Record systolic pressure when the Doppler device detects Korotkoff sounds.

Automated systems
Many types of automated systems are available. Some use oscillation; others detect sound or vessel wall movement (such as with a Doppler device), and still others use a microcomputer to interpret Korotkoff sounds.

Arterial catheter insertion sites

The doctor inserts an arterial catheter into the radial, brachial, or femoral artery. The radial and brachial arteries allow better access, permit freer patient movement, and are easier to observe and maintain.

The femoral artery, although larger and easier to palpate than the radial artery, typically is reserved for critically ill patients because a femoral line limits movement and is hard to maintain. Also, bleeding from a femoral site is harder to control, and active or occult bleeding into abdominal or thigh tissues may be difficult to assess.

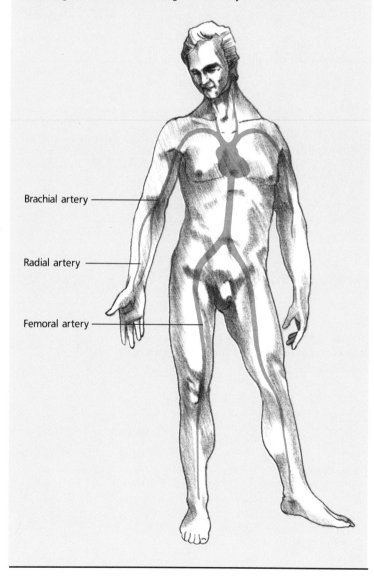

Brachial artery

Radial artery

Femoral artery

asepsis by wearing personal protective equipment throughout preparation.

Inflate the pressure bag to 300 mm Hg and check for air leaks. Then release the pressure.

Prepare the I.V. flush solution by adding the prescribed amount of heparin with an appropriate syringe and needle (unless the patient has a history of heparin sensitivity). Attach a medication label to the I.V. bag, noting the amount of heparin added, time, date, and your name or initials (depending on hospital policy).

Remove the transducer from the sterile package and attach the cable that will connect it with the bedside monitor. (Attaching the cable to the transducer helps prevent fluid from dampening the cable connections.) Make sure all connections of the pressure tubing and transducer are secure. Close the flow clamp on the pressure tubing set and spike the flush solution. Remove air from the flush solution by inverting the I.V. bag, opening the flow clamp, and squeezing. Then close the flow clamp and hang the I.V. bag on a pole at a height of approximately 2′ (60 cm), which applies approximately 45 mm Hg of pressure.

Gently squeeze the drip chamber until it is half filled with flush solution. Then open the flow clamp. Fill the pressure tubing and transducer system by activating the fast-flush release. The solution will run through the transducer and out through the transducer vent port. (Specific steps for flushing the transducer may vary. Be sure to follow the manufacturer's directions.)

Deliver the flush solution through the remaining tubing and stopcocks by turning the stopcocks. Activate the continuous flush device to remove all air. Replace all vented caps on stopcock side ports with nonvented or dead-end caps. Then mount the transducer on the patient or on an I.V. pole, depending on hospital policy.

Next, pressurize the I.V. flush solution. The amount of pressure to apply depends on the desired flow rate. Applying 300 mm Hg of pressure to a 3-ml flush device results in a flow rate of 3 ml/hour ($\pm$1 ml/hour); for a 30-ml flush device, applying 300 mm Hg results in a flow rate of 30 ml/hour ($\pm$10 ml/

hour). (For a pediatric patient, the procedure and equipment vary depending on where you work. So check your hospital's policy. The flush solution may be attached to a volumetric infusion pump or syringe pump to monitor and control volume administration more accurately.)

Set the alarms on the bedside monitor according to hospital policy.

Procedure

• Check the patient's history for an allergy or a hypersensitivity to iodine and the ordered local anesthetic.
• Maintain asepsis by wearing personal protective equipment throughout all procedures described below.

Inserting an arterial catheter

• Using a preassembled preparation kit, the doctor prepares and anesthetizes the insertion site. He covers the surrounding area with either sterile drapes or towels. The catheter is then inserted into the artery and attached to the fluid-filled pressure tubing.
• While the doctor holds the catheter in place, activate the fast-flush release to flush blood from the catheter. After each fast-flush operation, observe the drip chamber to verify that the continuous flush rate is as desired. A waveform should appear on the bedside monitor.
• The doctor may suture the catheter in place, or you may secure it with nonallergenic tape. Apply antimicrobial ointment and cover the insertion site with a dressing, as specified by hospital policy.
• Immobilize the insertion site. With a radial or brachial site, use an arm board and soft wrist restraint (if the patient's condition so requires). With a femoral site, assess the need for an ankle restraint; maintain the patient on bed rest, with the head of the bed raised no more than 15 to 30 degrees, to prevent the catheter from kinking. Level the zeroing stopcock of the transducer with the phlebostatic axis. Then zero the system to atmospheric pressure. (See Chapter 2.)
• Activate monitor alarms, as appropriate.
• Document the date of system setup so that all caregivers will know when to change the

components. Document systolic, diastolic, and mean pressure readings as well.

Obtaining a blood sample

• The specific procedure depends on whether an open or a closed sampling device is in place. (A closed device includes a reservoir to avoid exposure to air, eliminate the use of needles, and permit reinfusion of the discard or clearing volume.) (See *Closed arterial blood sampling system,* page 42.) Regardless of the type of device, be sure to follow the manufacturer's instructions closely.
• Wash your hands and maintain asepsis and universal precautions throughout the procedure. Explain the procedure to the patient to reduce his anxiety, and place a sheet protector under the site to be accessed.

From an open system. Follow these steps to collect a blood sample using an open system.
• Assemble the equipment, taking care not to contaminate the dead-end cap, stopcock, and syringes. Turn off or temporarily silence the monitor alarms, depending on hospital policy. (However, some hospitals require that alarms be left on.)
• Locate the stopcock nearest the patient. Open a sterile 4″ × 4″ gauze pad. Remove the dead-end cap from the stopcock and place it on the gauze pad.
• Insert the syringe for the discard sample into the stopcock. (This sample is discarded because it is diluted with flush solution.) Follow hospital policy on how much discard blood to collect. Usually, you'll withdraw 5 to 10 ml through a 5- or 10-ml syringe.
• Next, turn the stopcock off to the flush solution. Slowly retract the syringe to withdraw the discard sample. If you feel resistance, reposition the affected extremity and check the insertion site for obvious problems (such as catheter kinking). After correcting the problem, resume blood withdrawal. Then turn the stopcock halfway back to the open position to close the system in all directions.
• Remove the discard syringe and dispose of

ADVANCED EQUIPMENT

Closed arterial blood sampling system

Unlike an open arterial blood sampling system, a closed system has a reservoir, which doesn't allow air to enter the system during blood collection. It eliminates the use of needles and permits reinfusion of unused but collected arterial blood.

After the reservoir has been filled with blood, a syringe with an attached cannula is connected to the blood sampling site. Blood is withdrawn into the syringe. Once the syringe and cannula have been removed, the blood in the reservoir can be slowly reinfused.

The illustration shows the closed sampling system.

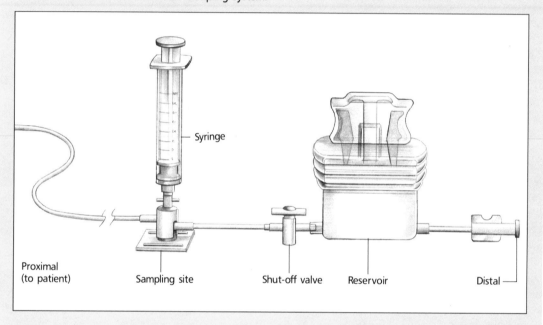

Proximal (to patient)   Sampling site   Shut-off valve   Reservoir   Distal

Syringe

the blood in the syringe, observing universal precautions.
• Place the syringe for the laboratory sample in the stopcock, turn the stopcock off to the flush solution, and slowly withdraw the required amount of blood. For each additional sample required, repeat this procedure. If the doctor has ordered coagulation tests, obtain blood for this sample from the final syringe to prevent dilution from the flush device.
• After you've obtained blood for the final sample, turn the stopcock off to the syringe and remove the syringe. Activate the fast-flush

release to clear the tubing. Then turn off the stopcock to the patient and repeat the fast flush to clear the stopcock port.
• Turn the stopcock off to the stopcock port and replace the dead-end cap. Reactivate the monitor alarms. Attach needles to the filled syringes and transfer the blood samples to the appropriate Vacutainers, labeling them according to your hospital's policy. Send all samples to the laboratory with appropriate documentation.
• Check the monitor for return of the arterial waveform and pressure reading.

From a closed system. Follow these steps to collect a blood sample using a closed system.
• Assemble the equipment, maintaining aseptic technique. Locate the closed-system reservoir and blood sampling site. Deactivate or temporarily silence monitor alarms. (However, some hospitals require that alarms be left on.)
• Clean the sampling site with an alcohol swab.
• Holding the reservoir upright, grasp the flexures and slowly fill the reservoir with blood over 3 to 5 seconds. (This blood serves as discard blood.) If you feel resistance, reposition the affected extremity and check the catheter site for obvious problems (such as kinking). Then resume blood withdrawal.
• Turn the one-way valve off to the reservoir by turning the handle perpendicular to the tubing. Using a syringe with attached cannula, insert the cannula into the sampling site. (Make sure the plunger is depressed to the bottom of the syringe barrel.) Slowly fill the syringe. Then grasp the cannula near the sampling site and remove the syringe and cannula as one unit. Repeat the procedure as needed to fill the required number of syringes. If the doctor has ordered coagulation tests, obtain blood for those tests from the final syringe to prevent dilution from the flush solution.
• After filling the syringes, turn the one-way valve to its original position, parallel to the tubing. Now smoothly and evenly push down on the plunger until the flexures lock in place in the fully closed position and all fluid has been reinfused. The fluid should be reinfused over a 3- to 5-second period. Then activate the fast-flush release to clear blood from the tubing and reservoir.
• Clean the sampling site with an alcohol swab. Reactivate the monitor alarms. Using the blood transfer unit, transfer blood samples to the appropriate Vacutainers, labeling them according to your hospital's policy. Send all samples to the laboratory, with appropriate documentation.

Changing arterial line tubing
• Wash your hands and follow universal precautions. Assemble the new pressure monitoring system.

• Consult hospital policy and procedure to determine how much tubing length to change.
• Inflate the pressure bag to 300 mm Hg and check it for air leaks. Then release the pressure.
• Prepare the I.V. flush solution and prime the pressure tubing and transducer system (as described under "Preparing the equipment," page 39). At this time, add both medication and tubing labels. Apply 300 mm Hg of pressure to the system. Then hang the I.V. bag on a pole.
• Place the sheet protector under the affected extremity. Remove the dressing from the catheter insertion site, taking care not to dislodge the catheter or cause vessel trauma. Turn off or temporarily silence the monitor alarms. (However, some hospitals require that alarms be left on.)
• Turn off the flow clamp of the tubing segment that you will change. Disconnect the tubing from the catheter hub, taking care not to dislodge the catheter. Immediately insert new tubing into the catheter hub. Secure the tubing and then activate the fast-flush release to clear it.
• Reactivate the monitor alarms. Apply an appropriate dressing.
• Level the zeroing stopcock of the transducer with the phlebostatic axis, and zero the system to atmospheric pressure.
• Document the date of system setup.

Removing an arterial line
• Consult hospital policy to determine if you are permitted to perform this procedure.
• Explain the procedure to the patient.
• Assemble all equipment. Wash your hands. Observe universal precautions, including wearing personal protective equipment, for this procedure.
• Document the systolic, diastolic, and mean blood pressures. If a manual, indirect blood pressure has not been assessed recently, obtain one now to establish a new baseline.
• Turn off the monitor alarms. Then turn off the flow clamp to the flush solution.
• Carefully remove the dressing over the insertion site. Remove any sutures, using the suture removal kit, and then carefully check that all sutures have been removed.
• Withdraw the catheter using a gentle, steady

motion. Keep the catheter parallel to the artery during withdrawal to reduce the risk of traumatic injury.

• Immediately after withdrawing the catheter, apply pressure to the site with a sterile 4″ × 4″ gauze pad. Maintain pressure for at least 10 minutes (longer if bleeding or oozing persists). Apply additional pressure to a femoral site or if the patient has coagulopathy or is receiving anticoagulants.

• Cover the site with an appropriate dressing and secure the dressing with tape. If stipulated by hospital policy, make a pressure dressing for a femoral site by folding in half four sterile 4″ × 4″ gauze pads, and apply the dressing. Cover the dressing with a tight adhesive bandage; then cover the bandage with a sandbag. Maintain the patient on bed rest for 6 hours with the sandbag in place.

• If the doctor has ordered a culture of the catheter tip (to diagnose a suspected infection), gently place the catheter tip on a 4″ × 4″ sterile gauze pad. Once the patient's bleeding is under control, hold the catheter over the sterile container. Using sterile scissors, cut the tip so it falls into the sterile container. Label the specimen and send it to the laboratory.

• Observe the site for bleeding. Assess and document circulation in the extremity distal to the site by assessing color, pulses, and sensation. Repeat this assessment every 15 minutes for the first 4 hours, every 30 minutes for the next 2 hours, then hourly for the next 6 hours.

Interpretation of findings

Normal arterial pressure varies with age and, to some extent, with the assessment method. After age 18, normal pressure ranges from 95/60 to 140/90 mm Hg; in older adults, it may measure 140/70 to 160/90 mm Hg. MAP normally ranges from 70 to 105 mm Hg.

Although an isolated measurement may provide important diagnostic information (for example, indicating severe hypotension or hypertension), you should consider blood pressure *trends* more important. Also, to avoid inaccurate conclusions, be sure to interpret values in light of the patient's clinical status and other hemodynamic findings. For instance, a patient with reduced cardiac output may maintain normal blood pressure through compensation, increasing resistance by peripheral vasoconstriction. Similarly, a patient with decreased resistance and increased blood flow may have normal blood pressure despite a severely compromised status. (See *Relating blood pressure to flow and resistance*.)

Blood pressure abnormalities

Abnormally low blood pressure, or hypotension, may reduce blood flow to the heart and other vital organs. It occurs when flow or resistance decreases. Causes of low blood flow include decreased cardiac output, absolute volume deficit, and relative volume deficit with volume remaining in the periphery. The major cause of decreased resistance is increased arterial tree radius (such as from vasodilation resulting from vasodilators or sepsis).

Abnormally high blood pressure, or hypertension, increases the heart's work load. When prolonged, it causes macrovascular and microvascular alterations that may threaten end-organ function. High blood pressure occurs when blood flow or resistance increases. Causes of increased flow include increased cardiac output and volume overload. Arterial vasoconstriction is the primary cause of increased resistance.

Normally, the heart rate rises slightly and blood pressure falls slightly when the patient moves suddenly from a lying or sitting position. In some cases, however, the blood pressure drop is severe. Called orthostatic (postural) hypotension, this phenomenon is most common in patients with hypovolemia, ineffective vasoconstriction, or inability to increase the heart rate (such as from a heart muscle problem, beta blocker or calcium channel blocker therapy, or autonomic nervous system dysfunction).

Direct versus indirect pressure readings

In critically ill patients, blood pressure readings obtained directly may differ by up to 14 mm Hg from those obtained indirectly. However, in patients with low blood flow, hypovolemia, or vasoconstriction, a differential of

Relating blood pressure to flow and resistance

When interpreting your patient's blood pressure reading, always consider his clinical status and other hemodynamic values. Keep in mind that the body can compensate for abnormalities in blood flow or vascular resistance. Consequently, blood pressure may remain normal even in a critically ill patient—until compensatory mechanisms are exhausted.

All three patients in the profiles below have normal blood pressure, yet two of them are severely compromised. Compare their hemodynamic values to these normal values:
• Cardiac output: 4 to 8 liters/minute
• Heart rate: 60 to 100 beats/minute
• Blood pressure: 90/60 to 140/90 mm Hg
• Mean arterial pressure (MAP): 70 to 105 mm Hg

Normal flow and resistance
Mark Bryson, age 42, was admitted for open-heart surgery. Before the operation, the doctor inserted an arterial line. Mr. Bryson's hemodynamic values are within the normal range:
• Cardiac output: 6.2 liters/minute
• Heart rate: 83 beats/minute
• Blood pressure: 122/76 mm Hg
• MAP: 91 mm Hg

Increased flow, decreased resistance
Peter West, age 24, was injured in a motor vehicle accident 1 week ago. He now has sepsis caused by a lacerated spleen and femur fracture. He's able to maintain a normal blood pressure because of increased cardiac output.
• Cardiac output: 12.2 liters/minute
• Heart rate: 116 beats/minute
• Blood pressure: 104/66 mm Hg
• MAP: 79 mm Hg

Decreased flow, increased resistance
Anna Wallace, age 62, had a massive anterior myocardial infarction 2 days ago. Although Ms. Wallace's cardiac output is diminished, she's able to maintain a normal blood pressure because of peripheral vasoconstriction.
• Cardiac output: 2.6 liters/minute
• Heart rate: 104 beats/minute
• Blood pressure: 102/76 mm Hg
• MAP: 85 mm Hg

---

up to 60 mm Hg may occur. Consequently, you should not attempt to validate a directly obtained reading by measuring pressure indirectly. If you have doubts about the blood pressure reading obtained through direct measurement, check the system for proper functioning rather than relying on indirect measurement.

Arterial waveform interpretation
Observing the pressure waveform on the monitor can enhance assessment of arterial pressure. An abnormal waveform may reflect an arrhythmia (such as atrial fibrillation) or other cardiovascular problems, such as aortic stenosis, aortic insufficiency, pulsus alternans, or pulsus paradoxus. (See *Interpreting arterial pressure waveforms,* pages 46 and 47.)

Nursing considerations
• Make sure that the position of the patient is documented when each blood pressure reading is obtained. This is important for determining trends. If the patient's blood pressure reading changes, you will need to assess whether the pressure changed because of a change in patient condition, a response to an intervention, or simply a change in patient position.
• Change the pressure tubing every 2 to 3 days, according to hospital policy.
• Change the dressing at the catheter site at intervals specified by your hospital. Regularly assess the site for signs of infection, such as redness and swelling. Notify the doctor immediately if you note any such signs.

(Text continues on page 49.)

Interpreting arterial pressure waveforms

Arterial waveforms reflect changes in left ventricular function and pressure and resistance in the systemic arterial tree. By observing the waveform, you may detect such conditions as aortic stenosis, atrial fibrillation, pulsus alternans, and pulsus paradoxus.

Normal waveform

A normal arterial waveform has four distinct components. *Peak systolic pressure* reflects pressure in the left ventricle during systole, which starts with the opening of the aortic valve. When aortic pressure exceeds left ventricular pressure, the aortic valve closes. On the waveform, the *dicrotic notch* indicates aortic valve closure. *Diastolic pressure* reflects vessel recoil, or the degree of arterial vasoconstriction. The *anacrotic notch,* indicating the first phase of ventricular systole (isovolumetric contraction), precedes aortic valve opening. (With peripheral arterial monitoring, the anacrotic notch normally doesn't appear.)

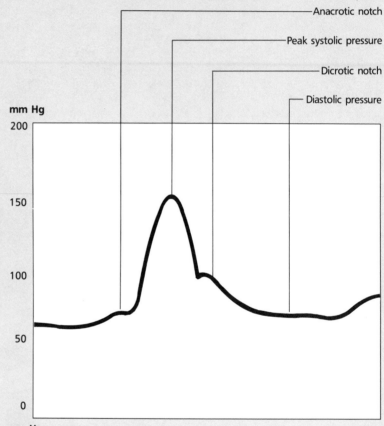

Aortic stenosis

In *aortic stenosis*, you'll see a small pulse wave with delayed peak systolic pressure. This lower systolic pressure results from slowed ventricular ejection through the stenotic aortic valve. Frequently, the dicrotic notch is not well-defined because of the abnormal closure of the valve leaflets. Because the systolic pressure is lower, these patients have a narrow pulse pressure.

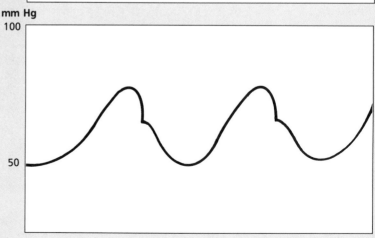

Atrial fibrillation
In *atrial fibrillation*, the amplitude varies because of the characteristic irregular rhythm.

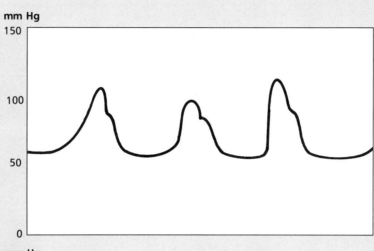

Pulsus alternans
In *pulsus alternans*, the waveform shows regular, alternating amplitudes of peak systolic pressure. These waveforms reflect an increased pooling of blood in the pulmonary vasculature, due to low intrathoracic pressure during inspiration, indicated by lower systolic pressure. Upon expiration, the higher systolic pressure results from a shunting of the pooled blood in the pulmonary bed to the left side of the heart.

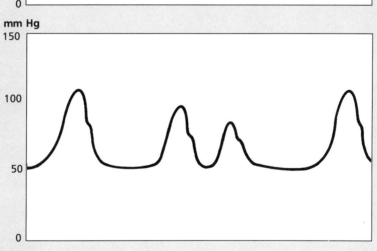

Pulsus paradoxus
In *pulsus paradoxus,* systolic pressure varies by more than 10 mm Hg from inspiration to expiration. This usually results from alterations in venous return to the right side of the heart and changes in intrathoracic or intrapericardial pressures.

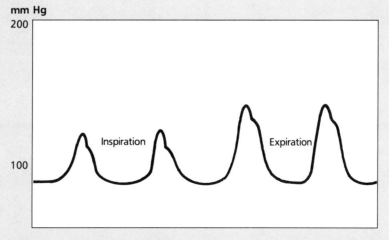

Handling arterial pressure monitoring problems

Insertion of an arterial line may cause various complications, some of them life-threatening. This chart lists possible causes for each complication, along with preventive and corrective measures.

COMPLICATION	POSSIBLE CAUSES	NURSING MEASURES
Arterial bleeding	• Loose connections • Oozing around catheter insertion site • Catheter dislodgment	• Check entire system for secure connections during each shift. • Assess for oozing around catheter insertion site every hour. • Immobilize catheter insertion site to prevent accidental catheter dislodgment. If catheter dislodges, immediately apply direct pressure, assess vital signs, follow standing orders for fluid administration, and notify doctor. • Notify doctor of any ecchymosis or hematoma. With a femoral line, assess for these problems lateral and posterior to insertion site.
Infection	• Failure to maintain aseptic technique during arterial line insertion, setup or maintenance of pressure system, tubing changes, or blood sample withdrawal • Failure to change components of pressure system as often as required • Contamination of multidose heparin vial	• Use careful aseptic technique during all procedures involving monitoring system or insertion site. • Assess for signs of local infection every hour. Report suspicious signs to doctor. • Assess patient's vital signs and evaluate for signs and symptoms of systemic infection. Notify doctor if vital signs change or if signs or symptoms of infection occur. • Change tubing, flush solution, and dressing according to hospital policy. The Centers for Disease Control and Prevention recommends changing I.V. components every 48 hours and changing the flush solution bag every 24 hours. • Use only single-dose heparin vials.
Air embolism	Entry of air into system, such as during initial setup and priming, catheter insertion, catheter dislodgment, accidental disconnection of pressure setup, open stopcocks, or inadvertent emptying of flush solution bag	• Check entire system for secure connections during each shift. • Remove all air from line during initial setup. • Immobilize insertion site to prevent accidental catheter dislodgment. • Make sure all stopcocks are in proper position. • Check I.V. bag for remaining I.V. flush solution. • Assess patient for signs of air embolism, such as decreased blood pressure; weak, rapid pulse; cyanosis; and loss of consciousness. If these signs occur, turn patient onto left side so air entering heart is absorbed in pulmonary artery. Notify doctor, and implement standing orders, as appropriate.
Arterial spasm or thrombosis	• Arterial trauma • Improper maintenance of flush solution or pressure system • Patient history of hypercoagulability	• Immobilize insertion site to prevent arterial wall irritation. • Every hour, check extremity distal to insertion site for color, pulses, sensation, movement, and temperature. Notify doctor of any changes. • If arterial spasm occurs, administer lidocaine, as ordered. • If thrombosis occurs, discontinue arterial line, as ordered and permitted. Prepare for arteriotomy and Fogarty catheterization, if ordered.

• Stay alert for signs and symptoms of other complications, such as arterial bleeding, air embolism, arterial spasms, and thrombosis. (See *Handling arterial pressure monitoring problems*.)

• Carefully document the amount of flush solution infused to avoid hypervolemia and volume overload, and to ensure accurate assessment of the patient's fluid status. Keep in mind that a patient with an indwelling arterial catheter receives fluid not just through the constantly circulating flush solution but also from fast flushes. Typically, a fast flush is performed after rezeroing and releveling the transducer (usually every 4 hours), after withdrawing blood samples through the arterial line, to maintain catheter patency and, possibly, to correct a positional catheter (such as one whose bevel is resting against the arterial wall).

• Be aware that erroneous pressure readings may result from a catheter that is clotted or positional; improper calibration, leveling, or zeroing of the monitoring system; loose connections; addition of extra stopcocks or extension tubing; or inadvertent entry of air into the system. If the catheter lumen clots, the flush system may be improperly pressurized. Regularly assess the amount of flush solution in the I.V. bag, and maintain 300 mm Hg of pressure in the pressure bag.

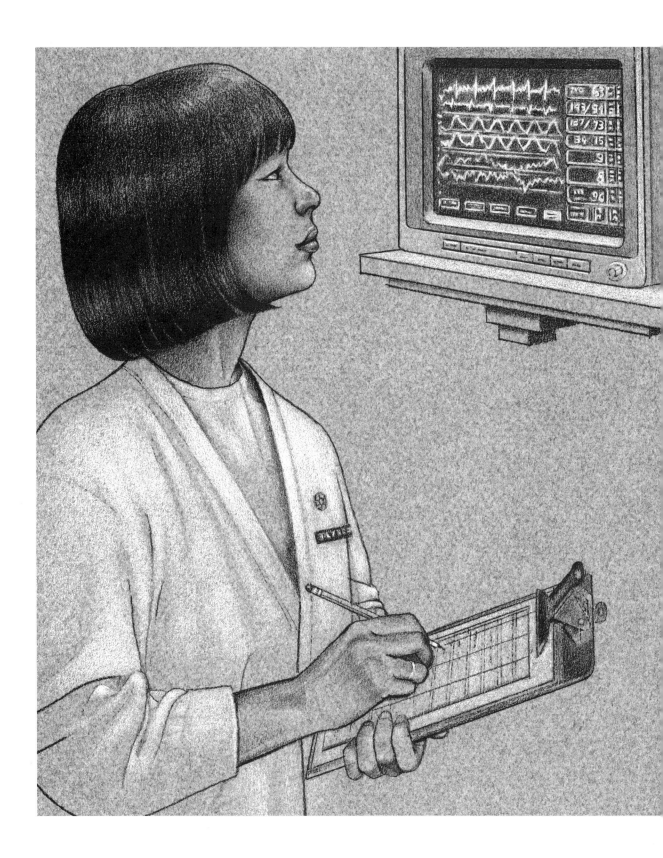

CHAPTER 4

Monitoring pulmonary artery and central venous pressures

Obtaining accurate hemodynamic information is essential when caring for acutely ill patients. Pulmonary artery pressure (PAP) and central venous pressure (CVP) monitoring makes diagnosis easier, helps evaluate the patient's response to therapy, and predicts patient prognosis. During the last 20 years, technological advances have taken PAP and CVP monitoring from the catheterization laboratory to the patient's bedside.

To ensure accurate measurement of these pressures and optimal patient care, you must be thoroughly familiar with the underlying physiologic principles and the procedural aspects of hemodynamic monitoring. This chapter provides that knowledge base. It begins with a discussion of cardiac physiology and its application to PAP and CVP monitoring. Then it describes how to prepare for and implement monitoring, interpret pressure readings and waveforms, maintain the monitoring system, and ensure high-quality patient care through-out monitoring.

Physiology

The heart's ability to act as a pump in meeting metabolic tissue needs is closely regulated. Ideally, the body can compensate for increased tissue demands. However, stress or cardiovascular alterations threaten normal compensation.

The major factors affecting cardiac performance are heart rate, preload, afterload, and contractility. Each plays an important role in maintaining oxygen delivery to tissues. Heart disease or circulatory compromise may affect one or more of these factors as the body attempts to maintain adequate cardiac performance.

Two-sided pump

Although a top-to-bottom perspective of the heart aids electrocardiogram (ECG) interpretation, you'll understand hemodynamic monitoring better if you think of the heart as a two-sided pump. The right and left sides each have their own structures and functions and generate pressure separately. (See *Structures of the heart.*) For optimal cardiac performance, both sides as well as the coupling structures they share must be competent and function together sequentially.

Right side
The right side of the heart consists of the right atrium and right ventricle. The right atrium receives deoxygenated venous blood from the systemic vasculature and myocardial muscle. Major vessels opening into the right atrium include the superior vena cava, which drains venous blood from the top half of the body; the inferior vena cava, which drains venous blood from the bottom half; and the coronary sinus, which drains venous blood from the heart itself.

The right ventricle receives venous blood from the right atrium through the tricuspid

valve. Because this ventricle dilates as venous return increases, it's considered a volume pump. It also propels blood through the pulmonic valve into the pulmonary artery, filling the pulmonary vasculature. Like the right side of the heart, the pulmonary vascular bed is compliant and has low pressure; consequently, little pressure from the right ventricle is required to propel the blood into the pulmonary vascular bed.

Left side
The left side of the heart pumps blood through all vessels except those leading to and from the lungs. Thus, it's larger and thicker than the right side. The left atrium receives oxygenated blood from pulmonary vessels through four pulmonary veins. From the left atrium, blood exits through the mitral valve and enters the left ventricle.

The left ventricle pumps blood through the aortic valve into the aorta and the remainder of the systemic vascular bed. As resistance to ejection increases, the left ventricle increases its contractile force. More pressure is required to fill the systemic circulation than the pulmonary circulation. Thus, the left side of the heart is considered a high-pressure system.

Coupling structures
Although the right and left sides differ in function, they're linked by various coupling structures—the pulmonary artery, pericardium, interventricular septum, and coronary arteries. When the left and right sides and all coupling structures are competent, the heart functions not as two separate pumps but as one integrated, two-sided pump. If these structures undergo changes, one or both ventricles may become dysfunctional.

Pulmonary artery
The pulmonary artery acts as the conduit between the right and left sides. The pulmonary capillary bed, which lies between the two sides, can sequester large amounts of blood. Measuring pressure changes for both sides of the heart may reveal changes in sequestering capacity.

Structures of the heart

When discussing anatomy in relation to hemodynamic monitoring, the heart is described as two separate pumps, right and left. Each has its own function and pressure. The right side of the heart includes the superior and inferior vena cavae, right atrium, right ventricle, tricuspid and pulmonic valves, and pulmonary artery. The left side includes the left atrium, left ventricle, aorta, and mitral and aortic valves.

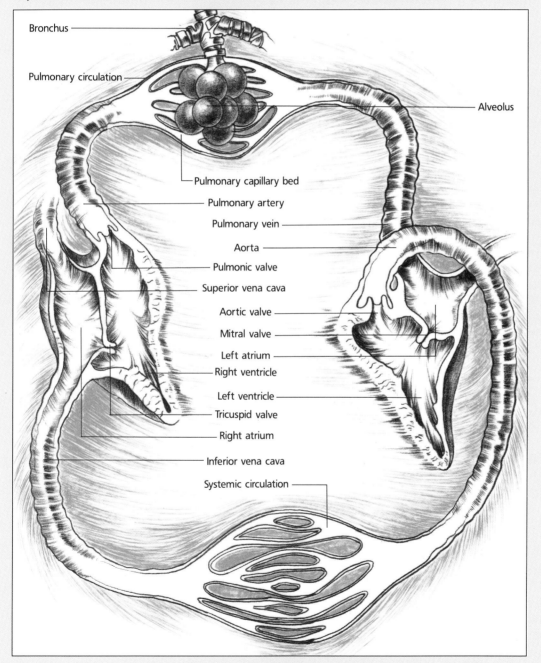

Bronchus

Pulmonary circulation

Alveolus

Pulmonary capillary bed

Pulmonary artery

Pulmonary vein

Aorta

Pulmonic valve

Superior vena cava

Aortic valve

Mitral valve

Left atrium

Right ventricle

Left ventricle

Tricuspid valve

Right atrium

Inferior vena cava

Systemic circulation

Pericardium

The rigid sac encasing both ventricles, the pericardium helps restrict ventricular relaxation and dilation during diastole. If one ventricle becomes dilated, such as from heart failure, the pericardium restricts further dilation and causes the other ventricle to encroach onto the opposite side.

Interventricular septum

Like a partition, the interventricular septum separates the ventricles. It serves as the posterior wall of the right ventricle and the anterior wall of the left ventricle. Changes in this shared mobile wall may cause undesired effects in one or both ventricles.

Coronary arteries

The coronary arteries arise from the root of the aorta, just above the aortic valve. Traveling along the exterior of the heart, they traverse the appropriate sulci, their distal branches penetrating the myocardium and endocardium. Their location affects blood flow during the cardiac cycle.

The coronary arteries include the right coronary artery (RCA) and left coronary artery (LCA) and their branches. More arterial branches supply blood to the left ventricle than the right ventricle because it is larger. The RCA supplies the anterior wall of the right ventricle and posterior one-third of the interventricular septum; its posterior descending branch supplies the posterior wall of the left ventricle.

The LCA has two major branches. The *circumflex artery*, which lies in the atrioventricular sulcus between the left atrium and left ventricle, supplies the lateral and posterior walls of the left ventricle. The *left anterior descending (LAD) artery* supplies the anterior wall of the left ventricle and a portion of the right ventricle. Because the RCA and LAD artery both supply blood to the ventricles, disease in either artery may affect both ventricles.

Coronary perfusion. Perfusion of both major coronary arteries requires adequate diastolic pressure in the aortic root. The coronary arteries perfuse the left ventricle primarily during diastole. During systole, ventricular wall stress increases, raising resistance to the extent that little blood enters the endocardium. However, the right ventricle, with less muscle mass than the left, undergoes less wall stress during systole. Thus, its resistance is lower and it receives more blood from the RCA at this time. Wall stress diminishes during ventricular diastole, allowing perfusion.

Circulatory system

Blood takes two separate paths through the body. In the *systemic circulation,* blood flows from the left ventricle to all parts of the body except the lungs, then to the right atrium. In the *pulmonary circulation,* blood flows from the right ventricle through the lungs to the left atrium. Pulmonary circulation has low resistance to blood flow, whereas systemic circulation has high resistance to blood flow.

Cardiac cycle

The cardiac cycle — one complete heartbeat — consists of systole (contraction) and diastole (relaxation) of both atria, followed by contraction and relaxation of both ventricles. The atria and ventricles act in a nearly synchronized manner. During ventricular systole, diastole occurs in the atria, and vice versa. The sequence is the same for both sides of the heart.

Typically, the ECG has been used to evaluate cardiac activity during systole and diastole. With hemodynamic monitoring, however, you can correlate the electrical activity shown on the ECG with the mechanical events shown by intracardiac waveforms. Because electrical activity precedes mechanical activity, the ECG waveform precedes the pressure waveform when the two are recorded simultaneously. The interval between the electrical and mechanical events is called *electromechanical coupling,* or the *excitation-contraction phase.* (See *Comparing the electrical and mechanical cardiac cycles.*)

Systole

Ventricular systole has three phases. During the *isovolumetric (isometric) contraction* phase, the ventricles contract in response to ventricular depolarization (indicated by the QRS complex on the ECG). Ventricular depolarization causes muscle fibers to shorten, leading to elevated pressure in the ventricles. As pressure increases, all heart valves are closed. Most of the oxygen supplied to the myocardium is consumed during the isovolumetric phase.

During the second phase of systole, *rapid ventricular ejection,* right ventricular pressure exceeds PAP and left ventricular pressure exceeds aortic pressure. Consequently, the aortic and pulmonic valves open, propelling blood out of the ventricles. Muscle fibers shorten even more, contributing to blood propulsion. During this phase, 80% to 85% of the blood volume is ejected. The sharp uprise in the waveform correlates with the ST segment on the ECG waveform.

As pressure begins to equalize, *reduced ventricular ejection* begins and blood ejection becomes more gradual. The atria, now in diastole, receive more blood from pulmonary and venous inflow, causing atrial pressure to rise (recorded as the *v* wave on the atrial pressure waveform). At the end of this phase, the pulmonary artery and aorta contain most of the blood ejected from the ventricles. PAP and aortic pressure slightly exceed ventricular pressure and blood starts to flow backward into the ventricles. As ventricular systole ends, ventricular pressure drops and the semilunar valves close. Reduced ventricular ejection correlates with the T wave on the ECG.

Diastole

The continuum of pressure changes within the heart and great vessels leads to the transition from systole to diastole. Like systole, diastole follows an electrical event—in this case, repolarization—and has three phases.

During *isovolumetric relaxation,* the first phase, the ventricles relax, causing a dramatic drop in ventricular pressure (indicated by the diastolic "dip" on the pressure waveform). This phase correlates with the period following the T wave on the ECG.

Comparing the electrical and mechanical cardiac cycles

These waveforms show the interval between the heart's electrical activity, shown by the electrocardiograph (ECG) waveform, and the mechanical activity of systole and diastole, shown by the right atrial and right ventricular pressure waveforms.

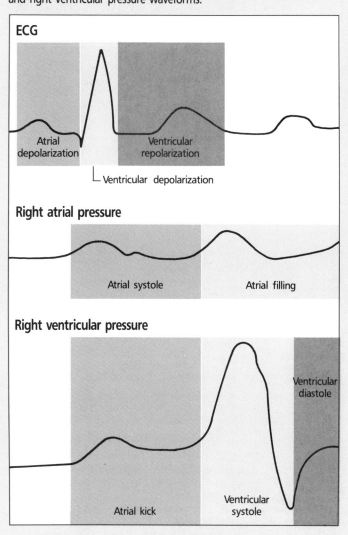

As tension leaves the myocardium, ventricular pressure drops below atrial pressure. In response, the atrioventricular (AV) valves open, leading to the next phase, *rapid ventricular filling,* during which approximately two-thirds of

Mechanical activity during the cardiac cycle

As these illustrations show, physiologic changes within the heart and vessels result in the successive phases of ventricular systole and diastole.

Isovolumetric phase
Systole begins with the isovolumetric phase (shown below). At this time, all valves are closed and the majority of oxygen is consumed. This phase is followed by rapid ventricular ejection, characterized by opening of the pulmonic and aortic valves and ejection of 80% to 85% of blood from the ventricles.

Reduced ventricular ejection
During the third systolic phase, reduced ventricular ejection, blood is ejected more slowly. With pulmonary and venous inflow, the atria (now in diastole) receive more blood. As atrial pressure rises, ventricular pressure falls and the semilunar valves close.

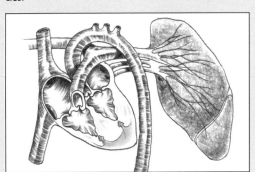

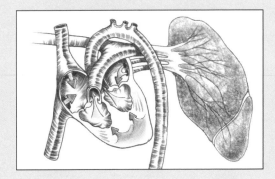

the blood volume moves passively from the atria to the ventricles.

During the next phase, *slow filling*, more atrial blood enters the ventricle through forceful atrial contraction (called atrial kick or atrial contribution). In sinus or atrial heart rhythms, atrial systole ejects the remaining one-third of the blood volume into the ventricle (producing the *a* wave on the pressure waveform). On the ECG, the slow filling phase corresponds to the PR interval.

At the end of diastole *(end diastole),* volume or pressure in the atria and ventricles should be equal. Immediately after diastole ends, more blood enters the ventricles. Ventricular pressure now exceeds atrial pressure, causing the AV valves to close. The cycle will then repeat. (See *Mechanical activity during the cardiac cycle.*)

Pulmonary artery pressure monitoring

Continuous pulmonary artery pressure (PAP) and intermittent pulmonary artery wedge pressure (PAWP) measurements provide important information about left ventricular function and preload. You can use this information not only for monitoring but also for aiding diagnosis, refining your assessment, guiding interventions, and projecting patient outcome.

Nearly all acutely ill patients are candidates for PAP monitoring — especially those who are hemodynamically unstable, who need fluid management or continuous cardiopulmonary assessment, or who are receiving multiple or frequently administered cardioactive drugs. PAP monitoring also is crucial for patients with

Isovolumetric relaxation
Diastole begins with isovolumetric relaxation. During this phase, all valves are closed and ventricular pressure continues to decline.

Rapid ventricular filling
Rapid ventricular filling, the next diastolic phase, occurs as ventricular pressure falls below atrial pressure and the atrioventricular (AV) valves open. Approximately two-thirds of the blood volume now enters the ventricles.

End diastole
As forceful atrial contraction propels more blood into the ventricle, the slow filling phase begins. At the end of this phase (end diastole), the remaining blood volume enters the ventricles. With ventricular pressure now exceeding atrial pressure, the AV valves begin to close.

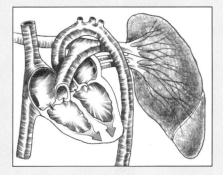 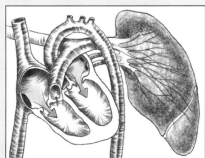 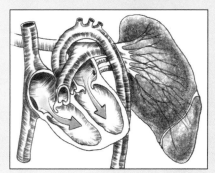

shock, trauma, pulmonary or cardiac disease, or multiorgan disease.

The original PAP monitoring catheter, which had two lumens, was invented by two doctors, Swan and Ganz. The device still bears their name but is commonly referred to as a pulmonary artery (PA) catheter. Current versions have up to six lumens, allowing you to gather additional hemodynamic information. Besides distal and proximal lumens used to measure pressures, a PA catheter has a balloon inflation lumen that inflates the balloon for PAWP measurement and a thermistor connector lumen that allows cardiac output measurement. Some catheters also have a pacemaker wire lumen that provides a port for pacemaker electrodes and measures continuous mixed venous oxygen saturation. (See *PA catheter: From basic to complex*, page 58.)

Fluoroscopy usually isn't required during catheter insertion because the catheter is flow directed, following venous blood flow from the right heart chambers into the pulmonary artery. Also, the pulmonary artery, right atrium, and right ventricle produce characteristic pressures and waveforms that can be observed on the monitor to help track catheter tip location. Marks on the catheter shaft, with 10-cm gradations, assist tracking by showing how far the catheter has been inserted.

The PA catheter is inserted into the heart's right side with the distal tip lying in the pulmonary artery. Left-sided pressures can be assessed indirectly.

During ventricular systole, the tricuspid and mitral valves are closed and the pulmonic and aortic valves are open. The higher pressure generated by the right ventricle during contraction is transmitted to the catheter tip located in the pulmonary artery. With the balloon de-

ADVANCED EQUIPMENT

PA catheter: From basic to complex

Depending on the intended uses, a pulmonary artery (PA) catheter may be simple or complex. The basic PA catheter has a distal and proximal lumen, a thermistor, and a balloon inflation gate valve. The *distal lumen,* which exits in the pulmonary artery, monitors PA pressure. Its hub usually is marked "PA distal" or is color-coded yellow. The *proximal lumen* exits in the right atrium or vena cava, depending on the size of the patient's heart. It monitors right atrial pressure and can be used as the injected solution lumen for cardiac output determination and infusing solutions. The proximal lumen hub usually is marked "Proximal" or is color-coded blue.

The *thermistor,* located about 1½" (4 cm) from the distal tip, measures temperature (aiding core temperature evaluation) and allows cardiac output measurement. The thermistor connector attaches to a cardiac output connector cable, then to a cardiac output monitor. Typically, it's red.

The *balloon inflation gate valve* is used for inflating the balloon tip with air. A stopcock connection, typically color-coded red, may be used.

Additional lumens

Some PA catheters have additional lumens used to obtain other hemodynamic data or permit certain interventions. For instance, a *proximal infusion port,* which exits in the right atrium or vena cava, allows additional fluid administration. A *right ventricular lumen,* exiting in the right ventricle, allows fluid administration, right ventricular pressure measurement, or use of a temporary ventricular pacing lead.

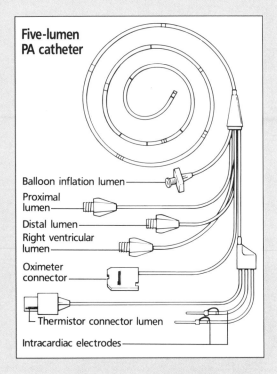

Five-lumen PA catheter

Balloon inflation lumen
Proximal lumen
Distal lumen
Right ventricular lumen
Oximeter connector
Thermistor connector lumen
Intracardiac electrodes

Some catheters have additional right atrial and right ventricular lumens for atrioventricular pacing. A *right ventricular ejection fraction fast-response thermistor,* with PA and right ventricular sensing electrodes, allows volumetric and ejection fraction measurements. Fiber-optic filaments, such as those used in pulse oximetry, exit into the pulmonary artery and permit measurement of continuous mixed venous oxygen saturation.

flated, the catheter records pulmonary artery systolic pressure, which reflects right ventricular systolic pressure.

During ventricular diastole, the tricuspid and mitral valves are open, the ventricles are filling with blood from their respective atria, and the pulmonic and aortic valves are closed.

With the balloon still deflated, pulmonary artery diastolic pressure (PADP) is recorded. After the pulmonic valve closes, the right ventricle continues to relax, causing a lower diastolic

pressure in the right ventricle than in the pulmonary artery. Right ventricular end-diastolic pressure (RVEDP) is less than PADP. The proximal lumen of the catheter exits in the right atrium or vena cava. During this phase, with a competent tricuspid valve, the RVEDP is reflected back to the right atrium. Therefore, right atrial pressure (RAP) is equal to RVEDP.

Because no obstruction normally exists between the pulmonary artery and the left atrium, the pressure recorded during diastole is virtually the same as left atrial pressure (LAP). With a pressure range of 6 to 20 mm Hg, this pressure is nearly the same as left ventricular end-diastolic pressure (LVEDP). PADP, LAP, and LVEDP are thus roughly equal, with PADP slightly higher than LAP by 1 to 4 mm Hg.

By inflating the balloon, the catheter floats downstream into a more distal branch of the pulmonary artery. Once the balloon lodges, the catheter is wedged. Because of the absence of valves between the pulmonic and mitral valves, and because the pulmonary capillary bed is a compliant system, an unrestricted vascular channel now exists between the catheter tip in the pulmonary artery through the pulmonary vascular bed, the pulmonary vein, the left atrium, the open mitral valve, and into the left ventricle. The distal lumen is now monitoring left ventricular filling pressure or LVEDP more closely.

This pressure—usually referred to as pulmonary artery wedge pressure (PAWP)—is also known as left atrial filling pressure, pulmonary capillary wedge pressure, pulmonary artery occlusion pressure, or the wedge. The importance of PAWP is that normally it closely approximates the pressure in the left ventricle during end diastole and provides a means of measuring left ventricular preload.

No specific contraindications for PAP monitoring exist. However, some patients undergoing PAP monitoring require special precautions. These include elderly patients with pulmonary hypertension, those with left bundle-branch block, and those for whom a systemic infection would be life-threatening.

Equipment

Equipment depends partly on the type of monitoring required. For PAP or intermittent RAP monitoring, gather a single-pressure line and transducer. For continuous CVP or RAP monitoring, obtain an additional transducer.

Typically, equipment includes a bedside monitor, an oscilloscope, pressure modules, and a pressure monitoring kit appropriate to the type of monitoring ordered. The kit usually includes pressure tubing, a flush device, an I.V. drip chamber, and a disposable transducer. A percutaneous introducer, used to insert the catheter, may be available individually or may be part of a prepackaged kit. The introducer should be at least one-half size larger than the catheter; in some cases, an introducer one size larger is used to make the side port more available for infusion.

Also obtain an I.V. solution bag; 500 to 1,000 ml of dextrose 5% in water or 0.9% sodium chloride solution; 1 to 2 units/ml of heparin flush solution; an I.V. pole with transducer mount; a pressure bag or continuous pressure device with gauge; a leveling device; a sterile basin with sterile water or sterile 0.9% sodium chloride solution; povidone-iodine ointment; a sterile gauze dressing or an occlusive dressing; tape; and sterile gloves, masks (for you and the doctor to wear during catheter insertion), and gowns (optional, depending on hospital infection control policy).

The doctor will choose a PA catheter of the appropriate design for the type of monitoring required. A sterile contamination sheath (sometimes included in the introducer kit) covers the external portion of the catheter.

Preparation
Preparing the patient

Check the patient's chart for heparin sensitivity, which contraindicates adding heparin to the flush solution. If the patient is alert, explain the procedure to him to reduce his anxiety. Mention that the catheter will monitor pressures from the pulmonary artery and heart. Reassure him that the catheter poses little danger and rarely causes pain. Tell him that if pain occurs at the introducer insertion site, the doctor will order an analgesic or a sedative.

Be sure to tell the patient and his family not to be alarmed if they see the pressure waveform on the monitor "move around." Explain that the cause usually is artifact.

Position the patient at the proper height and angle for effective catheter insertion. If the doctor will use a superior approach for percutaneous insertion (most commonly using the internal jugular or subclavian vein), place the patient flat or in a slight Trendelenburg position. Remove the patient's pillow to help engorge the vessel and prevent air embolism. Turn his head to the side opposite the insertion site.

If the doctor will use an inferior approach to access a femoral vein, position the patient flat. Be aware that with this approach, certain catheters are harder to insert and may require more manipulation.

Preparing the equipment

To obtain reliable pressure values and clear waveforms, the pressure monitoring system and bedside monitor must be properly calibrated and zeroed. Make sure that the monitor has the correct pressure modules; then calibrate it according to the manufacturer's instructions. (For details on calibration, see Chapter 2.)

Turn the monitor on before gathering the equipment to give it sufficient time to warm up. Be sure to check the operations manual for the monitor you're using; some older monitors may need 20 minutes to warm up.

Prepare the pressure monitoring system according to hospital policy. Hospital guidelines also may specify whether to mount the transducer on the I.V. pole or tape it to the patient and whether to add heparin to the flush solution. To treat any complications from catheter insertion, make sure to have emergency resuscitation equipment on hand (defibrillator, oxygen, and supplies for intubation and emergency drug administration).

Prepare a sterile field for insertion of the introducer and catheter. (A bedside tray may be sufficient.) For easier access, place the tray on the same side as the insertion site.

Procedure

• Maintain aseptic technique and use universal precautions throughout catheter preparation and insertion.
• Wash your hands. Clean the insertion site with a povidone-iodine ointment and drape it appropriately.
• Put on a mask. Help the doctor put on a sterile mask, gown, and gloves.

Preparing the catheter

• Open the outer packaging of the catheter, revealing the inner sterile wrapping. Using aseptic technique, the doctor opens the inner wrapping and picks up the catheter. Take the catheter lumen hubs as he hands them to you.
• To remove air from the catheter and verify its patency, flush the catheter. In the more common flushing method, you connect the syringes aseptically to the appropriate pressure lines and then flush them before insertion. This method makes pressure waveforms easier to identify on the monitor during insertion.

Alternatively, you may flush the lumens after catheter insertion with sterile I.V. solution from sterile syringes attached to the lumens. Leave the filled syringes on during insertion.
• If the system has multiple pressure lines (such as a distal line to monitor PAP and a proximal line to monitor RAP), make sure that the distal PA lumen hub is attached to the pressure line that will be observed on the monitor. Inadvertently attaching the distal PA line to the proximal lumen hub will prevent the proper waveform from appearing during insertion.
• Observe the diastolic values carefully during insertion. Make sure that the scale is appropriate for lower pressures. A scale of 0 to 25 or 0 to 50 mm Hg (more common) is preferred. (With a higher scale, such as 0 to 100 or 0 to 250 mm Hg, waveforms will appear too small and the location of the catheter tip will be hard to identify.)
• To verify integrity of the balloon, the doctor inflates it with air (usually 1.5 cc) before handing you the lumens to attach to the pressure monitoring system. He then observes for symmetrical shape. He also may submerge it in a small sterile basin filled with sterile water and observe for bubbles, which indicate a leak.

Inserting the catheter

• Assist the doctor as he inserts the introducer to gain access to the vessel. He may perform a cutdown or (more commonly) insert the catheter percutaneously, such as with a modified Seldinger technique. (See *Percutaneous catheter insertion: Modified Seldinger technique.*)
• After the introducer is placed and the cathe-

Percutaneous catheter insertion: Modified Seldinger technique

Safer and simpler than a cutdown procedure, the modified Seldinger technique has become the most common method for inserting a pulmonary artery catheter into a peripheral vessel. The doctor usually inserts the catheter into the internal jugular or subclavian vein (superior approach) or a femoral vein (inferior approach).

Using the right internal jugular vein creates a direct line into the right atrium, promoting catheter insertion. Using the subclavian vein has certain drawbacks. In some patients, the subclavian is tortuous, possibly leading to internal kinking of the introducer sheath or catheter. Also, the lung apices are above the clavicle level, so using the subclavian vein may cause a small pneumothorax.

The steps described below are common to all approaches used for percutaneous catheter insertion. However, some steps may vary slightly, depending on the equipment used and on the doctor's preference.

Preparation
• Position the patient appropriately for the insertion site selected.
• Wash your hands thoroughly. Then both you and the doctor must put on a gown, gloves, and a mask.
• Drape the patient and insertion site with a fenestrated drape or sterile towels.

Procedure
• Clean the insertion site with povidone-iodine swabs or gauze.
• The doctor raises a skin wheal at the insertion site by injecting 1% lidocaine using a 25G needle.

• Using a 22G needle and syringe, the doctor will locate the vessel he wishes to use. He'll leave the needle and syringe in place. He will then place a thin-walled, 18G needle or an over-the-needle catheter next to the 22G locating needle. (The doctor may prefer a specific type of locating needle. However, the steps are basically the same for all needles. For best results, find out the doctor's preference in advance.)
• As the doctor advances the catheter, he also aspirates for blood. When blood flows freely, he pulls out the locating needle.
• The doctor inserts the tip of the guide wire through the catheter or needle hub and advances it into the vessel to the desired depth.
• While holding the guide wire in place, the doctor pulls back the introducing needle.
• The doctor enlarges the insertion site with the point of a #11 scalpel. Then he inserts the dilator through the introducer sheath and threads the introducer (with the dilator) over the end of the guide wire. Using a twisting motion, he advances it through the skin and subcutaneous tissue, then into the vessel.
• When the dilator is within the vessel, the doctor advances the sheath. Then, holding the sheath in place, he removes the guide wire and dilator.
• The doctor aspirates blood from the side arm to remove all air from the sheath and side arm. He then flushes the side arm with sterile solution and attaches it to the I.V. solution tubing.
• The doctor may suture the catheter in place to help maintain it in the proper position. You may then apply ointment to the insertion site and cover it with an appropriate occlusive dressing.

ter lumens are flushed, the doctor inserts the catheter through the introducer. In the internal jugular or subclavian approach, he inserts the catheter into the end of the introducer sheath with the balloon deflated, directing the curl of the catheter toward the patient's midline.
• As insertion begins, observe the bedside monitor for waveform variations. (See *Normal PA waveforms,* page 62.)
• When the catheter exits the end of the intro-

ducer sheath and reaches the junction of the superior vena cava and right atrium (at the 15- to 20-cm mark on the catheter shaft), the monitor shows oscillations that correspond to the patient's respirations. The balloon is then inflated with the recommended volume of air to allow normal blood flow and to aid catheter insertion.
• Using a gentle, smooth motion, the doctor advances the catheter through the heart

Normal PA waveforms

During pulmonary artery (PA) catheter insertion, the monitor shows various waveforms as the catheter advances through the heart chambers.

Right atrium
When the catheter tip enters the right atrium, the first heart chamber on its route, a waveform like the one shown below appears on the monitor. Note the two small upright waves. The *a* waves represent left atrial contraction; the *v* waves, increased pressure or volume in the left atrium during left ventricular systole.

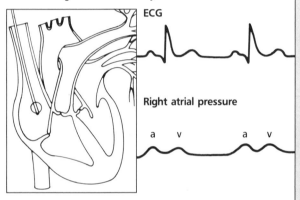

Pulmonary artery
The catheter then floats into the pulmonary artery, causing a waveform like the one shown below. Note that the upstroke is smoother than on the right ventricular waveform. The dicrotic notch indicates pulmonic valve closure.

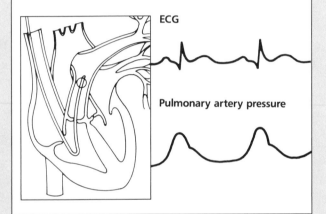

Right ventricle
As the catheter tip reaches the right ventricle, you'll see a waveform with sharp systolic upstrokes and lower diastolic dips.

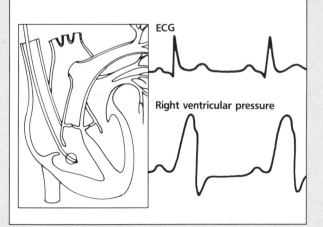

PAWP
Floating into a distal branch of the pulmonary artery, the balloon wedges where the vessel becomes too narrow for it to pass. The monitor now shows a pulmonary artery wedge pressure (PAWP) waveform (also called a wedge tracing), with two small uprises from left atrial systole and diastole. Once the waveform is seen, the balloon is deflated and the catheter is left in the pulmonary artery.

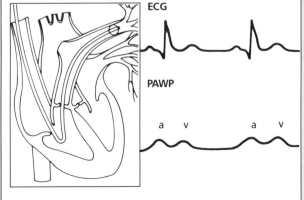

chambers, moving rapidly to the pulmonary artery because prolonged manipulation here may reduce catheter stiffness. When the mark on the catheter shaft reaches 15 to 20 cm, the catheter enters the right atrium. The waveform shows two small, upright waves; pressure is low (from 2 to 4 mm Hg). Read pressure values in the mean mode because systolic and diastolic values are similar.

• The doctor advances the catheter into the right ventricle, working quickly to minimize irritation. The waveform now shows sharp systolic upstrokes and lower diastolic dips. Depending on the size of the patient's heart, the catheter should reach the 30- to 35-cm mark. (The smaller the heart, the less catheter length will be needed to reach the right ventricle.) Record both systolic and diastolic pressures. Systolic pressure normally ranges from 15 to 25 mm Hg; diastolic pressure, 0 to 8 mm Hg.

• As the catheter floats into the pulmonary artery, note that the upstroke from right ventricular systole is smoother, and systolic pressure is nearly the same as right ventricular systolic pressure. Record systolic, diastolic, and mean pressures (typically from 8 to 15 mm Hg). A dicrotic notch on the diastolic portion of the waveform indicates pulmonic valve closure.

Wedging the catheter

• To obtain a wedge tracing, the doctor lets the inflated balloon float downstream with venous blood flow to a smaller, more distal branch of the pulmonary artery. Here, the catheter lodges, or wedges, causing occlusion of right ventricular and PA diastolic pressures. The tracing resembles the right atrial tracing because the catheter tip is recording LAP. The waveform shows two small uprises. Record PAWP in the mean mode (usually between 6 and 12 mm Hg).

A PAWP waveform, or wedge tracing, appears when the catheter has been inserted 45 to 50 cm. (However, in a large heart, a longer catheter length — up to 55 cm — typically is required. A catheter should never be inserted more than 60 cm.) Usually, 30 to 45 seconds elapse from the time the doctor inserts the introducer until the wedge tracing appears.

• The doctor deflates the balloon, and the catheter drifts out of the wedge position and into the pulmonary artery, its normal resting place.

• If the appropriate waveforms don't appear at the expected times during catheter insertion, the catheter may be coiled in the right atrium and ventricle. To correct this problem, deflate the balloon. To do this, unlock the gate valve or turn the stopcock to the ON position and then detach the syringe from the balloon inflation port. Back pressure in the pulmonary artery causes the balloon to deflate on its own. (Active air withdrawal may compromise balloon integrity.) To verify balloon deflation, observe the monitor for return of the PA tracing.

• Typically, the doctor orders a portable chest X-ray to confirm catheter position.

• Apply a sterile occlusive dressing to the insertion site.

• Document the date and time of catheter insertion, the doctor who performed the procedure, the catheter insertion site, pressure waveforms and values for the various heart chambers, balloon inflation volume required to obtain a wedge tracing, any arrhythmias occurring during or after the procedure, type of flush solution used and its heparin concentration (if any), type of dressing applied, and the patient's tolerance for the procedure. Remember to initial and date the dressing.

Obtaining intermittent PAP values

• After inserting the catheter and recording initial pressure readings, record subsequent PAP values and monitor waveforms. These values will be used to calculate other important hemodynamic indices. To ensure accurate values, make sure that the transducer is properly leveled and zeroed.

• If possible, obtain PAP values at the end of expiration (when the patient completely exhales). At this time, intrathoracic pressure approaches atmospheric pressure and has the least effect on PAP. If you obtain a reading during other phases of the respiratory cycle, respiratory interference may occur. For instance, during inspiration, when intrathoracic pressure drops, PAP may be false-low because the negative pressure is transmitted to the catheter. During expiration, when intrathoracic pressure rises, PAP may be false-high.

For patients with a rapid respiratory rate and subsequent variations, you may have trouble identifying the end of expiration. The monitor displays an average of the digital readings obtained over time, as well as those readings obtained during a full respiratory cycle. If possible, obtain a printout. Use the averaged values obtained through the full respiratory cycle. To analyze trends accurately, be sure to record values at consistent times during the respiratory cycle.

Taking a PAWP reading
• PAWP is recorded by inflating the balloon and letting it float in a distal artery. Some hospitals allow only doctors or specially trained nurses to take a PAWP reading because of the risk of pulmonary artery rupture—a rare but life-threatening complication. If your hospital permits you to perform this procedure, do so with extreme caution and make sure that you're thoroughly familiar with intracardiac waveform interpretation.
• To begin, verify that the transducer is properly leveled and zeroed. Detach the syringe from the balloon inflation hub. Draw 1.5 cc of air into the syringe and then reattach the syringe to the hub. Watching the monitor, inject the air through the hub slowly and smoothly. When you see a wedge tracing on the monitor, immediately stop inflating the balloon. Never inflate the balloon beyond the volume needed to obtain a wedge tracing.

Take the pressure reading at the end of expiration. Note the amount of air needed to change the PA tracing to a wedge tracing (normally, 1.25 to 1.5 cc). If the wedge tracing appeared with injection of less than 1.25 cc, suspect that the catheter has migrated into a more distal branch (requiring repositioning). If the balloon is in a more distal branch, the tracings may move up the oscilloscope, indicating that the catheter tip is recording balloon pressure rather than PAWP. This may lead to pulmonary artery rupture.

Removing the catheter
• To assist the doctor, inspect the chest X-ray for signs of catheter kinking or knotting. (In some states, you may be permitted to remove a PA catheter yourself under an advanced collaborative standard of practice.)
• Obtain the patient's baseline vital signs and note the ECG pattern.
• Explain the procedure to the patient. Place the head of the bed flat, unless ordered otherwise. If the catheter was inserted using a superior approach, turn the patient's head to the side opposite the insertion site. Gently remove the dressing.
• The doctor will remove any sutures securing the catheter. However, if he wants to leave the introducer in place after catheter removal, he will not remove the sutures used to secure it.
• Turn all stopcocks off to the patient. (You may turn stopcocks on to the distal port if you wish to observe waveforms. However, use caution because this may cause air embolism.)
• The doctor puts on sterile gloves. After verifying that the balloon is deflated, he withdraws the catheter slowly and smoothly. If he feels any resistance, he will stop immediately.
• Watch the ECG monitor for arrhythmias.
• If the introducer was removed, apply pressure to the site and check it frequently for signs of bleeding. Dress the site again as necessary. If the introducer is left in place, observe the diaphragm for any blood backflow. Such backflow verifies the integrity of the hemostasis valve.
• Return all equipment to the appropriate location. You may turn off the bedside pressure modules but leave the ECG module on.
• Reassure the patient and his family that he will be observed closely. Make sure that he understands that the catheter was removed because his condition has improved and he no longer needs it.
• Document the patient's tolerance for the procedure and note any problems encountered during catheter removal.

Interpretation of findings
Normal right ventricular systolic pressure measures 15 to 25 mm Hg; normal right ventricular diastolic pressure, 0 to 8 mm Hg. However, keep in mind that few acutely ill patients have normal values. Therefore, consider pressure trends and variations from baseline pressure values more important than isolated values.

Many patients with low output also have low blood pressure and signs of poor tissue perfusion. Hemodynamic monitoring can help identify the underlying cause of low output. For instance, blood pressure, cardiac output, and PAWP typically are low in a patient with hypovolemia. In contrast, a patient in cardiogenic shock typically has low blood pressure and cardiac output but high PAWP.

Right ventricular infarction also is characterized by low blood pressure and cardiac output. Because the dysfunction is on the right side, elevated RAP suggests increased right ventricular filling pressures. Unless the left ventricle is involved, PAWP will be normal or even below normal. Cardiac tamponade may produce similar values: decreased blood pressure, reduced cardiac output, and elevated right-sided pressures.

Obtaining right ventricular volumetric pressure values can enhance diagnosis. In cardiac tamponade, for instance, end-diastolic volume is low; with right ventricular infarction or failure, end-diastolic volume is high.

Hemodynamic data also help distinguish cardiac from pulmonary dysfunction. Such conditions as pulmonary hypertension elevate PAP regardless of the underlying cause. If PAP elevations result from cardiac dysfunction, treatments to enhance cardiac function will reduce PAP. Because the wedged catheter more accurately assesses left ventricular function, expect normal PAWP unless the patient has left ventricular disease.

Because PAWP reflects left atrial filling pressures, an occlusion between the catheter tip and left ventricle can lead to inaccurate readings. Causes of such an occlusion include mitral valve stenosis, left atrial myxoma, and pulmonary disease.

In certain conditions, LVEDP may exceed PAWP. When LVEDP is markedly high, as when severely decreased compliance causes pressures above 25 mm Hg, PAWP declines—partly because the pulmonary vascular bed has greater compliance and inadequately reflects the high pressures. Aortic regurgitation also may increase LVEDP from backward pressure. In the early stages, this backward pressure may not reflect all the way back to the left atrium and the wedge.

Lung zones
The lung zone in which the catheter tip is lodged can affect the PAWP value—both under normal circumstances and when the patient is receiving positive end-expiratory pressure (PEEP) treatment. Lung zones are identified by the relationships among inflow pressure (PAP), outflow pressure (pulmonary venous pressure), and surrounding alveolar pressure.

In zone 1, alveolar pressure exceeds PAP and pulmonary venous pressure. As a result, no blood flows from the compressed pulmonary capillary beds. However, because the PA catheter is flow directed, the tip probably will not rest in this zone.

Alveolar pressure also exceeds pulmonary venous pressure in zone 2. However, arterial pressure is sufficient to allow blood flow. Usually, PAWP readings are accurate when the catheter tip is lodged in this zone. However, with high PEEP levels, alveolar pressure may increase; the higher surrounding pressure transmits back to the catheter, possibly causing inaccurate PAWP values.

Zone 3 is the best location for recording PAWP. Here, pulmonary venous pressure exceeds surrounding alveolar pressure and all capillaries are open. The catheter tip usually rests below the level of the left atrium (verified by a lateral chest X-ray).

Waveform analysis
Such analysis helps differentiate cardiac tamponade from constrictive pericarditis. In both conditions, ventricular and atrial diastolic pressures are equal and hemodynamic changes may precede the patient's clinical signs and symptoms. However, the pressure waveforms differ. With cardiac tamponade, higher diastolic pressure causes loss of the *y* descent in the right atrial waveform. With constrictive pericarditis, pericardial rigidity causes rapid diastolic filling, which leads to an exaggerated *y* descent. (See *Interpreting abnormal PA waveforms,* page 66.)

Interpreting abnormal PA waveforms

Observing the pressure waveforms on the bedside monitor can help you detect hemodynamic changes. In cardiac tamponade, for instance, expect absence of the *y* descent on the right atrial waveform. In constrictive pericarditis, expect exaggerated *y* descents (representing decreased left atrial pressure at the end of ventricular systole). Acute mitral insufficiency typically causes a regurgitant *v* wave during atrial filling on the pulmonary artery wedge pressure (PAWP) recording. The descent represents reduced left atrial pressure after left atrial contraction. Ventricular septal defect causes an elevation in the *v* wave during a PAWP recording — the result of increased blood volume from the left ventricle.

Cardiac tamponade

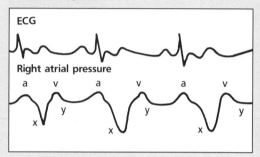

Constrictive pericarditis

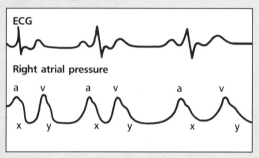

Acute mitral insufficiency

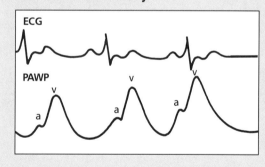

Ventricular septal defect

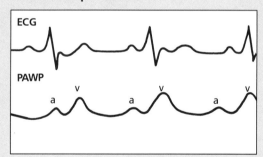

Spurious findings

Certain mechanical and technical factors may cause inaccurate values. These include improper transducer positioning, electrical interference, and balloon overwedging (overuse of the balloon to the point that its integrity is compromised, giving inaccurate values). However, a thorough understanding of the technical aspects of the monitoring system can help prevent or solve these problems. (See *Detecting catheter migration,* pages 68 and 69.)

Nursing considerations

• Advise the patient to use caution when moving about in bed to avoid dislodging the catheter.

• As ordered, arrange for daily chest X-rays to detect any catheter movement. A lateral view is preferable because it shows the catheter tip relative to the level of the left atrium. Because a lateral chest X-ray is hard to perform in the critical care unit, arrange for an anteroposterior view.

• Be aware that heparin flush solution is required to maintain patency of the catheter lu-

TROUBLESHOOTING

Unintended wedge or overdamped tracing

If you see an unintended wedge tracing (as shown in the second tracing below) or an overdamped tracing on your patient's pulmonary artery (PA) pressure monitor, assume the catheter is wedged. With partial wedging, the tracing will be unclear; PA systolic pressure may be lower than baseline and PA diastolic pressure may be higher. With complete wedging, you'll see a typical wedge tracing.

To correct the problem, detach the syringe to verify that air has been removed from the balloon. If the tracing still shows a wedge, attempt to reposition the catheter. For instance, turn the patient (or ask him to turn), ask him to cough, or aspirate and then flush the distal port. If these measures don't restore a PA tracing, notify the doctor immediately.

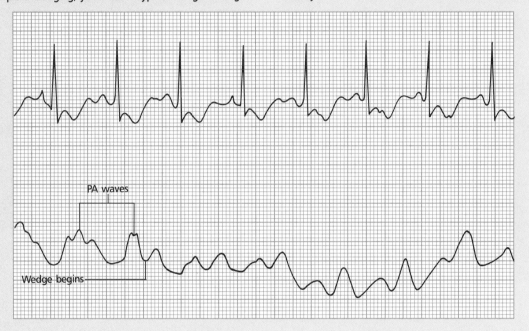

men during continuous PAP monitoring.
• Never leave the balloon inflated because this may cause pulmonary infarction. To determine if the balloon is inflated, check the monitor for a wedge tracing, which indicates inflation. (A PA tracing confirms balloon deflation.)
• If you suspect the catheter is wedged (for instance, if the monitor shows a wedge tracing or an overdamped tracing), take appropriate steps to reposition it. (See *Unintended wedge or overdamped tracing.*)
• Never inflate the balloon with more than the recommended air volume (specified on the

catheter shaft) because this may cause loss of elasticity or balloon rupture. With appropriate inflation volume, the balloon floats easily through the heart chambers and rests in the main branch of the pulmonary artery, producing accurate waveforms. If the patient has a suspected left-to-right shunt, use carbon dioxide to inflate the balloon, as ordered, because it diffuses more quickly than air. Never inflate the balloon with fluids because they may not be able to be retrieved from inside the balloon, preventing deflation.

(Text continues on page 70.)

Detecting catheter migration

A pulmonary artery (PA) catheter helps establish baseline hemodynamic indices and can optimize the patient's cardiac performance. But one potential complication of a PA catheter is that it can migrate and cause serious problems, such as pulmonary infarction. Although PA waveforms and arterial oxygen saturation (SaO_2) and venous oxygen saturation ($S\bar{v}O_2$) values can tell you when a catheter has migrated, they can be misinterpreted, as in the case of Harold Ogden, age 62.

Preoperative care

Mr. Ogden was admitted to the hospital for femoropopliteal bypass surgery to treat a popliteal artery obstruction. He had a history of two myocardial infarctions and vascular insufficiency.

On preoperative examination, Barbara Sendak, RN, assessed a grade III murmur, loudest at the apex. She suspected mitral regurgitation. Twenty-four hours before surgery, the doctor inserted a fiber-optic PA catheter.

Between 12 p.m. and 2 p.m., hemodynamic values were measured and recorded. (They're shown in the chart on page 69.)

Reviewing the 12 p.m. values, Ms. Sendak noted that Mr. Ogden's pulmonary artery pressure (PAP) and pulmonary artery wedge pressure (PAWP) were elevated and that his PAWP exceeded his diastolic PAP—a finding requiring further investigation.

Because the patient wasn't receiving positive end-expiratory pressure (PEEP), Ms. Sendak knew that his increased PAWP wasn't the result of catheter tip migration caused by PEEP therapy. She recalled that Mr. Ogden had a grade III murmur, presumably indicating mitral regurgitation. This disorder commonly causes an elevated *v* wave on the wedge tracing. Assuming the elevated *v* waves and high PAWP resulted from the mitral regurgitation, she did not investigate the abnormality any further.

An hour later, after obtaining the 1 p.m. values, Ms. Sendak noted that Mr. Ogden's $S\bar{v}O_2$ value had risen. Typically, $S\bar{v}O_2$ reflects the balance between oxygen supply and demand. If oxygen supply decreases or demand increases, $S\bar{v}O_2$ drops—and vice versa. However, she knew of no apparent reason why Mr. Ogden's oxygen demand would decrease. So she focused on increased oxygen supply as the only possible explanation for increased $S\bar{v}O_2$. However, she also noted that the values reflecting oxygen supply—cardiac output and SaO_2—had either remained virtually unchanged or decreased from the baseline values.

By 2 p.m., Mr. Ogden's values showed that his condition was deteriorating rapidly. His heart and respiratory rates had increased, his respirations became more labored, and his SaO_2 dropped. His $S\bar{v}O_2$ also declined markedly, indicating insufficient oxygen delivery to meet oxygen demands.

On closer review of Mr. Ogden's values and intracardiac waveforms, Ms. Sendak concluded that his PA catheter had migrated farther into the pulmonary artery, becoming mechanically wedged. In fact, wedging caused a pulmonary infarction, reflected by decreased SaO_2 and increased respiratory rate (which indicated impaired pulmonary gas exchange).

Conclusion

This case demonstrates the importance of accurately identifying PA waveforms and recognizing the significance of SaO_2 and $S\bar{v}O_2$ values when caring for a patient with a PA catheter. When a PA catheter migrates to a distal site, SaO_2 exceeds $S\bar{v}O_2$. By 1 p.m., the patient's $S\bar{v}O_2$ had risen, although no significant increase in oxygen delivery had occurred. At that time, the catheter was mechanically wedged. However, because the wedge tracing had giant *v* waves, it closely resembled the PA tracing. Therefore, Ms. Sendak failed to recognize it as a wedge tracing. She also should have suspected migration of the PA catheter to a more distal location because of the narrowing gap between systolic and diastolic PAP.

Hemodynamic values

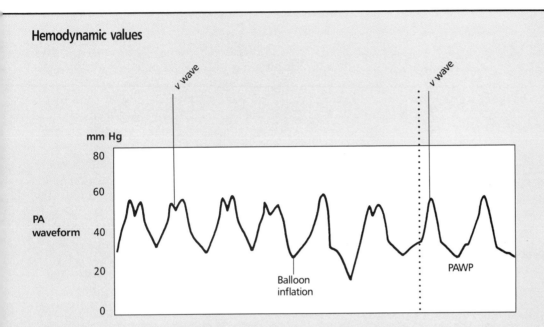

	12 p.m.	1 p.m.	2 p.m.
Heart rate	80 beats/minute	88 beats/minute	110 beats/minute
Respiratory rate	22 breaths/minute	22 breaths/minute	28 breaths/minute (labored)
SaO₂	97%	95%	89%
Cardiac output	5.9 liters/minute	5.2 liters/minute	6 liters/minute
PAWP	29 mm Hg	29 mm Hg	29 mm Hg
Systolic/diastolic PAP	45/22 mm Hg	44/28 mm Hg	44/38 mm Hg
SvO₂	66%	80%	54%

Complications of pulmonary artery catheterization

Although all invasive procedures carry inherent risks, pulmonary artery (PA) catheter insertion rarely causes complications. You can further reduce the risk by using proper technique when assisting with catheter insertion and removal and when caring for and maintaining the line.

PA perforation
This complication most commonly occurs in elderly patients with pulmonary hypertension. Using caution when inserting and wedging the catheter helps reduce the risk. Distal catheter migration also may cause PA rupture.

Pulmonary infarction
This complication may result from prolonged wedging, catheter migration, thromboembolism, or air embolism caused by balloon rupture.

Local or systemic infection
Failure to use aseptic technique during catheter insertion or maintenance may cause infection and subsequent septicemia. To help prevent this complication, be sure to follow the guidelines for invasive lines issued by the Centers for Disease Control and Prevention.

Catheter knotting
During insertion, the catheter may become knotted in the right ventricle as it is looped. The doctor will use special care when removing a knotted catheter.

Cardiac arrhythmias
Ventricular arrhythmias may occur during insertion or if the catheter tip slips into the right ventricle. Ensuring proper catheter placement may prevent arrhythmias. Also, lidocaine administration helps reduce the cardiac irritability that can lead to an arrhythmia.

Heparin-induced thrombocytopenia
Patients with heparin sensitivity or coagulopathy may suffer thrombocytopenia if heparin is applied to the catheter tip or added to the flush solution. Unless ordered, avoid adding heparin to the flush solution of such patients.

• To ensure patient safety, take precautions to prevent catheter migration. Made of radio-opaque polyvinylchloride, the catheter softens after insertion; if it migrates too far into a distal branch of the pulmonary artery, it may become mechanically wedged.

To prevent migration, during insertion the doctor may retract the catheter 3/8″ to 3/4″ (1 to 2 cm), reinflate the balloon with 1.5 cc of air and check for a wedge tracing, then deflate it. Retraction reduces the risk of catheter migration by minimizing any redundant loops in the right ventricle.

• If your hospital permits you to withdraw the catheter from a wedge to a PA position, use proper technique to prevent PA infarction. First, make sure that the balloon is deflated. Next, slowly and smoothly withdraw the catheter approximately 3/8″ to 3/4″ (1 to 2 cm) while watching the monitor. When you see a PA tracing, stop withdrawing. Then reinflate the balloon slowly and note the amount of air needed to obtain a wedge tracing. If less than 1 cc of air was required, deflate the balloon again, withdraw the catheter another 3/8″, and check for a PA tracing. If you still need a minimal amount of air to obtain a wedge tracing, notify the doctor. The catheter may have migrated distally.

• Be aware that the catheter may slip back into the right ventricle. Because the tip may irritate the ventricle, be sure to detect this problem promptly by checking the monitor for a right ventricular waveform. Also note the pressure values; systolic PAP will remain the same but diastolic pressure will drop below its previous value.

If a right ventricular waveform appears, inflate the balloon to induce the catheter to float into the pulmonary artery. You may also try changing the patient's position to change catheter location. If these maneuvers fail to correct the problem, the doctor may attempt to advance the catheter again — but only if the exposed catheter segment has remained sterile. If not, the doctor may withdraw the catheter and replace it with a new one.

• To minimize valvular trauma, make sure that the balloon is deflated whenever the catheter is withdrawn from the pulmonary artery to the right ventricle or from the right ventricle to the right atrium.

• Care for the insertion site according to hospital policy and Centers for Disease Control and Prevention (CDC) standards. Assess the site regularly for signs of infection, such as redness. Also assess for other complications. (See *Complications of pulmonary artery catheterization.*)

The CDC recommends changing the dressing whenever it's moist or every 24 to 48 hours, re-dressing the site according to your hospital's policy, changing the catheter every 72 hours, changing the pressure tubing every 48 hours, and changing the flush solution every 24 hours. However, these recommendations were issued in 1982. Since then, some hospitals have maintained closed-pressure monitoring systems for longer than the recommended times with no increase in infection rates. Nonetheless, before departing from CDC recommendations, determine your hospital's policy.

Central venous pressure monitoring

In this procedure, the doctor inserts a catheter through a vein and advances it until its tip lies in or near the right atrium. Because no major valves lie at the junction of the vena cavae and right atrium, pressure at the end of diastole reflects back to the catheter. When connected to a manometer, the catheter measures central venous pressure (CVP), an index of right ventricular function.

CVP monitoring helps you assess cardiac function, evaluate venous return to the heart, and indirectly gauge how well the heart is pumping. The central line also provides access to a large vessel for rapid, high-volume fluid administration and allows frequent blood withdrawal for laboratory samples. In patients with normal left ventricular function, CVP monitoring also helps evaluate the response to fluid administration. However, CVP values don't correlate directly to left ventricular function or true right ventricular preload. Therefore, CVP monitoring has limited value in analyzing trends in volume status.

CVP monitoring can be done *intermittently* or *continuously.* The catheter is inserted percutaneously or using a cutdown method. Typically, a single CVP line is used for intermittent pressure readings. To measure the patient's volume status, a disposable plastic water manometer is attached between the I.V. line and the central catheter with a three- or four-way stopcock. CVP is recorded in centimeters of water (cm H_2O) or millimeters of mercury (mm Hg) read from manometer markings.

Equipment
For intermittent CVP monitoring
Gather a disposable CVP manometer set, leveling device (such as a rod from a reusable CVP pole holder or a carpenter's level or rule), additional stopcock (to attach the CVP manometer to the catheter), extension tubing (if needed), I.V. pole, I.V. solution, I.V. drip chamber and tubing, dressing materials, and tape.

For continuous CVP monitoring
Gather a pressure monitoring kit with disposable pressure transducer; leveling device; bedside pressure module with oscilloscope; continuous I.V. flush solution; 1 unit/1 to 2 ml of heparin flush solution; and pressure bag.

For withdrawing blood samples through the central line
Gather the appropriate number of syringes for the ordered tests, plus a 5- or 10-ml syringe for the discard sample. (Syringe size depends on the tests ordered.) If the central line is used only intermittently, also obtain a syringe with 0.9% sodium chloride solution and a syringe with heparin flush solution.

For removing a central venous catheter
Gather sterile gloves, suture removal set, sterile gauze sponges, iodophor ointment, dressing, and tape.

Preparation

Gather equipment. Explain the procedure to the patient to reduce his anxiety.

Procedure

Assist the doctor as he inserts the central venous catheter. (The procedure is similar to that used for PAP monitoring [see Procedure in "Pulmonary artery pressure monitoring," page 60], except that the catheter is advanced only as far as the superior vena cava.)

Obtaining intermittent CVP readings with a water manometer

• With the central line in place, position the patient flat. Align the base of the manometer with the previously determined zero reference point by using a leveling device. Because CVP reflects right atrial pressure, you must align the right atrium (the zero reference point) with the zero mark on the manometer. To find the right atrium, locate the fourth intercostal space at the midaxillary line. Mark the appropriate place on the patient's chest so that all subsequent recordings will be made using the same location.

If the patient can't tolerate a flat position, place him in semi-Fowler's position. When the head of the bed is elevated, the phlebostatic axis remains constant but the midaxillary line changes. Use the same degree of head elevation for all subsequent measurements.

• Attach the water manometer to an I.V. pole or place it next to the patient's chest. In either case, make sure that the zero reference point is level with the right atrium. (See *Measuring CVP with a water manometer.*)

• Verify that the water manometer is connected to the I.V. tubing. Typically, markings on the manometer range from −2 to 38 cm H_2O. However, markings may differ from one manufacturer to the next, so be sure to read the manufacturer's directions before setting up the manometer and obtaining readings.

• Turn the stopcock off to the patient and slowly fill the manometer with I.V. solution until the fluid level is 10 to 20 cm H_2O higher than the patient's expected CVP value. Don't overfill the tube because fluid that spills over

the top can become a source of contamination.

• Turn the stopcock off to the I.V. solution and open to the patient. The fluid level in the manometer will drop. Once the fluid level comes to rest, it will fluctuate slightly with respirations. Expect it to drop during inspiration and to rise during expiration.

• Record CVP at the end of inspiration, when intrathoracic pressure has a negligible effect. Depending on the type of water manometer you're using, note the value either at the bottom of the meniscus or at the midline of the small floating ball.

• After you've obtained the CVP value, turn the stopcock to resume the I.V. infusion. Adjust the I.V. drip rate as required.

• Place the patient in a comfortable position.

• Document the patient's tolerance for the procedure.

Performing continuous CVP monitoring with a water manometer

• Make sure that the stopcock is turned so that the I.V. solution port, CVP column port, and patient port are open.

• Be aware that with this stopcock position, infusion of the I.V. solution increases CVP. Therefore, expect higher readings than those taken with the stopcock turned off to the I.V. solution. If the I.V. solution infuses at a constant rate, CVP will change as the patient's condition changes, although the initial reading will be higher. Assess the patient closely for changes.

Performing continuous CVP monitoring with a pressure monitoring system

• Make sure that the central line or the proximal lumen of a PA catheter is attached to the system. (If the patient has a central line with multiple lumens, one lumen may be dedicated to continuous CVP monitoring and the other lumens used for fluid administration.)

• Set up a pressure transducer system (as described in Chapter 2). Connect noncompliant pressure tubing from the CVP catheter hub to the transducer. Then connect the flush solution container to a flush device.

• To obtain values, position the patient flat. If

Measuring CVP with a water manometer

To ensure accurate central venous pressure (CVP) readings, make sure the manometer base is aligned with the patient's right atrium (the zero reference point). The manometer set usually contains a leveling rod to allow you to determine this quickly.

After adjusting manometer position, examine the typical three-way stopcock, as shown here. By turning it to any position shown, you can control the direction of fluid flow. Four-way stopcocks also are available.

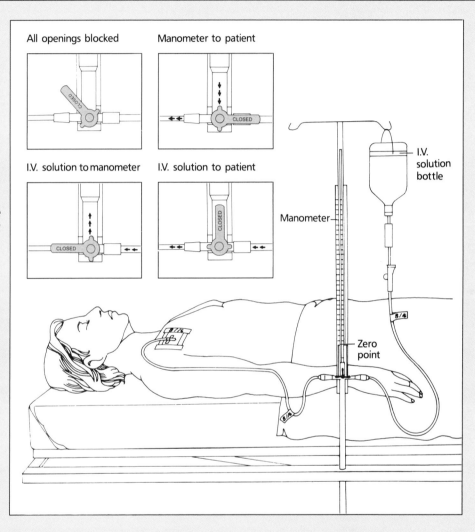

he can't tolerate this position, use semi-Fowler's position. Locate the level of the right atrium by identifying the phlebostatic axis. Zero the transducer, leveling the transducer air-fluid interface stopcock with the right atrium. Read the CVP value from the digital display on the monitor and note the waveform. Both the numerical value and the waveform provide valuable information about the patient's status.

(See *CVP waveform*, page 74.) Be sure to document the patient's position; then use this position for all subsequent readings.

Obtaining blood samples through a central line
• Wash your hands and maintain aseptic technique throughout the procedure.
• To prevent entry of air into the bloodstream,

CVP waveform

In this normal central venous pressure (CVP) waveform, obtained with a pressure monitoring system, the *a* wave falls within the PR interval of the accompanying electrocardiogram waveform.

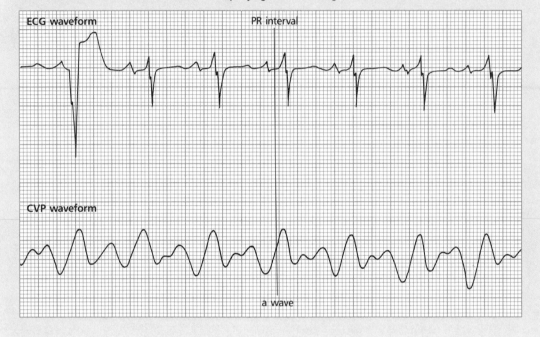

position the patient flat if the catheter was inserted using a superior approach (such as through a jugular or subclavian vein).
• As appropriate, attach a stopcock to the end of the catheter or use a heparin lock device.
• To ensure accurate laboratory values, remove I.V. solution from the inner lumen of the catheter by collecting a discard sample of approximately 5 ml. Dispose of this sample according to hospital policy.
• Withdraw blood for the laboratory samples from the stopcock or heparin lock attachment. The amount to withdraw depends on the test ordered.
• After withdrawing blood, flush the central line with I.V. solution and restart the infusion. If using a heparin lock device, flush the line by attaching a separate syringe of sterile solution (usually 0.9% sodium chloride solution). As ordered, add heparin to the solution to prevent

clotting of the catheter lumen.
• Alternatively, you may use a closed system to obtain blood samples through a CVP line. This method reduces the risk of contamination caused by disconnecting the line and allows reinfusion of the discard sample. Recent health care protection standards recommend using a closed system that eliminates needles, preventing inadvertent needle sticks. (For details on withdrawing blood through a closed system, see Chapter 3.)

Removing a central line
• You may assist the doctor in removing a central line. (In some states, a nurse is permitted to remove the catheter with a doctor's order or when acting under advanced collaborative standards of practice.)
• If the head of the bed is elevated, take measures to minimize the risk of air embolism dur-

ing catheter removal. For instance, place the patient in Trendelenburg's position if the line was inserted using a superior approach. If the patient can't tolerate this position, position him flat.
• Turn the patient's head to the side opposite the catheter insertion site. The doctor removes the dressing and exposes the insertion site. If sutures are in place, he removes them carefully.
• Turn the I.V. solution off.
• The doctor pulls the catheter out in a slow, smooth motion and then applies pressure to the insertion site.
• Clean the insertion site, apply iodophor ointment, and cover it with a dressing, as ordered.
• Assess the patient for signs of respiratory distress, which may indicate air embolism.
• Document the date and time of catheter removal, the type of dressing applied, and the patient's tolerance for the procedure.

Interpretation of findings
Normal CVP ranges from 5 to 10 cm H_2O.

Any condition that alters venous return, circulating blood volume, or cardiac performance may affect CVP. If circulating volume increases (such as with increased venous return to the heart), CVP increases. If circulating volume decreases (such as with reduced venous return), CVP drops.

Specific causes of increased CVP include volume overload, hepatic disease, depressed cardiac function (which decreases forward blood flow and leads to backward congestive heart failure), vasoconstriction, cardiac tamponade, chronic or acute pulmonary hypertension, and PEEP therapy. Backward heart failure, such as from inadequate pumping or low cardiac output, also leads to a rise in CVP. Specific causes of decreased CVP include volume deficit (as occurs from hemorrhage or dehydration), sepsis, and certain shock states that cause venous pooling.

CVP also is affected by changes in left ventricular function or the pulmonary vascular bed. However, in critically ill patients, CVP measurement may not accurately reflect these changes.

Because CVP may fluctuate, you should analyze values for trends rather than attaching great significance to isolated values. Also, be sure to interpret CVP values in conjunction with the patient's clinical status and history. For instance, in a patient with a chronic pulmonary disorder (such as cor pulmonale), an above-normal CVP value may not reflect acute failure.

Nursing considerations
• As ordered, arrange for daily chest X-rays to check catheter placement.
• Care for the insertion site as stipulated by hospital policy. Typically, you'll change the dressing every 24 to 48 hours.
• Be sure to wash your hands before performing dressing changes and to use aseptic technique and sterile gloves when re-dressing the site. When removing the old dressing, observe for signs of infection, such as redness, and note any patient complaints of tenderness. Apply ointment and then cover the site with a sterile gauze dressing or a clear occlusive dressing.
• After the initial CVP reading, reevaluate readings frequently to establish a baseline for the patient. Authorities recommend obtaining readings at 15-, 30-, and 60-minute intervals to establish a baseline.
• If the patient's CVP value fluctuates by more than 2 cm H_2O, suspect a change in the patient's clinical status and report this finding to the doctor.
• Change the I.V. solution every 24 hours and the I.V. tubing every 48 hours, according to hospital policy. Expect the doctor to change the catheter every 72 hours. Label the I.V. solution, tubing, and dressing with the date, time, and your initials. Document the same information in the patient's chart.

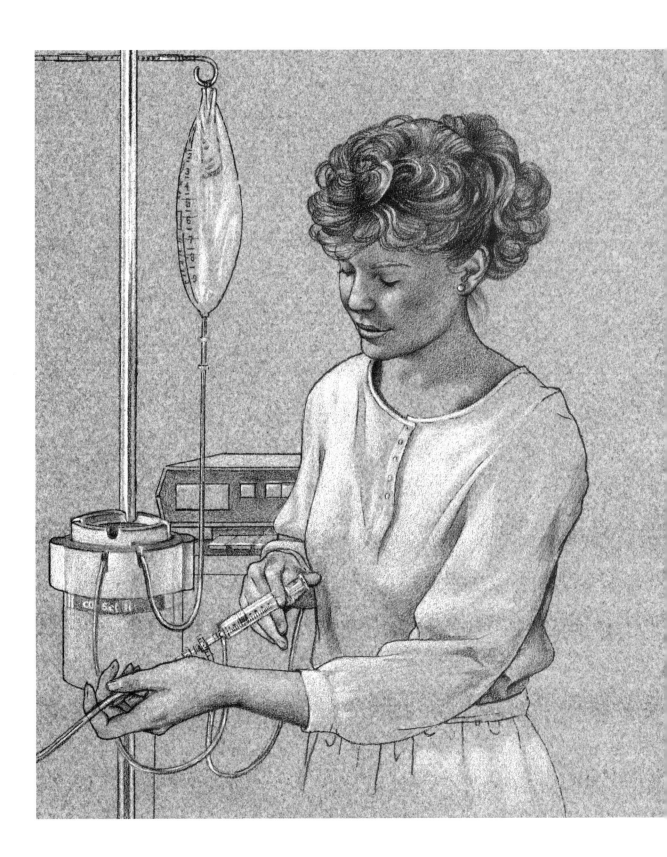

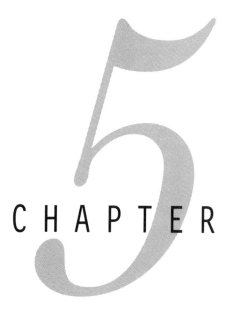

CHAPTER 5

Monitoring cardiac output

A key indicator of cardiac function, cardiac output refers to the volume of blood pumped every minute from the left ventricle into the systemic circulation. The actual measurement of cardiac output is the product of stroke volume (the volume of blood expelled with each heartbeat) multiplied by the heart rate (the number of heartbeats per minute).

Cardiac output delivers oxygenated hemoglobin to the cells. When cardiac output is too low, inadequate amounts of oxygen are delivered to the tissues, resulting in anaerobic metabolism. Various conditions can cause diminished cardiac output, including myocardial infarction (MI), cardiomyopathy, cardiac tamponade, acidosis, and hypoxia.

As cardiac output increases, so does myocardial oxygen demand. This can stress the heart, especially when myocardial oxygen delivery is compromised, such as in arteriosclerosis. Cardiac output may also rise in hyperdynamic conditions, such as sepsis, or when tissue oxygen demand is elevated, such as during exercise or stress.

Monitoring a patient's cardiac output requires skillful application of sophisticated techniques. To carry out the step-by-step procedures used to measure cardiac output, you'll need to understand the role of cardiac output in the overall function of the heart.

This chapter begins by reviewing the physiology of cardiac output. It continues with coverage of the key methods used to measure cardiac output and your role in these procedures.

Physiology

Cardiac output is the product of heart rate and stroke volume. The amount of blood ejected from the ventricle with each heartbeat (normal range = 60 to 100 ml/heartbeat), stroke volume is determined by ventricular filling (preload), resistance to ventricular ejection (afterload), and myocardial contractility. In a healthy heart, if stroke volume decreases, the heart rate will increase to maintain adequate cardiac output. But when the heart is damaged or the heart rate is too high, cardiac output drops because ventricular filling time is reduced.

Heart rate

At a normal heart rate, the ventricles contract (systole) for one-third of the cardiac cycle and relax (diastole) for two-thirds. Systole occurs over a relatively constant duration, so changes in heart rate primarily affect diastolic time. The ventricles fill with blood during diastole, meaning that changes in heart rate significantly affect diastolic filling. As the heart rate decreases, stroke volume usually increases (and vice versa), thus maintaining adequate blood flow. However, a heart rate that exceeds the usual range of 60 to 100 beats/minute can adversely affect cardiac output.

Elevated heart rates reduce ventricular filling time and coronary artery perfusion time, while increasing myocardial oxygen demand. When the heart rate rises, diastolic filling time

is shortened. Beyond a limit—usually more than 170 beats/minute in nondiseased hearts—the ventricles may not have adequate time to fill before the next systolic ejection. And because the coronary arteries fill during diastole, an increased heart rate causes less blood flow (or oxygen delivery) to the myocardium at a time when its oxygen demand is high.

Slow heart rates may also decrease cardiac output. When the heart beats too slowly, the ventricles can overfill. A compromised heart, which may occur following an MI, may be incapable of pumping the increased volume to maintain an adequate cardiac output.

Changes in heart rhythm may also affect cardiac output. Under normal circumstances, atrial contraction occurs just before ventricular contraction, contributing an additional 30% to ventricular volume. This phenomenon is called atrial contribution or atrial kick. Conditions which disrupt atrial contraction, such as junctional rhythm or atrial fibrillation, reduce ventricular filling and thus stroke volume.

Stroke volume

Three factors determine stroke volume: preload, afterload, and contractility.

Preload

Ventricular wall tension at the end of diastole, preload stretches the myofibrils. The more the myofibrils are stretched, the harder and faster they snap back, strengthening the heart's contraction and increasing cardiac output. But myofibrils have their limits, and excessive stretching weakens the heart's ability to contract with sufficient force.

Preload is primarily determined by venous return to the heart. But since ventricular wall tension can't be directly measured, and the technology to measure end-diastolic volume has only recently been developed, preload is estimated by the pressure in the ventricle at end diastole. Central venous pressure is an estimate of right ventricular preload; pulmonary artery wedge pressure, an estimate of left ventricular preload.

The relationship between end-diastolic pressure and actual volume depends on ven-

Understanding cardiac output

Cardiac output equals the heart rate multiplied by the stroke volume. The stroke volume, in turn, refers to the amount of blood ejected from the ventricle in 1 minute.

To better understand how stroke volume affects cardiac output and thus cardiac performance, consider the Frank-Starling law. Describing the relationship between myocardial muscle length and the force of contraction, this law states that the more you stretch the muscle fiber in diastole, or the more volume in the ventricle, the stronger the next contraction will be in systole. The law also says that this phenomenon will occur until a physiologic limit has been reached. Once that limit has been reached, the force of contraction will begin to decline, regardless of the increase in fiber stretch. This principle is represented by the curve at right.

In the heart, this ability to increase the force of contraction converts an increase in venous return to an increase in stroke volume. Stroke volume must match venous return or the heart will fail. The three determinants of stroke volume are preload, afterload, and contractility.

Preload

Preload refers to the amount of myocardial fiber stretch at the end of disatole. It also refers to the amount of volume in the ventricle at this phase. The relationship between end-diastolic volume and end-diastolic pressure depends on the compliance of the muscle wall. With normal compliance, relatively large increases in volume create relatively small increases in pressure, whereas in a noncompliant ventricle, a greater pressure is generated with little increase in volume. Enhanced compliance of the ventricle allows for large changes in volume with little rise in pressure.

Frank-Starling curve

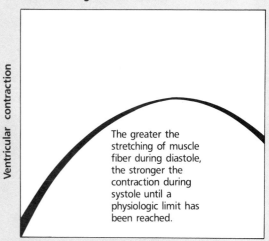

The greater the stretching of muscle fiber during diastole, the stronger the contraction during systole until a physiologic limit has been reached.

Afterload

Afterload is the resistance, impedance, or pressure that the ventricle must overcome to eject its blood volume. It's determined by the volume and mass of blood ejected, the size and wall thickness of the ventricle, and the impedance of the vasculature.

Afterload has an inverse relationship to ventricular function. As resistance to ejection rises, the force of contraction diminishes, resulting in a reduced stroke volume.

Contractility

Contractility refers to the heart's inherent ability to temporarily shorten its myocardial muscle fibers without altering the length of the fibers. Contractility is influenced by the effect of the sympathetic nervous system on the heart, increases in heart rate, metabolic changes, and drug therapy.

tricular wall compliance. In a compliant ventricle, large changes in volume result in small changes in pressure. In a noncompliant ventricle, small changes in volume result in greater changes in pressure. (See *Understanding cardiac output*.)

Either increased or reduced preload may be detrimental to cardiac output. Conditions such as hypovolemia or peripheral vasodilation (causing venous pooling) result in inadequate ventricular filling and weak ventricular contraction. Hypervolemia or a very slow heart rate

Calculating vascular resistance

When you calculate vascular resistance, you're actually calculating afterload – the resistance the ventricle must overcome to eject its blood volume. But why calculate this measurement? One reason would be if your patient's cardiac output is abnormal and you want to help detect the cause, and thus guide effective treatment.

Calculating systemic vascular resistance
Systemic vascular resistance (SVR) is normally 800 to 1,200 dynes/second/cm⁵. You can calculate this measurement using the following equation, in which MAP refers to the mean arterial pressure; RAP, the right atrial pressure; and CO, cardiac output.

$$SVR = \frac{(MAP - RAP) \times 80}{CO}$$

Calculating peripheral vascular resistance
Peripheral vascular resistance (PVR) is normally less than 250 dynes/second/cm⁵. You can calculate this measurement using the following equation, in which MPAP refers to the mean pulmonary artery pressure and PAWP indicates the pulmonary artery wedge pressure.

$$PVR = \frac{(MPAP - PAWP) \times 80}{CO}$$

may cause overfilling of the ventricles and can lead to heart failure. The amount of blood ejected from the heart (stroke volume) must match the venous return (preload), or the heart will fail.

Afterload

Afterload refers to the resistance that the ventricles must work against to eject their blood volume. Afterload depends on ventricular size and wall thickness, the volume of blood ejected, and resistance of the blood vessels.

Afterload is estimated by systemic vascular resistance (left ventricular afterload) and pulmonary vascular resistance (right ventricular afterload). Resistance is calculated from the pressures at the beginning and end of the circuit, and the blood flow through the circuit. (See *Calculating vascular resistance.*)

Afterload is inversely related to ventricular function. In other words, as resistance to ejection increases, the force of contraction and thus the stroke volume decrease. The diminished stroke volume will be more pronounced in a diseased heart, which can't generate enough force to overcome the increased resistance. Causes of increased afterload include aortic valve stenosis, arteriosclerosis, hypertension, and increased systemic vascular resistance from catecholamine stimulation or hypovolemia.

The mediators released in septic or anaphylactic shock cause massive vasodilation and decreased afterload, which causes elevated cardiac output. In such cases, the heart is pumping against no resistance. A severely decreased afterload affects the isovolumetric contraction phase of the cardiac cycle, decreasing contractile strength and stroke volume.

Contractility

The ventricle's ability to contract depends on how much the myofibrils are stretched at the end of diastole. The more myofibrils are stretched, the more forceful the contraction, causing larger amounts of blood to be ejected with greater force.

Numerous other factors influence the strength of myocardial contraction, including sympathetic stimulation, metabolic influences (such as acidosis or hypoxia), and drugs. Myocardial contractility can't be directly measured, but indicators of contractility include stroke volume index and ventricular work indices. The ventricular function curves show the relationship among contractility, preload, and afterload. (See *Measuring ventricular stroke work indices.*)

Cardiac output measurement

Measuring cardiac output – the amount of blood ejected by the heart – helps evaluate cardiac function. The most widely preferred method for calculating this measurement is the bolus thermodilution technique. Based on the earlier indicator-dilution method, thermodilution uses cold, instead of a contrast dye, as the indicator. The thermodilution technique is accurate and can be performed at the patient's bedside, making it the most practical method for clinical use. You'll use it to evaluate the cardiac status of critically ill patients or those with suspected cardiac disease. (For other techniques used to measure cardiac output, see *Determining cardiac output using the Fick and indicator-dilution methods,* page 82.)

To measure cardiac output, a quantity of solution colder than the patient's blood is injected into the right atrium via a port on a pulmonary artery (PA) catheter. This indicator solution mixes with the blood as it travels through the right ventricle into the pulmonary artery, and a thermistor on the catheter registers the change in temperature of the flowing blood. A computer then plots the temperature change over time as a curve and calculates flow based on the area under the curve.

The area under this bell-shaped curve, sometimes called a "washout" curve, is inversely proportional to the flow rate or cardiac output. In slowly flowing blood, only a small amount of blood dilutes the cold indicator; thus, the peak amplitude of the curve and temperature change over time will be greater. Conversely, the area under a curve generated from a high cardiac output will be less, because of greater dilution of the indicator and a smaller peak temperature change.

Requirements for thermodilution use

For the thermodilution technique to yield accurate cardiac output measurements, certain conditions must be met. You must accurately measure the amount and temperature of the injectate. If any injectate is lost from the system, such as when the solution leaks from the syringe or the solution is warmed, the measured cardiac output will be falsely high. The injectate must also be thoroughly mixed with

Measuring ventricular stroke work indices

If cardiac output is low and you have determined that the patient's preload and afterload are normal, you can go one step further by checking the patient's ventricular contractility. Ventricular contractility is estimated at the bedside by calculating right and left ventricular stroke work indices.

Right ventricular stroke work index
This index, which is abbreviated RVSWI, is normally 7 to 12 g/minute/m^2/beat. You can calculate this index using the following equation, in which SVI refers to the stroke volume index; MPAP, the mean pulmonary artery pressure; and CVP, the central venous pressure.

$$RVSWI = SVI \times (MPAP - CVP) \times 0.0136$$

Left ventricular stroke work index
This index, which is abbreviated LVSWI, is normally 35 to 85 g/minute/m^2/beat. You can calculate this index using the following equation, in which MAP refers to the mean arterial pressure and PAWP indicates the pulmonary artery wedge pressure.

$$LVSWI = SVI \times (MAP - PAWP) \times 0.0136$$

the patient's blood as it passes through the heart. Recirculation will also yield inaccurate cardiac measurements.

Although the thermodilution method has advantages, it also has certain limitations and can lead to complications. This technique requires an indwelling thermodilution PA catheter, which may increase the risk of cardiac arrhythmia, pulmonary infarction, pulmonary artery rupture, infection, and sepsis. And because measuring cardiac output requires injecting several fluid boluses, one after the other, some patients may be susceptible to fluid overload. Finally, since bolus cardiac output measurement requires manual fluid injections, data can't be obtained continuously, and any procedural errors will affect the accuracy of the cardiac output measurements.

The decision to use iced or room-tempera-

Determining cardiac output using the Fick and indicator-dilution methods

Besides bolus thermodilution, two other techniques can be used to measure cardiac output: the Fick method and the indicator-dilution method. Although these two older methods may be highly accurate, their use is usually confined to research projects or the cardiac catheterization laboratory.

Fick method

Often used as a standard by which other cardiac output measurement methods are evaluated, the Fick method measures the blood's oxygen content before and after it passes through the lungs.

By determining the amount of oxygen taken up from every 100 ml of blood during one passage through the tissues and the total volume of oxygen taken up by the body during a period of time (the body's oxygen consumption), you can calculate the number of 100-ml increments that passed through the body during that time.

For example, if 5 cc of oxygen is taken up from 100 ml of blood, and 300 cc of oxygen is taken up in 1 minute, then 60 increments of 5 cc of oxygen must have flowed through the tissues during that minute, indicating a cardiac output of 6 liters/minute.

Measuring cardiac output by the Fick method requires venous and arterial blood samples to determine the arterial and venous oxygen difference. Oxygen consumption – the amount of air entering the lungs each minute – is calculated using a spirometer. Next, cardiac output (CO) is calculated:

$$CO = \frac{\text{oxygen consumption (cc/min)}}{\text{arterial oxygen content (cc/min)} - \text{venous oxygen content (cc/min)}}$$

Indicator-dilution method

In this method, dye is injected into the right superior vena cava or right atrium. A blood sample is then taken from a peripheral arterial site to measure the concentration of the dye. Cardiac output is calculated by dividing the quantity of the dye by the mean concentration and time in minutes.

This method is particularly helpful in detecting intracardiac shunts and valvular regurgitation, but measurements are not accurate if these conditions are already present. The indicator-dilution method is more accurate in high cardiac output states.

ture injectate should be based on your hospital's policy, as well as your patient's status. The accuracy of the bolus thermodilution technique depends on the computer being able to differentiate the temperature change caused by the injectate in the pulmonary artery and the temperature changes in the pulmonary artery. Because iced injectate is colder than room-temperature injectate, it provides a stronger signal to be detected.

Typically, however, room temperature injectate is more convenient and provides equally accurate measurements. Iced injectate may be more accurate in patients with high or low cardiac outputs, hypothermic patients, or when smaller volumes of injectate must be used (3 to 5 ml), such as in patients with volume restrictions, or in children.

Equipment

To measure cardiac output using the thermodilution method, you'll need a thermodilution PA catheter in position. You'll also use a cardiac output computer and cables (or a module for the bedside cardiac monitor), and you'll need a closed or open injectate delivery system. Make sure you also have a 10-ml syringe, a 500-ml bag of dextrose 5% in water or 0.9% sodium chloride solution, and crushed ice and water if the iced injectate is used. (See *Closed injectate delivery system.*)

The newer bedside cardiac monitors measure cardiac output continuously, using either an invasive or a noninvasive method. If your bedside monitor doesn't have this capability, you'll need a stand-alone cardiac output com-

ADVANCED EQUIPMENT

Closed injectate delivery system

This illustration shows the equipment needed to measure cardiac output using a closed injectate delivery system. First, an iced or room-temperature solution is injected into the proximal or right atrium port of the pulmonary artery catheter.

A computer then calculates the cardiac output from temperature changes in the injected material in the proximal lumen and the temperature in the pulmonary artery. The thermistor on the catheter tip measures the temperature in the pulmonary artery. The computer displays the cardiac output as a digital readout.

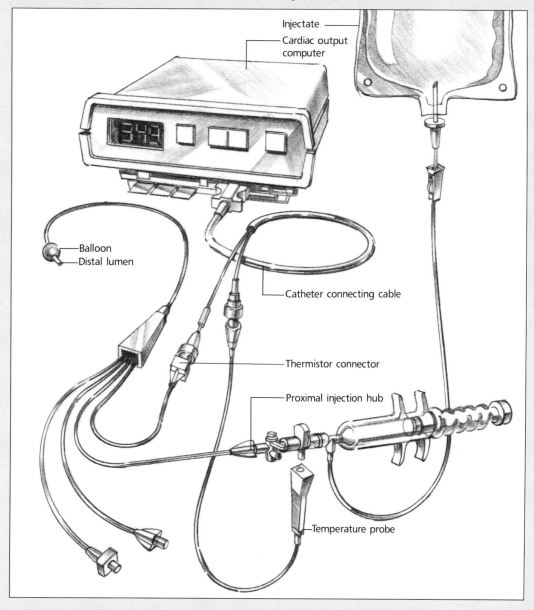

Measuring cardiac output continuously

Cardiac output can be measured and charted continuously using either an invasive or a noninvasive method. Invasive methods generally produce more accurate results, but may be poorly tolerated depending on the patient's condition. Because of their questionable accuracy, noninvasive techniques are not recommended for monitoring critically ill patients.

Invasive method

The Edwards Critical-Care Vigilance Monitor and the IntelliCath Continuous Cardiac Output Pulmonary Artery Catheter form a system that combines the use of indicator-dilution principles with advanced signal-processing technology. The catheter has a thermal filament located in the area adjacent to the usual port for bolus thermodilution injections. Small energy pulses are infused directly into the blood in a random, repeating, on-off pattern (input data).

The resulting blood temperature changes are detected at the thermistor in the pulmonary artery (output data). The input data (energy) and output data (temperature changes) are then entered into a complex mathematical equation to generate what is equivalent to an indicator-dilution curve. Cardiac output is calculated from the area under the curve.

The continuous cardiac output value is displayed in the upper left corner of the monitor. This value is updated every 30 to 60 seconds and represents an average of the previous 3 to 6 minutes of data. The cardiac output is plotted on the trend graph illustrating changes over time.

The Vigilance system offers fluid-free, hands-free, continuous cardiac output monitoring. Measurement results are comparable to the bolus thermodilution technique. The patient's cardiac output performance is displayed without your intervention, eliminating potential sources of user-induced error.

Noninvasive method

Several systems use a noninvasive method of determining stroke volume and cardiac output called electrical bioimpedance. With these systems, several electrodes are placed on the patient's thorax to apply an alternating electrical current. The thoracic tissue's resistance to the current is inversely related to the thoracic blood content. Using this technique, you can measure cardiac output on a beat-to-beat basis, or intermittently at a selected frequency.

The transtracheal Doppler (ABCOM) device is another method of continuous, noninvasive cardiac output measurement and can be used with patients who must be intubated. The special endotracheal tube incorporates an ultrasound transducer that measures blood velocity and aortic diameter in the ascending aorta. These measurements are used by the system to calculate cardiac output continuously. Readings are updated every few seconds.

Vigilance monitor and IntelliCath

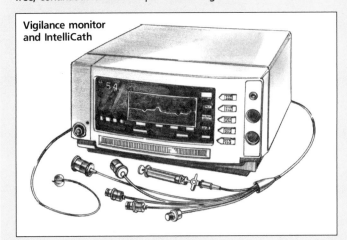

Transtracheal Doppler device

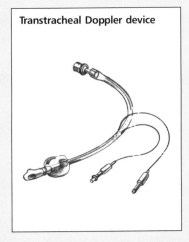

puter. (See *Measuring cardiac output continuously.*)

Preparation
To measure cardiac output, you'll need to prepare both your patient and the necessary equipment.

Preparing the patient
Make sure your patient is in a comfortable position. Advise him not to move during the procedure, as movement can cause error in measurement. Explain to him that the procedure will help determine how well his heart is pumping, and that he will feel no discomfort.

Preparing the equipment
Wash your hands thoroughly, and assemble the equipment at your patient's bedside. Insert the closed injectate system tubing into the 500-ml bag of I.V. solution. Connect the 10-ml syringe to the system tubing and prime the tubing with I.V. solution until it's free of air. Then clamp the tubing. The steps that follow differ, depending on whether you're using an iced- or room-temperature injectate delivery system.

Iced injectate closed delivery system. After clamping the tubing, place the coiled segment into the Styrofoam container and add crushed ice and water to cover the entire coil. Let the solution cool for 15 to 20 minutes. Next, connect the primed system to the stopcock of the proximal injectate lumen of the PA catheter. Then connect the temperature probe from the cardiac output computer to the closed injectate system's flow-through housing device. Connect the cardiac output computer cable to the thermistor connector on the PA catheter and verify the blood temperature reading. Finally, turn on the cardiac output computer and enter the correct computation constant, as provided by the catheter's manufacturer. The constant is determined by the volume and temperature of the injectate as well as the size and type of catheter. (With children, you'll need to adjust the computation constant to reflect a smaller volume and a smaller catheter size.)

Room-temperature injectate closed delivery system. After clamping the tubing, connect the primed system to the stopcock of the proximal injectate lumen of the PA catheter. Next, connect the temperature probe from the cardiac output computer to the closed injectate system's flow-through housing device. Connect the cardiac output computer cable to the thermistor connector on the PA catheter and verify the blood temperature reading. Finally, turn on the cardiac output computer and enter the correct computation constant, as provided by the catheter's manufacturer. The constant is determined by the volume and temperature of the injectate as well as the size and type of catheter.

Procedure
The steps you follow to measure cardiac output will vary somewhat, again depending on whether you use an iced or a room-temperature injectate closed delivery system.

Iced injectate closed delivery system
• Unclamp the I.V. tubing and withdraw 5 ml of solution into the syringe. (With children, use 3 ml or less.)
• Inject the solution to flow past the temperature sensor while observing the injectate temperature that registers on the computer. Verify that the injectate temperature is between 43° F and 54° F (6° C and 12° C).
• Verify a PA waveform on the cardiac monitor.
• Withdraw exactly 10 ml of cooled solution before reclamping the tubing.
• Turn the stopcock at the catheter injectate hub to open a fluid path between the injectate lumen of the PA catheter and syringe.
• Press the START button on the cardiac output computer or wait for the INJECT message to flash.
• Inject the solution smoothly within 4 seconds, making sure that it doesn't leak at the connectors.
• If available, analyze the contour of the thermodilution washout curve on a strip chart recorder for a rapid upstroke and a gradual, smooth return to baseline. (See *Analyzing thermodilution cardiac output curves*, pages 86 and 87.)

Analyzing thermodilution cardiac output curves

Monitoring thermodilution curves can provide helpful information for analyzing cardiac output, particularly when data is scattered or produces unexpected results, in which case specific types of curves can indicate specific problems.

Normal output curve

A typical thermodilution curve is smooth and characterized by a rapid upswing and peak, followed by a gradual return to baseline. The shape of the upslope depends primarily on the indicator injection rate. The downslope of the curve is a function of flow rate and stroke volume. This particular curve, at right, reflects normal cardiac output.

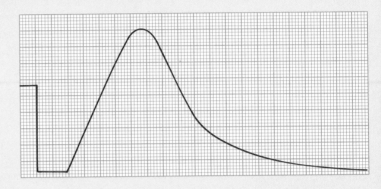

Low and high output curves

When analyzing thermodilution curves, you should look at the curve amplitude and the area beneath it, which reflects cardiac output. The level of cardiac output is inversely proportional to the area you see beneath the thermodilution curve. This means that a greater area beneath the curve implies lower cardiac output, while a smaller area beneath the curve corresponds to higher cardiac output.

For example, the curve at right, with a larger area beneath it, reflects low cardiac output, in this case 3.7 liters/minute. The second curve, with a smaller area beneath it, reflects a higher cardiac output, in this case 7.5 liters/minute.

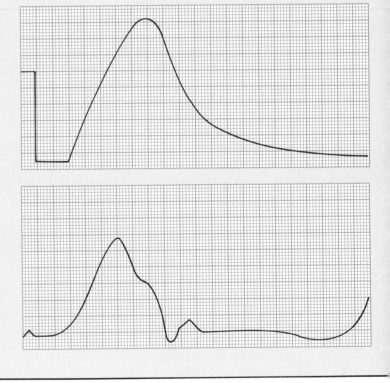

• Wait 1 minute between injections and repeat the procedure until three values are within 10% to 15% of the median value. Compute the average, and record the patient's cardiac output.

• Return the stopcock to its original position and make sure the injectate delivery system tubing is clamped.
• Verify the presence of a PA waveform on the cardiac monitor.

Curves reflecting improper technique

Thermodilution injections should be given smoothly and rapidly—usually 10 ml in less than 4 seconds. If the patient has normal cardiac output, the resulting curve should have a clean, smooth shape with a rapid upswing and slightly prolonged downslope. In this particular case, however, the injection technique was slow and uneven, as reflected by the curve. The expected cardiac output was 3 liters/minute. However, because of the exaggerated curve area resulting from poor injection technique, the output was too low—2.4 liters/minute.

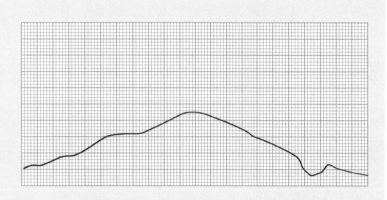

Inconsistent curves

Curves resulting from a set of injections of similar injectate temperature and volume may not appear consistent in shape and size.

Although these two curves were shot consecutively using the same injectate volume and temperature, they look different. This patient was on an intra-aortic balloon pump and was having ventricular arrhythmias. If you were not already aware of the patient's arrhythmias from the electrocardiogram, you could not depend on the curves to make this diagnosis. However, the obvious irregularities in the curves point to some concurrent problem (if cardiac output is stable, consecutive curves should not vary more than 15%).

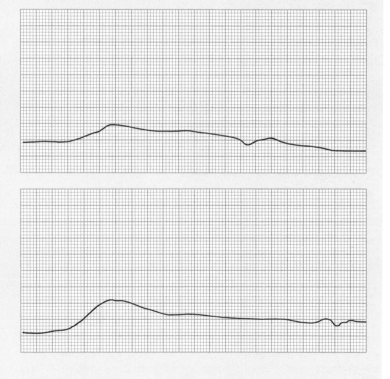

Room-temperature injectate closed delivery system

• Verify the presence of a PA waveform on the cardiac monitor.
• Unclamp the I.V. tubing and withdraw exactly 10 ml of solution. Reclamp the tubing.
• Turn the stopcock at the catheter injectate hub to open a fluid path between the injectate lumen of the PA catheter and the syringe.
• Press the START button on the cardiac output

How cardiac output can be altered

Cardiac output is affected by four determinants: heart rate, preload, afterload, and contractility. If one of these factors is compromised, a patient may report breathing problems, palpitations, or other symptoms of cardiac distress. By correlating a patient's history with his current vital signs and cardiac monitor readings, you can determine the reason for altered cardiac output. Consider the cases of the four patients described below.

Increased heart rate

Ellen Marcheskie, a 27-year-old schoolteacher with a history of mitral valve prolapse, was admitted complaining of palpitations and dizziness. After you set up a cardiac monitor, you noted that she had supraventricular tachycardia, with a rate of 180 beats/minute. This tachyarrhythmia originated above the ventricles—in the sinoatrial node, atrial tissue, or atrioventricular junction.

You knew that a normal heart rate ranges from 60 to 100 beats/minute. An accelerating heart rate usually increases cardiac output—until the heart beats too fast for its own good. Ms. Marcheskie's heart was beating so fast that you reasoned the left ventricle didn't have time to fill with enough blood to stretch the myocardium and produce a forceful contraction. The result? Decreased stroke volume *and* decreased cardiac output.

Increased preload

Mary Pugh, a 56-year-old homemaker with a long history of congestive heart failure, was admitted complaining of severe shortness of breath.

Ms. Pugh had been taking digoxin regularly. Her husband told you that at her daughter's wedding reception the day before, she ate two servings of chicken cordon bleu, a spicy salad, and a lot of salted vegetables, olives, and pickles. This dietary splurge exceeded Ms. Pugh's daily sodium restrictions, increasing her blood volume to the point where she was hypervolemic, and her weakened heart was paying the price.

Taking Ms. Pugh's vital signs, you discovered that her heart rate was 100 beats/minute; her blood pressure, 124/86 mm Hg; and her respirations, 30 breaths/minute. Your assessment revealed bilateral crackles in her lung bases and an S_3, caused by the increased blood volume entering the failing left ventricle early in diastole. You also noticed a left lateral displacement of the point of maximum impulse, jugular vein distention, pitting edema, decreased urine output, and lethargy.

Ms. Pugh told you she gained 2 lb in 1 day, a important sign of fluid retention. A gain of 1 kg (2.2 lb) equals an additional liter of fluid. You determined that Ms. Pugh's increased preload overstretched her myocardium, weakened her myocardial contractility, and reduced her cardiac output.

Decreased afterload

Ed Patrick, a 42-year-old waiter who suffered a myocardial infarction (MI) 8 years ago, was admitted with a pancreatic abscess. Mr. Patrick's abscess was drained in the operating room, and he was transferred to your unit. He was placed on mechanical ventilation, and an arterial line and pulmonary artery line were inserted.

Mr. Patrick stabilized with a blood pressure of 100/82 mm Hg, a pulse of 100 beats/minute, and a respiratory rate of 20 breaths/minute. You measured his cardiac output at 7 liters/minute. His pulmonary artery wedge pressure (PAWP) was 10 mm Hg; his central venous pressure (CVP), 3 mm Hg. He also had a systemic vascular resistance (SVR) of 1,200 dynes/second/cm⁵ (normal is 800 to 1,200 dynes/second/cm⁵).

Suddenly Mr. Patrick's temperature rose to 103° F (39.4° C), and you measured his heart rate at 130 beats/minute. His blood pressure fell to 82/60 mm Hg while his respirations increased

computer or wait for an INJECT message to flash.
• Then inject the solution smoothly within 4 seconds, making sure that the solution does not leak at the connectors.

• If available, analyze the contour of the thermodilution washout curve on a strip chart recorder for a rapid upstroke and a gradual, smooth return to the baseline.
• Repeat these steps until three values are

to 32 breaths/minute. His PAWP was now up to 12 mm Hg; his CVP dropped to 2 mm Hg; and his SVR had fallen off dramatically to only 500 dynes/second/cm^5. His cardiac output shot up to 10 liters/minute. After evaluating these measurements, you suspected that Mr. Patrick was in septic shock. You reasoned that his elevated temperature and the bacterial endotoxins caused massive vasodilation, drastically lowering his SVR. As a result, his cardiac output soared.

Increased contractility
Admitted with hyperthyroidism, 62-year-old Ruby Stone had a heart rate of 110 beats/minute and her pulses were bounding. You measured her blood pressure as 158/70 mm Hg. She complained of palpitations and told you she felt warm. Checking her chart, you noted that her triiodothyronine and thyroxine levels on admission were elevated, indicating an increase in thyroid function.

You knew that both increased and decreased contractility can lower cardiac output. Contractility is affected by the sympathetic nervous system and such pathologic states as an MI and hyperthyroidism. In Ms. Stone's case, abnormally strong contractions, caused by elevated stimulatory hormones, increased the work load of her heart. Consequently, you decided, myocardial oxygen consumption increased to the point where the supply no longer met the demand.

Conclusion
For each of the patients above, cardiac output was compromised by a different factor. But by quickly reviewing each patient's history and correlating it with the appropriate signs and measurements, you can determine whether heart rate, preload, afterload, or contractility was the cause. The faster you're able to do this, the faster your patient's cardiac output can return to normal.

within 10% to 15% of the median value. Compute the average, and record the patient's cardiac output.
• Then return the stopcock to its original position and make sure that the injectate delivery system tubing is clamped.
• Verify a PA waveform on the cardiac monitor.
• Discontinue cardiac output measurements when the patient is hemodynamically stable and weaned from his vasoactive and inotropic medications. You can leave the PA catheter inserted for pressure measurements.
• Disconnect and discard the injectate delivery system and the I.V. bag. Cover any exposed stopcocks with air-occlusive caps.
• Monitor the patient for signs or symptoms of inadequate perfusion, including restlessness; fatigue; changes in level of consciousness; decreased capillary refill time; pale, cool skin; diminished peripheral pulses; and oliguria.

Interpretation of findings
The normal range for cardiac output is 4 to 8 liters/minute. The adequacy of cardiac output for an individual is better assessed by calculating the individual's cardiac index (CI), adjusted for his body size.

To calculate your patient's CI, divide his cardiac output by his body surface area (BSA), a function of height and weight. For example, a cardiac output of 4 liters/minute may be adequate for a 65" 120-lb patient (normally a BSA of 1.59 and a CI of 2.5) but would be inadequate for a 74" 230-lb patient (normally a BSA of 2.26 and a CI of 1.8). Normal CIs for adults range from 2.5 to 4.2 liters/minute/m^2. (Normal CIs for infants and children range from 3.5 to 4 liters/minute/m^2; for pregnant women, 3.5 to 6.5 liters/minute/m^2; and for elderly adults, 2 to 2.5 liters/minute/m^2.) All hemodynamic indices may be adjusted to the patient's body size to determine if the measurement is normal.

Abnormal findings
An abnormally low CI indicates that the heart isn't pumping adequately. Cardiac output may decline because of altered heart rate, preload, afterload, or contractility. A patient with low cardiac output should receive treatment aimed at the underlying determinant. (See *How cardiac output can be altered*.)

An abnormally high CI may also be detrimental. Patients with limited myocardial oxygen reserve may be unable to meet the increased oxygen demand resulting from an elevated heart rate and increased contractility. Even when the body is at rest, the myocardium extracts 75% of the oxygen from blood flowing through the coronary arteries. Resting skeletal muscles, in comparison, extract only 25% of the oxygen from the arterial blood.

During stress or exercise, the balance between myocardial oxygen supply and oxygen demand is upset. The heart beats faster and contracts more forcefully, requiring more oxygen. Since myocardial oxygen extraction can increase only slightly above resting levels, the myocardium receives more oxygen through coronary artery dilation. In patients with coronary artery disease, fatty plaque and calcium deposits prevent the arteries from dilating to deliver more oxygenated blood to the myocardium. This imbalance between oxygen supply and demand can lead to myocardial ischemia.

Nursing considerations

• Many experts recommend injecting boluses at a fixed point in the respiratory cycle, such as at end expiration. This ensures a more stable baseline blood temperature prior to each injection, yielding less variation in repeated measurements. However, others believe that injections should not be timed with respiration because the practice can affect the measurement.
• Because accurate cardiac output measurement requires a stable baseline pulmonary artery temperature prior to injection, avoid giving bolus injections of fluid or medications just before measuring cardiac output. Concomitant infusions given at a continuous rate should not affect measurement accuracy.
• Measure cardiac output as often as necessary, depending on your patient's condition. You may need to provide hourly assessments for postoperative cardiac or post-MI patients, whereas stable patients may only require cardiac output measurements every 4 to 8 hours. Cardiac output should be measured after significant changes in heart rate, preload, afterload, or contractility, or after the patient has been given drugs.
• PA catheters are usually removed after 72 hours because the incidence of infection in-

creases significantly with longer indwelling times. For patients who still need hemodynamic monitoring, you can insert a new catheter in a new site for another 72 hours. Injectate delivery systems and I.V. solutions should be changed according to your hospital's policy.
• Record cardiac output, CI, and other hemodynamic values on the vital signs record in the patient's chart.
• When monitoring any patient parameter, make sure you evaluate trends rather than isolated values. For example, an hourly decrease in cardiac output by 0.1 liter/minute may seem insignificant from hour to hour. However, at the end of 24 hours, the cardiac output would have fallen by 2.4 liters/minute, which is a significant change in any patient.
• Add the fluid volume injected for cardiac output determinations to the total *intake* for the patient. Injectate delivery of 30 ml/hour will contribute 720 ml to the patient's 24-hour intake.
• After cardiac output measurement, make sure the clamp on the injectate bag is secured. This will prevent inadvertent delivery of the injectate to the patient.

Avoiding other complications

To limit your mistakes, which may result from inexperience or improper technique, watch for the following problems:

Injectate loss. This problem may occur when the injectate is warmed after the injectate temperature is measured, or when injectate leaks from the delivery system. Because cardiac output is calculated using a known amount of solution at a known temperature, any warming or loss of injectate will affect the computed cardiac output and thus the accuracy of the cardiac output measurement. Indicator loss will produce falsely high cardiac output readings. For every 0.1 ml (of a 10-ml volume) that is lost, a 1% error is introduced. To prevent injectate loss, carefully check for loose connections at the injection site where injectate may leak.

Injectate loss may also result from inaccurate measurement of the injectate or from changes in injectate temperature after the injectate has been registered by the cardiac output computer. Always measure the injectate volume carefully and make sure the syringe is free of air bubbles. Avoid handling the barrel of the syringe, especially with a bath injectate setup.

Certain conditions, such as right to left shunts and severe tricuspid regurgitation, may cause injectate loss between the injection port and where the temperature measurement is taken within the pulmonary artery.

Incorrect catheter placement. Correct catheter placement is essential for accurate cardiac output measurements. The tip of the PA catheter must be positioned in the right, left, or main pulmonary artery. To verify correct catheter placement, make sure the PA waveform is not damped prior to making measurements. A damped tracing may mean that the thermistor is not free-floating, which can cause incorrect cardiac output values.

Improper injection technique. To prevent errors in measurement, complete the injection within 4 seconds in a single, smooth motion. Irregular injections cause multiple peaks in the washout curve, resulting in inaccurate estimation of the area under the curve and thus an error in measurement.

If the injectate lumen of the catheter is blocked, boluses may be injected through other lines such as the venous infusion port on the PA catheter, introducer side port, or through any catheter that exits into a central vein or the right atrium. The injection port must be located beyond the introducer sheath to avoid retrograde flow and injectate loss.

Incorrect computation constant. The computation constant accounts for the gain of heat from the catheter tubing as injectate travels through the catheter into the blood. With some older monitors, the computation constant must be entered as a numerical value, whereas newer equipment calculates the value internally when you enter the injectate volume and catheter size. If you mistakenly use an incorrect computation constant, you can calculate the correct cardiac output by using a

---

How to correct an inaccurate computation constant

You may inadvertently enter an incorrect computation constant. Suppose, for example, you are using 5 ml of room-temperature injectate with a 7.5 French catheter. The computation constant as specified by the manufacturer is .294.

However, suppose the nurse before you was using 10 ml of room-temperature injectate and the cardiac output computer was set for a constant of .607. If you didn't change the constant and used 5 ml of injectate, the measured cardiac output (CO) would be 4 liters/minute, when the patient's actual CO is 1.9 liters/minute.

The following formula allows you to correct the CO value without making more injections:

$$\text{Correct CO} = 4 \text{ liters/minute} \times \frac{.294}{.607}$$
$$= \frac{1.18}{.607}$$
$$= 1.9 \text{ liters/minute}$$

---

correction formula. (See *How to correct an inaccurate computation constant.*)

Inadequate signal-to-noise ratio. The *signal*, or temperature change induced by a cold injection, must be distinguished from *thermal noise*, the normal temperature changes in the pulmonary artery, in order to produce accurate bolus thermodilution measurements. Thermal noise is created when blood returns to the heart from the superior and inferior vena cavae and is affected by muscle movement and ventilation.

To strengthen the signal, you can either increase the volume or lower the temperature of the injectate. Because a 10° C difference between injectate temperature and blood temperature is recommended, you may need to give iced injectate to hypothermic patients for accurate cardiac output measurement.

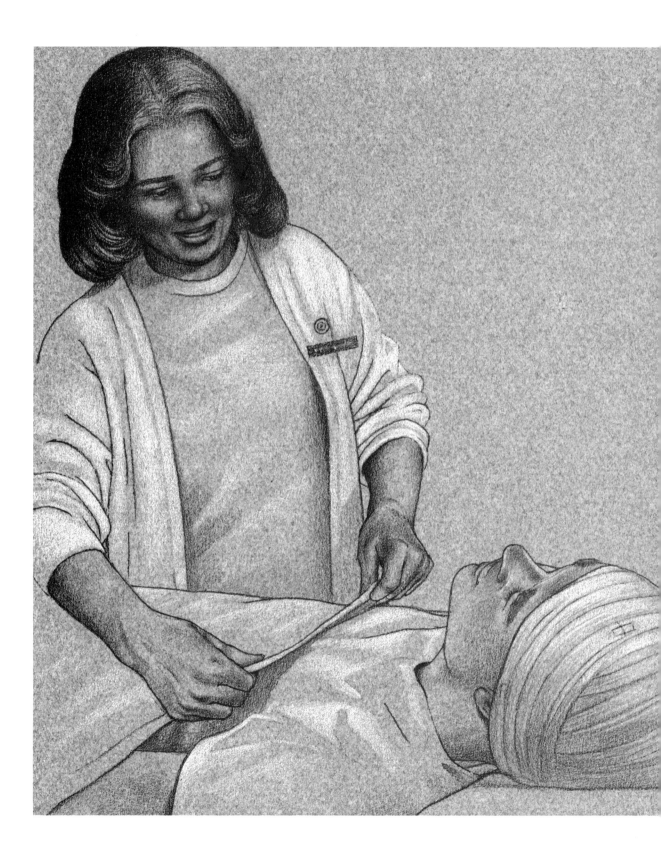

CHAPTER 6

Monitoring ICP and cerebral blood flow

Head injury and other neurologic conditions can cause increased intracranial pressure (ICP), or intracranial hypertension. By the time clinical signs of increased ICP appear, the condition usually has progressed and the patient has a poor prognosis.

Fortunately, ICP monitoring allows caregivers to detect ICP changes before clinical signs occur. The use of such monitoring has grown dramatically in the last 10 years as monitoring techniques have advanced and caregivers have become adept at recognizing and treating increased ICP. Accordingly, patient outcomes have improved. ICP monitoring is now common practice for high-risk patients.

Physiology

The cranial vault encases the brain, extracellular fluid (blood), and cerebrospinal fluid (CSF). Be-

PATHOPHYSIOLOGY

How poor compliance increases ICP

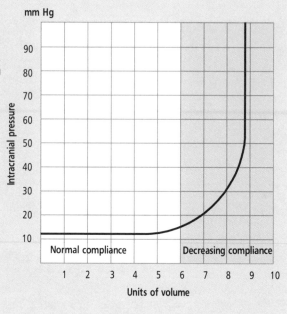

As this graph shows, normal compliance is indicated by the constant intracranial pressure (ICP) caused by the cranial vault maintaining a constant equilibrium. In decreased compliance, this equilibrium is disturbed, and a small volume increase can cause a sudden, sharp increase in ICP.

cause the cranium is rigid and can't expand, brain volume (about 1,400 ml), blood volume (150 ml), and CSF volume (150 ml) must remain nearly constant to maintain normal ICP. If one volume increases, another must decrease; otherwise, ICP rises.

Normally, several compensatory mechanisms help maintain ICP: CSF displacement from the ventricles, cerebral vasoconstriction, compression of the low-pressure venous system, and cerebral tissue shifting. When these mechanisms fail, ICP rises rapidly, leading to life-threatening decompensation.

Compliance

Compliance is the relationship between brain volume and ICP. With normal compliance, the cranial vault maintains a pressure equilibrium. With poor compliance, a small volume increase causes a large pressure increase. The relation-

ship between volume and pressure can be demonstrated in a patient who has an intraventricular catheter by placing a small volume of fluid in the catheter, then observing the corresponding ICP increase. This test shouldn't be performed if the patient's ICP is less than 25 mm Hg. (See *How poor compliance increases ICP.*)

The volume-pressure relationship differs in each patient. Factors affecting compliance include the degree of the volume increase, the duration over which the volume increases, and the overall size of the cranial vault. For example, an epidural hematoma causes a faster volume increase than an evolving brain tumor. Thus, ICP rises more rapidly in a patient with an epidural hematoma than in one with a brain tumor. However, in an elderly patient with an acute hematoma, ICP may rise relatively slowly because the cerebral atrophy that accompanies aging creates more space in the cranial vault.

Cerebral blood flow

The brain's cellular metabolism depends on an adequate supply of oxygen. Oxygen supply, in turn, hinges on adequate cerebral blood flow (CBF). An extensive capillary network provides blood to the brain, supplying it with 15% of the total resting cardiac output. Total CBF remains relatively constant, although the flow rate to specific regions fluctuates with metabolic tissue demands. Increased metabolism enhances local blood flow because oxygen tension decreases and carbon dioxide tension increases.

Cerebral perfusion pressure (CPP) serves as a rough index of CBF. You can determine CPP by subtracting the patient's ICP from his mean arterial pressure (MAP). In adults, CPP normally ranges from 70 to 100 mm Hg. Maintaining ICP relative to MAP ensures adequate CBF. Inadequate CPP results in ischemia, which progresses to neuronal hypoxia and cell death. When ICP and MAP are equal, CPP is 0 mm Hg and CBF ceases.

Autoregulation
In healthy people, autoregulation maintains CBF at near-normal levels despite a wide variation in MAP. This mechanism allows cerebral vessels to dilate or constrict to maintain a constant blood flow to cerebral tissues.

Autoregulation is achieved by pressure-related or metabolic factors. For instance, stretch receptors in arterioles respond to changes in blood pressure and ICP. The vasomotor tone that causes arteriolar constriction or dilation then maintains a nearly constant CBF. Metabolic autoregulation occurs from the accumulated by-products of cellular metabolism. The resulting acidosis leaves excesses of carbon dioxide and hydrogen ions, potent vasodilators.

Autoregulation may fail after brain injury. When this occurs, vasomotor tone diminishes and CBF depends on changes in systemic blood pressure.

ICP monitoring

Continuous ICP monitoring has become common practice in intensive care units (ICUs) that treat at-risk patients. It's most often used for trauma patients, who are susceptible to cerebral edema. Other likely candidates include patients with subarachnoid hemorrhage, tumors that obstruct the ventricular system, cerebral aneurysm, intracranial hemorrhage, or Reye's syndrome.

Thanks to the wide variety of ICP monitoring methods, few limitations on its use exist. The doctor typically chooses the system.

Each ICP monitoring system carries certain inherent risks. However, infection is always the most serious threat. Its incidence varies widely—from 11% to 64%. Its risk increases when an intraventricular catheter is used, when monitoring lasts more than 5 days, when the system is flushed, and when an open system is used.

To minimize the risk of infection, the doctor usually inserts the pressure sensor in the operating room. However, if aseptic technique can be ensured, insertion may take place in the emergency department or ICU. Skillful nursing care plays a key role in preventing infection or reducing the risk. For instance, you must use strict aseptic technique when setting up and maintaining the system.

Equipment
All ICP monitoring systems share three basic components: sensor, pressure transducer, and recording device. A sensor can be placed in the ventricle, subarachnoid space, epidural space, subdural space, or brain parenchyma. (See *Types of ICP monitoring,* pages 96 and 97.) The sensor transmits ICP changes to the transducer, which converts the impulses to electrical or light signals. A recording device converts the signals to visible tracings, which appear on an oscilloscope or are transferred to graph paper.

ICP monitoring sensors for the various types of ICP monitoring include the fiber-optic transducer-tipped catheter, intraventricular catheter, epidural or subdural sensor or cathe-

Types of ICP monitoring

Intraventricular catheter monitoring

In this procedure, which monitors intracranial pressure (ICP) directly, the doctor inserts a catheter into the lateral ventricle through a burr hole.

Although this method measures ICP most accurately, it carries the greatest risk of infection. This is the only type of ICP monitoring that allows evaluation of brain compliance and drainage of significant amounts of cerebrospinal fluid (CSF).

Contraindications usually include stenotic cerebral ventricles, cerebral aneurysms in the path of catheter placement, and suspected vascular lesions.

Subarachnoid screw monitoring

This procedure involves insertion of a special screw with a hollow bolt into the subarachnoid space through a twist-drill burr hole that's positioned in the front of the skull behind the hairline.

Placing the screw is easier than placing an intraventricular catheter, especially if a computed tomography scan reveals that the cerebrum has shifted or the ventricles have collapsed. This type of ICP monitoring also carries less risk of infection and parenchymal damage because the screw doesn't penetrate the cerebrum.

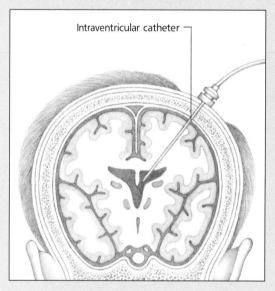

Intraventricular catheter

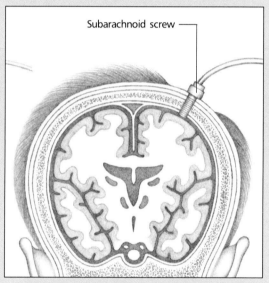

Subarachnoid screw

ter, and subarachnoid screw. Each device has its benefits and drawbacks.

Fiber-optic transducer-tipped catheter

The most advanced and versatile ICP monitoring device, the fiber-optic transducer-tipped catheter is a #4 French catheter that the surgeon implants in the ventricle, subarachnoid space, subdural space, or brain parenchyma. Certain placements allow CSF drainage to treat increased ICP.

A miniature transducer at the tip of the catheter has a mirrored diaphragm, which reflects pressure changes and produces changes in light intensity. The light is transmitted by fiber optics to an amplifier, which converts the light changes to electrical signals. These signals, in turn, produce oscilloscopic images. The recorder then displays mean ICP.

Calibrated by the manufacturer, the fiber-optic transducer-tipped catheter needs to be zeroed to atmospheric pressure only before insertion. The device can be connected to an ex-

Epidural sensor monitoring

The least invasive method with the lowest incidence of infection, this monitoring system uses a sensor inserted into the epidural space through a burr hole.

Unlike an intraventricular catheter or a subarachnoid screw, the sensor can't become occluded with blood or brain tissue. Accuracy is questionable, however, because the epidural sensor doesn't measure ICP directly from a CSF-filled space. Several types of sensors are available; some can be recalibrated repeatedly. Fiber-optic sensors must be calibrated before they're inserted.

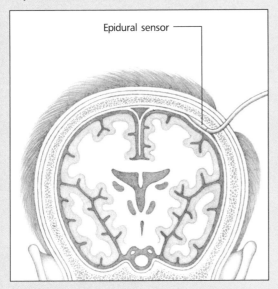

Epidural sensor

Intraparenchymal monitoring

In this procedure, the doctor inserts a catheter through a small subarachnoid bolt and, after puncturing the dura, advances the catheter a few centimeters into the brain's white matter. There's no need to balance or calibrate the equipment after insertion.

Although this method doesn't provide direct access to CSF, ICP measurements are accurate because brain tissue pressures correlate well with ventricular pressures. Intraparenchymal monitoring may be used to obtain ICP measurements in patients with compressed or dislocated ventricles.

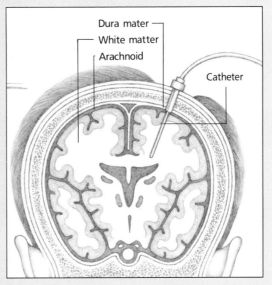

Dura mater
White matter
Arachnoid
Catheter

isting monitoring system in the ICU for trend analysis, or the amplifier can function as an independent monitor. The catheter also operates under battery power if necessary, such as for patient transport.

Intraventricular catheter

Implanted into the anterior horn (most common site) or posterior horn of the lateral ventricle, this Silastic catheter typically attaches to a drainage system with a stopcock for transducer attachment. Besides permitting ICP

monitoring, it allows CSF drainage to treat increased ICP. As a drawback, the intraventricular catheter poses the greatest risk of infection and inadvertent CSF loss.

Epidural or subdural sensor or catheter

Several systems can be used to monitor ICP in the epidural space. In one of the first epidural systems developed, the surgeon implants a fiber-optic sensor into the epidural space and then connects it to a monitor for a digital readout of mean ICP. The mechanism for pressure readings is the same as for the fiber-optic transducer-tipped catheter. Because this system isn't affected by environmental factors, it doesn't need to be recalibrated.

Alternatively, the surgeon may implant a pneumatic flow sensor in the epidural space. The pressure required to maintain airflow determines ICP. This type of sensor provides the most accurate epidural monitoring.

A Silastic catheter placed in the subdural space also can sense pressure changes. The catheter attaches to a transducer via a stopcock. The external setup is the same as for an intraventricular catheter. Subdural catheters are used most commonly after surgery.

Subarachnoid screw
In this method, the surgeon places a screw with a hollow bolt in a twist-drill burr hole in the skull and dura. The bolt attaches to a transducer, usually via a stopcock. Although easy to insert, this device may become blocked in patients with cerebral edema as the brain herniates through the bolt.

Preparation
Make sure that the patient or (if the patient is unconscious) a family member is fully informed about the procedures involved in ICP monitoring, and obtain a signed consent form. If the patient is awake, inform him that the surgeon will place a device inside his head to allow ICP monitoring. Mention that his head will be shaved beforehand and that a dressing will be placed over the site once the device is in place. Tell him that the monitoring system will restrict his movement. Reassure him that you'll assess him frequently.

Whenever possible, the doctor will insert the monitor in the operating room. If he must insert it in the emergency department or the ICU, be sure to use aseptic technique when preparing the area. Shave the insertion site; then clean it with an iodophor solution.

For insertion, the patient usually is positioned supine, with his head slightly elevated. With most systems, the monitoring device is placed on the right side anteriorly. However, if the monitor will be inserted during a craniotomy for hematoma or tumor removal, the sur-

gical site determines monitor placement.

If a separate transducer will be used, you'll probably have to prime the system completely before connecting it to the patient. Unlike the systems used to monitor other pressures, one used to monitor ICP lacks a periodic flow of fluid. It must be primed with fluid completely to eliminate air in the tubing, which can cause inaccurate pressure readings. Use preservative-free 0.9% sodium chloride solution to prime the tubing. Prime it from the point at which the pressure tubing attaches to the implanted device past both stopcocks to the drip chamber. You may attach the transducer at either stopcock. (See *Setting up an ICP monitoring system,* pages 100 and 101.) Be sure to maintain aseptic technique when setting up and maintaining the external components that will be attached to the implanted device.

The pressure tubing usually comes as a one-piece unit consisting of a short length of pressure tubing, a stopcock, and another length of pressure tubing. Attach the unit to the device to be implanted. The second length of tubing may have a distal stopcock before the drainage collection drip chamber.

When you've completed the setup, cover the system with a sterile towel until it's connected to the patient.

If the patient will have a subarachnoid screw, gather a short length of pressure tubing and a stopcock, or just a stopcock that fits directly onto the hollow bolt. Prime it completely with 0.9% sodium chloride solution, using aseptic technique.

If the patient will have a fiber-optic transducer-tipped catheter, preparation usually involves only zeroing the system immediately before catheter insertion. Follow the manufacturer's directions closely when zeroing the system to ensure accurate ICP values.

Procedure
• If the monitor will be inserted in the ICU or the emergency department, assist the surgeon as needed. Using aseptic technique, prepare an insertion tray with a twist drill and various needles, syringes, hemostats, and sutures.
• Position the patient flat or supine. The surgeon will work from the top of the bed.

• If a fiber-optic transducer-tipped catheter or an epidural sensor will be inserted, help the surgeon balance the system. As he holds the cable at the patient end, attach the monitor end to the cable and turn the monitor on. If mean pressure on the monitor doesn't read zero, adjust the system according to the manufacturer's guidelines until a zero appears.
• The surgeon inserts the monitor and sutures it in place to prevent accidental dislodgment. As he does this, observe the patient's vital signs and neurologic response (unless he has received a paralytic agent).
• Help the surgeon connect the transducer component to the implanted device. Then check the balance and calibration, following the directions supplied by the manufacturer of the bedside monitor. The monitor should display mean pressure.
• Be sure to make a hard copy of the initial ICP waveform to help you troubleshoot the system later, if needed.
• Clean the insertion site with an iodophor solution and apply a dry, sterile occlusive dressing over the site.
• Document the initial ICP reading, waveform, and neurologic findings at the time of monitor insertion.

Monitor removal
• The surgeon may discontinue ICP monitoring if the patient's ICP has been stable for 2 to 3 days or if he didn't require CSF drainage. Collect sterile gloves, a dry dressing, suture material, sterile scissors, and forceps for the surgeon.
• The surgeon removes the anchoring suture and then removes the monitoring device. He closes the insertion site with a suture and places a dry dressing over it.
• For the first 24 hours, observe the site frequently for CSF leakage. Also observe carefully for any sign of infection, including meningitis.
• For 2 to 3 days after monitor removal, maintain the site with sterile dressings.

Interpretation of findings
ICP fluctuates continuously as ventricular fluid patterns change. Normal ICP ranges from 4 to 15 mm Hg (or 50 to 200 mm H_2O). However,

trends are more important than isolated values. Whenever possible, correlate ICP trends with clinical findings. (See *Using an intraventricular catheter to monitor and treat ICP,* page 102.)

You may see four ICP waveform patterns on the monitor. The normal waveform indicates ICP between 4 and 15 mm Hg. It usually occurs continuously and indicates a normal ICP.

A waves are an ominous sign of intracranial decompensation and poor brain compliance. They may be sudden and transient, spiking from temporary rises in thoracic pressure or from any other condition that increases ICP beyond the brain's compliance limits. (Such activities as sustained coughing or straining with bowel movements can cause temporary rises in thoracic pressure.)

Typically, A waves denote cerebral ischemia and further brain injury. In pressure readings above 20 mm Hg, they presumably reflect permanent cell damage from hypoxia. A waves may be accompanied by changes in neurologic status, such as deterioration in level of consciousness, altered respiratory pattern, headache, nausea, vomiting, abnormal pupil reaction, and altered motor function.

B waves correlate with changes in respiration and may occur more frequently with decreasing compensation. Because B waves sometimes precede A waves, notify the doctor if your patient has frequent B waves.

Clinically insignificant, C waves may fluctuate with respirations. They reflect normal changes in systemic arterial pressure.

When assessing your patient's waveforms, focus mainly on A waves. The clinical significance of B and C waves remains unknown. (See *Interpreting ICP waveforms,* page 103.)

Nursing considerations
• Be sure to obtain ICP readings at consistent times every day. Make sure the patient's head is in the same position for each reading. Avoid stimulating him before obtaining a reading.
• Check for trends in ICP because these are a better indicator than isolated values. Also, be sure to correlate ICP increases with the patient's clinical condition and with any activity taking place around him. Many care activities

(Text continues on page 102.)

Setting up an ICP monitoring system

To set up an intracranial pressure (ICP) monitoring system, begin by opening a sterile towel. On the sterile field, place a 20-ml luer-lock syringe, an 18G needle, a 250-ml bag filled with 0.9% sodium chloride solution (with outer wrapper removed), and a disposable transducer. Put on sterile gloves and fill the 20-ml syringe with 0.9% sodium chloride solution from the I.V. bag. Remove the injection cap from the patient line and attach the syringe. Turn the system stopcock off to the short end of the patient line, and flush through to the drip chamber, as shown.

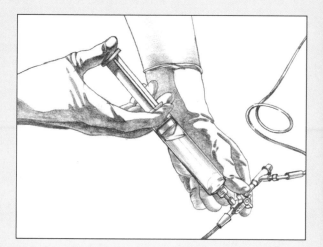

Loosen the dead end cap on the patient line. Turn the stopcock off to the long portion of the patient line, and flush with solution, as shown. Tighten the dead end cap, and turn the stopcock off to the patient line.

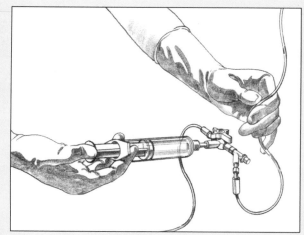

Attach the manometer to the I.V. pole at the head of the bed. Slide the drip chamber onto the manometer, and align the chamber to the zero point, as shown. Next, connect the transducer to the monitor. Put on a clean pair of sterile gloves. Keeping one hand sterile, turn the patient stopcock off to the patient.

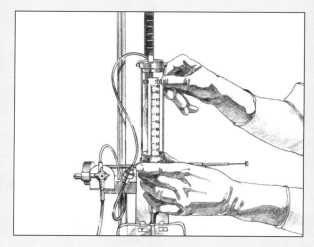

Align the zero point with the patient's head, level with the middle of the ear, as shown.

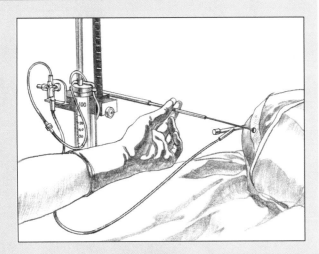

Lower the flow chamber to zero, and turn the stopcock off to the dead end cap, as shown at right. With a clean hand, balance the system according to monitor guidelines.

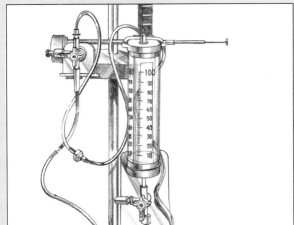

Turn the system stopcock off to drainage, and raise the flow chamber to the ordered height, as shown at right. Return the stopcock to the ordered position, and observe the monitor for the return of ICP patterns.

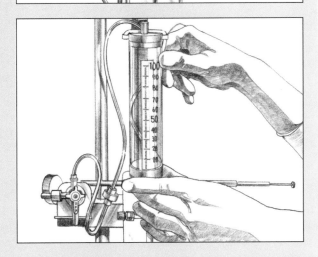

Using an intraventricular catheter to monitor and treat ICP

Besides allowing intracranial pressure (ICP) monitoring, an intraventricular catheter also allows cerebrospinal fluid (CSF) drainage to treat increased ICP before and after surgery. It's your responsibility to correlate pressure readings with changes in your patient's status, maximizing a positive outcome. Consider the case of Saul Miller, age 42.

Initial care
Mr. Miller was admitted to your unit after sudden onset of headache and loss of consciousness. A computed tomography scan taken just after his arrival showed a large subarachnoid hemorrhage with blood in the lateral and third ventricles.

After he was placed under your nursing supervision, you noted that Mr. Miller exhibited flexion withdrawal in reaction to pain and that his pupils were equal but reacted sluggishly to light.

The doctor then inserted an intraventricular catheter in the anterior horn of the right lateral ventricle to monitor Mr. Miller's ICP and drain CSF. Initially, ICP measured 15 mm Hg and CSF drainage was bloody.

Preoperative care
As ordered, you place the drip chamber at a height of 20 mm Hg and leave the system open to drain. For the first 8 hours, ICP ranges from 12 to 15 mm Hg. Then you note that no drainage appears in the collection chamber and that the ICP waveform has remained unchanged since catheter insertion.

During the next 8 hours, you document Mr. Miller's ICP at 15 to 24 mm Hg and observe approximately 5 ml of bloody drainage in the collection chamber. Assessing his neurologic status, you find that he now needs a greater stimulus to exhibit flexion withdrawal in reaction to pain. You report these findings to the doctor, who instructs

you to lower the drip chamber to a height of 12 mm Hg to promote ventricular drainage.

Over the next 24 hours, the intraventricular catheter drains a total of 300 ml of bloody fluid. Mr. Miller's ICP drops, hovering between 10 and 12 mm Hg. You now find that he has a brisker pupil response to light and can follow simple commands and express his complaints.

Surgery
After performing a four-vessel arteriogram that identifies an aneurysm of the middle cerebral artery, the doctor surgically clips the aneurysm and then returns Mr. Miller to your care with the intraventricular catheter in place.

Postoperative care
Ventricular monitoring and drainage continue for 3 days postoperatively. Mr. Miller's ICP values remain stable at 10 to 12 mm Hg. You report less than 50 ml of drainage over each 24-hour monitoring period. The doctor orders clamping of the catheter over a 24-hour period. Mr. Miller's ICP values and clinical status remain stable, and he no longer requires CSF drainage. On the fifth postoperative day, the doctor removes the catheter.

Conclusion
Mr. Miller's treatment shows how an intraventricular catheter helps to monitor and treat ICP. But more important, it demonstrates the importance of correlating ICP readings with subtle shifts in a patient's condition. You were alerted to changes in Mr. Miller's neurologic status by a decreased sensitivity to pain, an increase in ICP, and a decrease in drainage. You and the doctor were then able to intervene by lowering the drip chamber, causing the excess CSF to drain and the ICP to return to normal.

can cause a transient ICP increase. To avoid misinterpreting values, obtain an ICP reading before starting the care activity; then monitor for ICP changes as you perform care.
• Help assess the patient's brain compliance by observing his response to care. If ICP doesn't

return to baseline values within 4 minutes after the care activity ends, suspect reduced compliance. Alter your care to minimize its effect on ICP, and notify the doctor.
• If the patient has a fluid-filled monitoring system in place, ensure that all connections are

Interpreting ICP waveforms

You may see various types of intracranial pressure (ICP) waveforms on your patient's bedside monitor.

Normal waveform
A normal waveform shows a steep upward systolic slope, followed by a downward diastolic slope with a dicrotic notch.

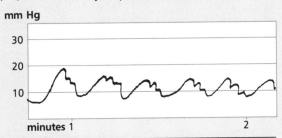

A waves
Commonly called plateau waves because of their shape, A waves may reach an amplitude of 50 to 100 mm Hg, last for 5 to 20 minutes, then drop sharply—signaling exhaustion of the brain's compliance mechanisms. A waves are the most clinically significant ICP waveforms.

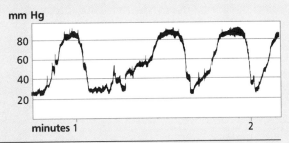

B waves
Sharp and rhythmic, with a sawtooth pattern, B waves may occur as frequently as every 1½ to 2 minutes and may reach an amplitude of 50 mm Hg.

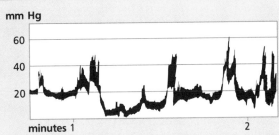

C waves
C waves are rapid and rhythmic, but not as sharp as B waves. They usually occur every 4 to 8 minutes and have an amplitude of about 20 mm Hg.

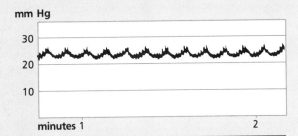

Waveform denoting equipment problem
A waveform that looks like the one shown here signals a transducer or monitor problem such as obstruction in the system. Determine if the transducer needs recalibrating.

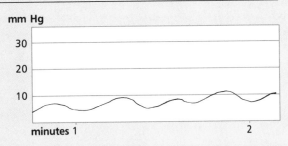

tight and the system is air-free. Air in the system can cause damped waveforms and alter ICP values. Zero the system at least every 8 hours and whenever you question its accuracy. Maintain the transducer at the level of the foramen of Monro.

• If the patient has an implanted catheter attached to a drainage system, maintain the height of the drip chamber at the ordered level so that the system drains at the desired pressure. When draining, carefully observe the fluid flowing into the drip chamber; drainage of more than 2 or 3 ml of fluid at a time may cause ventricular collapse. Assess the system's patency by observing drainage for color, clarity, blood, and sediment. Also note the amount of drainage over time.

• Observe the monitor insertion site every 8 hours for redness and drainage. If you see drainage, determine whether it's CSF by checking for a halo sign or testing drainage for glucose. Notify the doctor if you suspect CSF leakage because leakage increases the risk of infection.

• To help prevent infection, change the sterile dressing daily. After removing the old dressing, clean the site with an iodophor solution. Then apply a new sterile occlusive dressing.

• If the surgeon orders prophylactic antibiotic administration through an intraventricular catheter, monitor the patient's brain compliance. Instilling antibiotics into this type of catheter may compromise a patient with low compliance. Carefully observe how much ICP increases after antibiotic therapy; an increase of 5 mm Hg may suggest low compliance.

• Make sure all caregivers know that an ICP monitoring system is in place, especially if the patient has an intraventricular catheter (which may cause CSF loss).

• If the doctor has ordered CSF drainage, unplug the bed to prevent accidentally changing the level of the patient's head relative to the drainage bag. Minimize activities around the patient to avoid causing a rise in ICP. Turn alarm volumes low, keep bright lights to a minimum, and schedule diagnostic tests and procedures so the patient gets adequate rest and ICP can return to baseline between periods of stimulation. Alert all caregivers to use

sterile gloves when manipulating the dressing.

• Use aseptic technique when obtaining CSF specimens for culture and analysis. Ideally, you should obtain specimens from the port closest to the ventricle. Most systems have a stopcock or a Y-port just distal to the patient connection point. Clean the specimen site with iodophor solution; then withdraw CSF using a 3-ml syringe. To prevent undesired effects, don't withdraw more than 2.5 ml at once.

• Document all ICP and CPP trends and the condition of the monitoring site. If you see CSF leakage, document the amount and color.

CBF monitoring

Traditionally, caregivers have estimated cerebral blood flow (CBF) in neurologically compromised patients by calculating CPP. However, modern technology permits continuous regional blood flow monitoring at the bedside. A sensor placed on the cerebral cortex calculates CBF in the capillary bed by thermal diffusion. Thermistors within the sensor sense the temperature differential between two metallic plates — one heated, one neutral. This differential relates inversely to CBF: As the differential decreases, CBF increases — and vice versa. This monitoring technique yields important information about the effects of interventions on CBF. It also yields continuous real-time values for CBF, which are essential in conditions where compromised blood flow may put the patient at risk, such as ischemia and infarction. (See *Why monitor CBF?*)

CBF monitoring is indicated whenever CBF alterations are anticipated. It's used most commonly in patients with subarachnoid hemorrhage (in which a vasospasm may restrict blood flow), trauma associated with high ICP, or vascular tumors. Use of this new technology is likely to grow as practitioners become more familiar with the information it provides.

As with ICP monitoring, CBF monitoring may lead to infection. To help prevent this complication, administer prophylactic antibiotics, as ordered, and maintain a sterile dressing around the insertion site. CSF leakage, another

Why monitor CBF?

Cerebral blood flow (CBF) monitoring yields important information about the effects of interventions on CBF. By carefully correlating CBF with other assessment findings, you can detect complications and intervene promptly, improving the patient's chances of avoiding multiple deficits caused by reduced oxygen flow to the brain. Take, for example, the case of Edna Thompson, age 52.

Initial treatment
Ms. Thompson underwent a craniotomy to remove an aneurysm of the right middle cerebral artery and is still at risk for vasospasm. Anesthesia was not reversed at the completion of surgery. Postoperatively, she was admitted to your unit after a ventriculostomy and with a CBF monitor in place.

Care on your unit
When first assessing Ms. Thompson, you measure her pupils at 3 mm and note that they're reactive to light. But there are no other significant assessment findings. You also find that her intracranial pressure (ICP), measured by an intraventricular catheter, ranges from 12 to 15 mm Hg. CBF ranges from 40 to 65 ml/100 g/minute.

Eight hours after the patient arrived on your unit, you note that Ms. Thompson has begun to localize to painful stimulus—but more quickly with her right side than her left side. Her pupils continue to appear small and reactive to light. CBF values remain stable at 45 to 58 ml/100 g/minute, and ICP remains unchanged.

At the end of the first 24 hours of postoperative care, Ms. Thompson's CBF consistently measures 75 to 80 ml/100 g/minute. On assessment, you find that she can follow commands intermittently, her right and left extremities move equally, and her pupils are equal and react briskly to light.

During the second day of postoperative care, Ms. Thompson's CBF drops to 40 to 45 ml/100 g/minute, and her right extremities become weaker than her left. All other assessment findings remain unchanged. Other hemodynamic parameters show a normal fluid volume status.

You report these findings to the doctor, who then orders an albumin infusion. Over the next 3 hours, Ms. Thompson's CBF rises, remaining at 75 to 85 ml/100 g/minute, and she regains some strength in her left side.

Conclusion
By correlating the patient's reduced CBF with her extremity weakness and normal fluid volume status, you were able to intervene promptly. As a result, all parameters returned to baseline, demonstrating that the faster a health care team can respond to CBF decreases, the better the patient's prognosis.

---

potential complication, may occur at the sensor insertion site. To prevent leakage, the surgeon usually places an additional suture at the site.

Equipment
CBF monitoring requires a special sensor that attaches to a computer data system or to a small analog monitor that operates on a battery for patient transport. (See *CBF monitoring systems*, page 106.)

Preparation
Make sure that the patient or a family member is fully informed about the procedures involved in CBF monitoring, and obtain a consent form. If the patient will need CBF monitoring after surgery, inform him that a sensor will be in place for about 3 days postoperatively to measure CBF. Tell him that the insertion site will be covered with a dry sterile dressing. Mention that the sensor may be removed at the bedside.

No special equipment setup is needed. Depending on the type of system you're using, you may need to verify that a battery has been inserted in the monitor to allow CBF monitoring during patient transport to the ICU.

ADVANCED EQUIPMENT

CBF monitoring systems

To monitor cerebral blood flow (CBF) at the patient's bedside, you may use a monitor such as the one shown below. This monitor has a digital display; some also display waveforms. The CBF sensor, placed in the cerebral cortex, continuously measures cortical blood flow.

Bedside CBF monitor

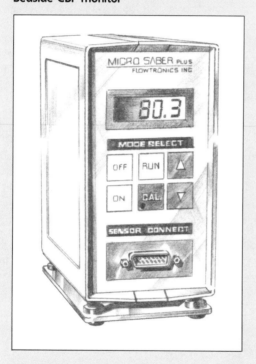

CBF sensor

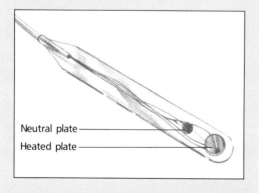

Neutral plate
Heated plate

Procedure

• The surgeon typically inserts the sensor in the operating room, during or at completion of a craniotomy. (Occasionally, he may place it through a burr hole.) He implants the sensor far from major blood vessels and verifies that the metallic plates have good contact with the brain surface. (See *Placing a CBF sensor.*)

• If ordered, attach the distal end of the sensor to the monitor. Once the sensor is in place, turn the monitor on. Turn the RUN/CAL switch to CAL, and adjust the ZERO ADJUST knob until the digital readout is 0.00. This calibrates the system. Then adjust the knob to the lock position, and turn the RUN/CAL switch to RUN.

• Document the baseline CBF value.

Monitor removal

• When the surgeon decides to discontinue monitoring (usually after 72 hours), gather a suture removal set and sterile gloves.

• The surgeon removes the anchoring suture and then gently removes the sensor from the insertion site. He closes the wound with a stitch.

• Carefully observe and document the condition of the site, and document leakage, if any.

Interpretation of findings

CBF fluctuates with the brain's metabolic demands, normally ranging from 60 to 90 ml/100 g/minute. However, the patient's neurologic condition dictates the acceptable range. For instance, in a patient in a coma, CBF may be half the normal value; in a patient in a barbiturate-induced coma with burst suppression on the electroencephalogram, CBF may be as low as 10 ml/100 g/minute. Vasospasm secondary to subarachnoid hemorrhage may result in CBF below 40 ml/100 g/minute. In an awake patient, CBF above 90 ml/100 g/minute may indicate hyperemia.

Nursing considerations

• Document CBF values hourly. Be sure to check for trends and correlate values with the patient's clinical status.

• Be aware that stimulation or activity may cause a 10% increase or decrease in CBF. If you note a 20% increase or decrease, suspect

Placing a CBF sensor

Typically, the surgeon inserts a cerebral blood flow (CBF) sensor during a craniotomy. He tunnels the sensor toward the craniotomy site and then carefully inserts the metallic plates of the thermistor to make sure that they continuously contact the surface of the cerebral cortex. After closing the dura and replacing the bone flap, he closes the scalp.

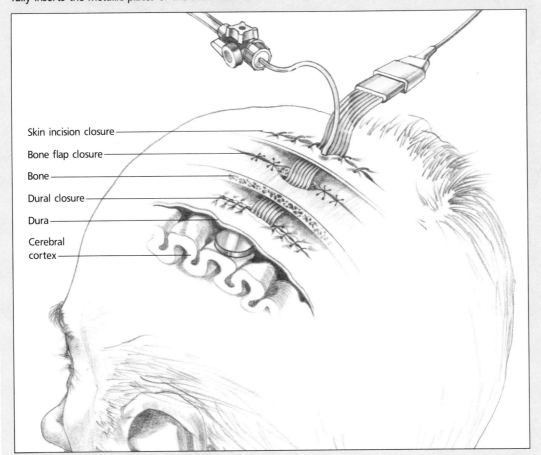

Skin incision closure

Bone flap closure

Bone

Dural closure

Dura

Cerebral cortex

poor contact between the sensor and the cerebral cortex. To correct this, turn the patient toward the side of the sensor or gently wiggle the catheter back and forth (using a sterile-gloved hand). To determine if these maneuvers have improved contact between the sensor and the cortex, observe the CBF value on the monitor as you perform them.

• If your patient has low CBF but no neurologic symptoms that indicate ischemia, suspect a fluid layer (a small hematoma) between the sensor and the cortex.

• To reduce the risk of infection, change the dressing at the insertion site daily. After cleaning the site with an iodophor solution (if ordered), apply a new dry sterile dressing. Be sure to use sterile technique during dressing changes. If ordered, administer prophylactic antibiotics. Observe the site for CSF leakage, which increases the risk of infection. (The surgeon may place an additional suture to prevent or stop such leakage.)

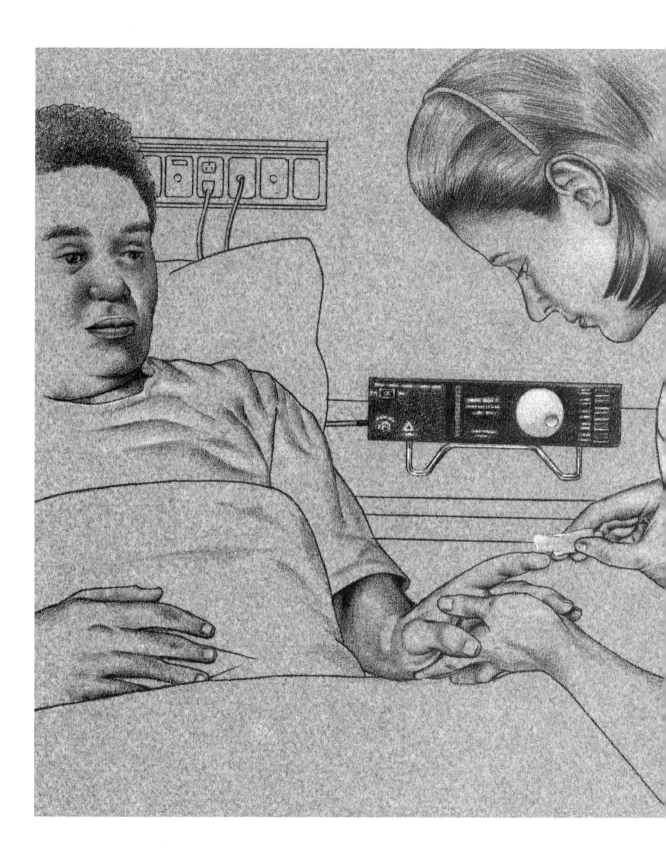

CHAPTER 7

Monitoring gas exchange

By supplying body cells with oxygen and eliminating excess carbon dioxide, gas exchange plays an essential role in sustaining life and promoting growth. Unfortunately, all hospital patients are at risk for altered gas exchange, an abnormality that can impede recovery from illness or injury and even cause death.

To monitor your patient's gas exchange, you need advanced skills and special training. For example, to assess oxygenation completely, you must evaluate many factors — oxygen content (oxygen saturation, hemoglobin, and oxygen tension), oxygen transport (oxygen content and cardiac output), and oxygen consumption (tissue oxygen demands). To do this, you must know how to set up various monitoring systems and interpret the results.

This chapter provides the up-to-date information you need. It reviews the factors that affect gas exchange, including respiratory control, oxygen transport and delivery, and lung ventilation and perfusion. Then it discusses the monitoring techniques that provide important data about your patient's oxygenation status: pulse oximetry, transcutaneous oxygen and carbon dioxide monitoring, end-tidal carbon dioxide monitoring, mixed venous oxygen saturation monitoring, bedside pulmonary function monitoring, and apnea monitoring. For each technique, the chapter explains how the equipment works, describes how to prepare for and carry out the procedure, and tells how to interpret the values supplied by the monitor.

Physiology

Gas exchange—the addition of oxygen and removal of carbon dioxide from pulmonary capillary blood—occurs during breathing, or ventilation. Breathing has two phases—*inspiration*, which moves air into the lungs, and *expiration*, which moves air out of the lungs.

Respiratory control
The brain, nerves, and various chemical and physical factors interact to regulate breathing and maintain ventilatory homeostasis.

Respiratory centers
Respiratory centers in the brain stem control respiratory rate and depth, adjust ventilation to meet the body's metabolic demands, innervate the diaphragm, and contain chemoreceptors that affect ventilation.

The *medullary respiratory center* controls respiratory rate and depth through the interaction of neurons that regulate inspiration and neurons that regulate expiration. These neurons also react to other impulses, such as from the *pons*. Regulating respiratory rhythm, the pons harmonizes the transition from inspiration to expiration through its interaction with the medullary respiratory center. The *apneustic center* within the pons stimulates inspiratory neurons in the medulla to trigger inspiration. These neurons, in turn, induce the *pneumotaxic center* (also in the pons) to inhibit the apneustic center and trigger expiration. (See *Innervation of respiratory structures.*)

Receptors
Various receptors contribute to ventilation. *Chemoreceptors* in the medullary respiratory center help regulate respiratory rate and depth in response to changes in oxygen, carbon dioxide, and pH in the blood. The *central chemoreceptor*, or carbon dioxide sensor, responds to carbon dioxide changes affecting hydrogen ion concentration in the cerebrospinal fluid (CSF). When CSF acidity rises, the central chemoreceptor stimulates the respiratory centers to increase respiratory rate and depth until the carbon dioxide level returns to normal. Conversely, lowered CSF acidity triggers the central chemoreceptor to decrease respiratory rate and depth until cellular metabolism produces more carbon dioxide.

Peripheral chemoreceptors in the carotid and aortic bodies stimulate respiratory centers in the brain stem to increase ventilation if the partial pressure of arterial oxygen (PaO_2) decreases. Ventilation normally increases when the PaO_2 falls below 50 mm Hg.

Reflex responses
The Hering-Breuer reflex, a protective mechanism, limits lung expansion. When the lungs expand, stretch receptors in the alveolar ducts trigger the flow of inhibitory messages to the respiratory center. In response, the diaphragm and intercostal muscles relax, allowing passive expiration.

Changes in arterial blood pressure also cause reflex respiratory responses by stimulating pressoreceptors in the aortic and carotid bodies. For instance, respirations reflexively slow when blood pressure suddenly rises and speed up when blood pressure suddenly falls.

Other stimuli
Fever may trigger the respiratory center to increase respirations, whereas a reduced temperature may lead to a decreased respiratory rate. Airway irritation causes receptors to induce coughing or sneezing. Sensory stimulation, such as sudden heat or cold, may cause a reaction—for example, a gasp—that affects respirations.

Innervation of respiratory structures

Higher brain centers as well as other sources stimulate respiratory centers in the pons and medulla. These centers then send impulses to various respiratory structures, altering respiratory patterns.

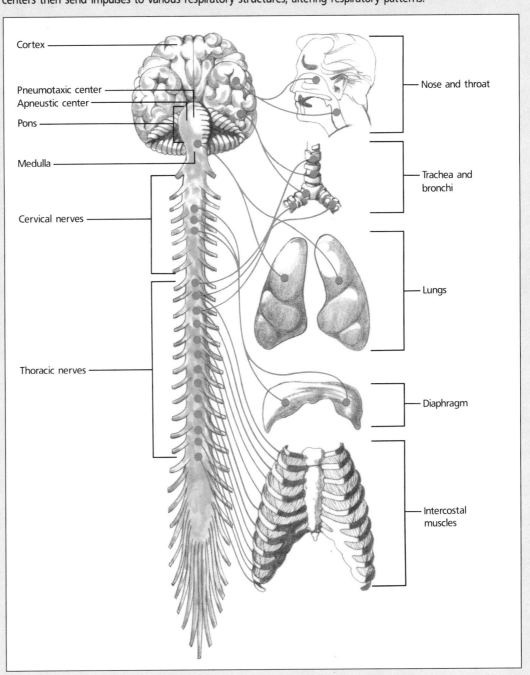

Cortex

Pneumotaxic center
Apneustic center
Pons

Medulla

Cervical nerves

Thoracic nerves

Nose and throat

Trachea and bronchi

Lungs

Diaphragm

Intercostal muscles

Physical factors

Physical factors, including resistance and compliance, also affect gas exchange.

Resistance. The three types of resistance — elastic, nonelastic, and airway — can challenge effective gas exchange and must be overcome to avoid compromising the patient's breathing.

Elastic resistance, the result of elastic lung fibers and the surface tension between alveolar air and the alveolar sac lining, allows the lungs to contract during expiration. Certain factors counteract lung elasticity — chest wall rigidity; negative intrathoracic pressure, which allows the lungs to expand with the chest wall; and surfactant, a lipoprotein that prevents alveolar collapse.

Nonelastic resistance results from forces that interfere with normal chest expansion. For instance, obesity, pregnancy, weight gain, and restrictive dressings inhibit downward thoracic expansion. These conditions compromise inspiration by increasing the work of breathing.

Airway resistance refers to resistance to airflow within the airway. The greater the airway resistance, the more pressure is needed to move air into and out of the lungs.

Airway resistance depends on airway radius, length, and flow rate. A 50% reduction in radius (such as from accumulated secretions) increases airway resistance 16-fold. Even a slight reduction in radius (such as from mucus or airway edema) may seriously impede airflow, particularly in neonatal and pediatric patients.

Airway resistance increases with airway length: The longer the airway, the higher the resistance. Long endotracheal tubes and breathing circuit tubing can elevate airway resistance and reduce airflow to the alveoli, increasing the work of breathing.

The airflow rate influences airway resistance through its effect on the airflow pattern. Turbulence, caused by a high flow rate, increases resistance, whereas laminar airflow, a linear pattern occurring at low flow rates, decreases resistance. However, an extremely low flow rate may prevent adequate alveolar ventilation. Ideally, the flow rate is low enough to produce a laminar airflow while effectively ventilating the alveoli.

Compliance. A measure of how easily the lung and chest wall expand during inspiration, compliance also affects the work of breathing. Changes in the lung's elastic and collagen fibers can increase or decrease lung compliance. Aging and such lung diseases as emphysema increase compliance, making the lungs easier to inflate. Other diseases, such as interstitial fibrosis, diminish compliance, making the lungs harder to inflate. Lung compliance relates inversely to airway resistance: As resistance increases, lung compliance decreases.

Gas exchange

The exchange of oxygen and carbon dioxide takes place at the alveolocapillary membrane, where the alveolus and pulmonary capillary meet. Gas exchange occurs by *diffusion,* a process in which gases move from an area of higher pressure to an area of lower pressure.

Partial pressures of gases

To understand how oxygen and carbon dioxide diffuse, you must be familiar with the concept of the partial pressure of gases. *Partial pressure,* or tension, refers to the pressure exerted by any one gas in a mixture of gases or in a liquid. Dalton's law states that the pressure exerted by a particular gas in a mixture of gases (such as the air that enters the lungs) corresponds to the sum of the partial pressures of the separate components. Within the body, changes in the partial pressures of oxygen and carbon dioxide provide the driving force for diffusion. (See *Understanding gas diffusion.*)

The rate and extent of gas diffusion depend largely on the pressure gradient — the differential in partial pressures between the two sides of a semipermeable membrane. Gas moves from a high-pressure area to a low-pressure area until pressures are equalized. Diffusion slows as the pressure gradient diminishes and pressures on each side of the membrane approach equilibrium.

The rate of blood flow through pulmonary capillaries, the hemoglobin level, the surface area available for gas exchange, and gas solu-

Understanding gas diffusion

The concept of diffusion draws on Dalton's law of partial pressures. This law states that in a mixture of gases, the pressure (tension) exerted by each gas is independent of the other gases and directly corresponds to the percentage of the total mixture that it represents.

Here's how Dalton's law works. Atmospheric air inspired at sea level exerts a pressure of 760 mm Hg against all parts of the body. Oxygen represents 21% of air and thus exerts a partial pressure (P_{O_2}) of 159 mm Hg, or 21% of 760 mm Hg. Carbon dioxide, a trace element of atmospheric air, has a partial pressure (P_{CO_2}) of 0.3 mm Hg. Nitrogen, making up 78% of air, has a partial pressure (P_{N_2}) of 596 mm Hg. Water vapor has a partial pressure (P_{H_2O}) of 5.7 mm Hg.

During inspiration, the upper respiratory tract warms and humidifies atmospheric air, increasing P_{H_2O} to 47 mm Hg. Partial pressures of the other gases decline because total pressure must remain at 760 mm Hg.

Before entering the alveoli, inspired air mixes with gas that wasn't exhaled on the previous expiration. Because this gas contains more carbon dioxide and less oxygen than inspired air, partial pressures change again.

The air that finally enters the alveoli for diffusion across the respiratory membrane goes through further partial pressure changes. However, it remains high in P_{O_2} and low in P_{CO_2}. On the other side of the respiratory membrane is deoxygenated blood from the right ventricle, which has a low P_{O_2} and high P_{CO_2}.

The differential in partial pressures of oxygen and carbon dioxide causes the two gases to cross the respiratory membrane toward the lower side of their respective pressure gradients. Oxygen diffuses into the blood, and carbon dioxide diffuses outward, equalizing gas pressures on both sides of the respiratory membrane.

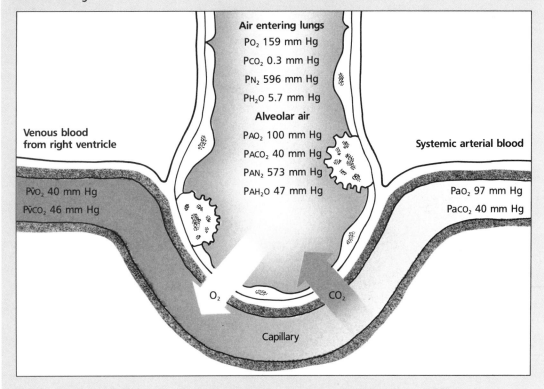

Air entering lungs
P_{O_2} 159 mm Hg
P_{CO_2} 0.3 mm Hg
P_{N_2} 596 mm Hg
P_{H_2O} 5.7 mm Hg

Alveolar air
P_{AO_2} 100 mm Hg
P_{ACO_2} 40 mm Hg
P_{AN_2} 573 mm Hg
P_{AH_2O} 47 mm Hg

Venous blood from right ventricle

$P_{\bar{v}O_2}$ 40 mm Hg
$P_{\bar{v}CO_2}$ 46 mm Hg

Systemic arterial blood

Pa_{O_2} 97 mm Hg
Pa_{CO_2} 40 mm Hg

O_2 CO_2

Capillary

Interpreting the oxyhemoglobin dissociation curve

Oxygen travels through the body in two forms: bound to hemoglobin molecules (97% to 98%) and dissolved in plasma (1% to 3%). The oxygen-hemoglobin combination is loose and reversible, which allows hemoglobin to pick up oxygen easily and release it to tissues. This relationship is expressed graphically by the oxyhemoglobin dissociation curve, which shows the percentage of hemoglobin bound with oxygen and the corresponding partial pressure of oxygen (PO_2).

This may seem like a complex concept, but all it really means is that certain factors affect how much oxygen is released from or picked up by hemoglobin. If the curve shifts to the right, oxygen is released more easily, so the hemoglobin is less saturated but more oxygen is available to tissues. Causes of a rightward shift include a decreased blood pH, an increased partial pressure of carbon dioxide in arterial blood ($PaCO_2$), an increased 2,3-diphosphoglycerate (DPG) level, and an increased body temperature.

A leftward shift indicates that oxygen is bound more tightly to hemoglobin, which is more saturated. This means less oxygen is available to tissues. A decreased body temperature, an increased blood pH, a decreased DPG level, and a decreased $PaCO_2$ contribute to a leftward shift.

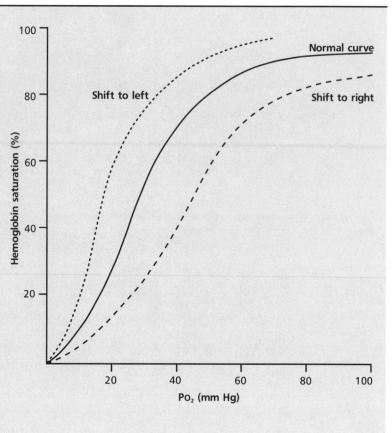

bility also affect diffusion. For instance, carbon dioxide diffuses across the alveolocapillary membrane about 20 times more easily than oxygen because it's more soluble.

Oxygen transport in blood
Roughly 98% of the oxygen in the blood is transported in a reversible chemical combination with hemoglobin (called oxyhemoglobin). Each hemoglobin molecule has four oxygen-binding sites. Unbound hemoglobin is called reduced, or deoxygenated, hemoglobin.

Oxygen saturation represents the percentage of hemoglobin saturated with oxygen; *oxygen content* reflects the actual amount of oxygen carried in the blood. Normal arterial oxygen saturation (SaO_2) is roughly 95% or

greater; normal mixed venous oxygen saturation ($S\bar{v}O_2$) is roughly 75%.

PaO_2 is the portion of oxygen dissolved in plasma. Normally, the partial pressure of oxygen (PO_2) of ambient air at sea level is about 159 mm Hg. After air enters the trachea and mixes with water vapor, PO_2 decreases. By the time oxygen diffuses from the alveoli to pulmonary capillaries, its partial pressure measures from 80 to 100 mm Hg. When oxygen reaches mixed venous blood, its partial pressure (now termed $P\bar{v}O_2$) measures 40 mm Hg.

Oxyhemoglobin dissociation curve
Hemoglobin saturation is closely linked with PO_2, as shown by the oxyhemoglobin dissociation curve. The S shape of this curve indicates

that the relationship isn't linear; a given increase or decrease in PO_2 doesn't always cause an equivalent rise or fall in hemoglobin saturation. The upper portion of the curve, where PO_2 is highest, is relatively flat. Oxygen readily binds, or associates, with hemoglobin when PO_2 is high. At PO_2 values between 60 and 100 mm Hg, oxygen saturation normally exceeds 90%.

The steep part of the oxyhemoglobin dissociation curve shows what happens in body tissues, where PO_2 is lower. As PO_2 drops below 60 mm Hg, hemoglobin saturation falls rapidly, even with small PO_2 decreases. Oxygen unloads (dissociates) from the hemoglobin molecule for use by tissues — ideally, to maintain aerobic metabolism. (See *Interpreting the oxyhemoglobin dissociation curve.*)

Shifts in curve
A change in blood pH, body temperature, the partial pressure of carbon dioxide in arterial blood ($PaCO_2$), or the 2,3-diphosphoglycerate (DPG) level will alter hemoglobin's affinity for oxygen, causing the oxyhemoglobin dissociation curve to shift to the left or right.

A rightward shift reflects decreased affinity. Less hemoglobin binds with oxygen for any given PO_2, making hemoglobin more likely to release oxygen to tissues. Causes of a rightward shift include decreased blood pH, increased body temperature, increased $PaCO_2$, and an increased DPG level. Clinical conditions that may cause such a shift include acidosis, fever, hypoventilation, and anemia.

A leftward shift represents an increased hemoglobin affinity for oxygen. As more hemoglobin binds with oxygen for any given PO_2, hemoglobin is less likely to release oxygen to tissues. Causes of a shift to the left include increased blood pH, decreased body temperature, reduced $PaCO_2$, and a decreased DPG level. Clinical conditions that may cause such a shift include alkalosis, hypothermia, hyperventilation, hypophosphatemia, and carbon monoxide poisoning. Fetal hemoglobin, normally present in neonates and infants, also has a greater affinity for oxygen and may cause a leftward shift.

Oxygen content
The total amount of oxygen in the blood equals the amount of oxygen bound to hemoglobin plus the amount of oxygen dissolved in plasma. Normally, arterial oxygen content is approximately 20 ml/dl of blood; normal mixed venous oxygen content measures approximately 15 ml/dl of blood. Because approximately 98% of oxygen is bound to hemoglobin, SaO_2 is an important index of oxygen content. The hemoglobin and PaO_2 values also may affect total oxygen content. (See *Determining oxygen content,* page 116.)

Oxygen delivery
Oxygen delivery (DO_2) — the amount of oxygen transported to tissues — is determined by total oxygen content and cardiac output. In a normal adult, approximately 1,000 ml of oxygen travels each minute through the arteries to the tissues. In addition, roughly 775 ml of oxygen returns to the right side of the heart and the lungs each minute. Any condition that compromises oxygen content or cardiac output can impair DO_2. (See *Calculating DO_2,* page 117.)

Oxygen consumption
Representing the difference between arterial and venous oxygen transport, oxygen consumption ($\dot{V}O_2$) reflects the amount of oxygen consumed by tissues per minute. In a healthy, resting state, overall $\dot{V}O_2$ amounts to roughly 25% of DO_2. When oxygen needs increase, such as during illness, tissues may extract more than 25% of the total amount of oxygen in an effort to support aerobic metabolism. When oxygen needs exceed oxygen supply, anaerobic metabolism may occur, possibly causing hypoxia.

Respiratory rate
Normally, the respiratory rate (breaths/minute) varies with age, activity and stress levels, and health status. An abnormal rate is cause for concern, especially when accompanied by respiratory distress. Respiratory rhythm and depth also are clinically important. Except in premature and newborn infants, the respiratory rate normally is regular. Recognizing abnormal respi-

Determining oxygen content

To determine the oxygen content of your patient's arterial and mixed venous blood, use the following equation:

$$\text{Oxygen content} = (1.34 \times \text{Hb} \times \text{So}_2) + (0.003 \times \text{Po}_2)$$

In this equation, 1.34 is the amount of oxygen carried by 1 g of hemoglobin, expressed in milliliters; Hb is the hemoglobin value; So_2 is the oxygen saturation value (of arterial or mixed venous blood); 0.003 is the solubility coefficient of oxygen; and Po_2 is the partial pressure of oxygen (in arterial or mixed venous blood).

The following examples show how the equation works to determine normal arterial oxygen content (Cao_2) and normal mixed venous oxygen content ($\text{C}\bar{\text{v}}\text{o}_2$).

Normal arterial oxygen content (Cao_2)
Assume Hb is 15 g; Sao_2, 97%; and Pao_2, 100 mm Hg.

$$\begin{aligned}
\text{Cao}_2 &= (1.34 \times 15 \times 0.97) + (0.003 \times 100) \\
&= 19.5 + 0.3 \\
&= 19.8 \text{ ml oxygen/dl blood}
\end{aligned}$$

Normal mixed venous oxygen content ($\text{C}\bar{\text{v}}\text{o}_2$)
Assume Hb is 15 g; $\text{S}\bar{\text{v}}\text{o}_2$, 75%; and $\text{P}\bar{\text{v}}\text{o}_2$, 40 mm Hg.

$$\begin{aligned}
\text{C}\bar{\text{v}}\text{o}_2 &= (1.34 \times 15 \times 0.75) + (0.003 \times 40) \\
&= 15.08 + 0.12 \\
&= 15.2 \text{ ml oxygen/dl blood}
\end{aligned}$$

Below-normal Sao_2 or Hb values decrease arterial oxygen content, as the following examples show.

Decreased arterial oxygen content (Cao_2)
Assume Sao_2 is decreased to 80%.

$$\begin{aligned}
\text{Cao}_2 &= (1.34 \times 15 \times 0.80) + (0.003 \times 100) \\
&= 16.08 + 0.3 \\
&= 16.38 \text{ ml oxygen/dl blood}
\end{aligned}$$

In this next example, Hb is decreased to 9 g.

$$\begin{aligned}
\text{Cao}_2 &= (1.34 \times 9 \times 0.97) + (0.003 \times 100) \\
&= 11.7 + 0.3 \\
&= 12 \text{ ml oxygen/dl blood}
\end{aligned}$$

In the following example, both values are decreased: Sao_2 is 80%; Hb is 9 g.

$$\begin{aligned}
\text{Cao}_2 &= (1.34 \times 9 \times 0.80) + (0.003 \times 100) \\
&= 9.65 + 0.3 \\
&= 9.95 \text{ ml oxygen/dl blood}
\end{aligned}$$

ratory patterns can provide valuable clues about a patient's respiratory status. (See *Recognizing common respiratory patterns,* page 118.)

Lung volumes and capacities
Adequate gas exchange depends on normal amounts of air exchanged in breathing. These air volumes and capacities can be measured to evaluate a patient's ventilatory adequacy.

Ventilation, expressed as volume per unit of time, is determined by respiratory frequency (f) and tidal volume (V_T), the volume of air inspired or expired with each normal breath. In the normal adult, V_T measures 10 to 15 ml/kg of body weight. For example, in a patient weighing 70 kg, V_T should be approximately 700 ml. Minute volume (MV) is the product of respiratory frequency and V_T ($\text{MV} = \text{f} \times \text{V}_\text{T}$). Thus, in a patient who breathes 20 times/minute and has a V_T of 1,000 ml, MV is approximately 20,000 ml/minute.

Dead space
Approximately one-third of the V_T (3 to 5 ml/kg of body weight) never reaches the alveoli and thus doesn't participate in gas exchange with blood. This air is contained in the *anatomic dead space* (the conducting airways, such as the nose, mouth, pharynx, larynx, trachea, and large bronchi).

Alveolar (physiologic) dead space refers to alveolar areas with reduced perfusion. Lung disease or impaired blood flow to the lungs may significantly increase alveolar dead space. Total dead-space volume is the sum of anatomic and alveolar dead-space volume.

Mechanical dead space results from excessive breathing circuit tubing of a mechanical ventilator, which is external to the patient. The tubing should be minimized to prevent airway resistance and reduce the risk of rebreathing exhaled gas.

Alveolar ventilation
Alveolar ventilation refers to the volume of air that reaches the alveoli and takes part in gas exchange with blood—roughly two-thirds of the V_T, or the difference between V_T and

dead space. This volume relates directly to $PaCO_2$: As the rate of alveolar ventilation increases, carbon dioxide removal rises. As the rate of alveolar ventilation declines, carbon dioxide removal likewise decreases.

Ventilation-perfusion ratio

For effective gas exchange, the alveoli must receive adequate oxygen and the pulmonary capillaries must receive sufficient blood flow. Moreover, ventilation ($\dot{V}$) and perfusion ($\dot{Q}$) must occur in a specific ratio. An abnormal $\dot{V}/\dot{Q}$ ratio may alter PaO_2, impairing oxygenation of body tissues. (See *Ventilation-perfusion spectrum,* page 119.)

Ideally, ventilation and perfusion would be perfectly matched in all lung units, producing a $\dot{V}/\dot{Q}$ ratio of 1. However, this doesn't happen even in the normal, healthy lung. Alveoli are ventilated at a rate of about 4 liters/minute, and pulmonary capillaries are perfused with approximately 5 liters of blood/minute. This creates a normal $\dot{V}/\dot{Q}$ ratio of 4:5, or 0.8. Because dependent lung portions have the most blood flow and the upper lobes receive more ventilation than the lower lobes, the $\dot{V}/\dot{Q}$ ratio differs from one lung region to another.

Shunting

When some alveoli are perfused but not ventilated, shunting occurs. This condition, which decreases the $\dot{V}/\dot{Q}$ ratio, prevents gas exchange in the affected lung region. Blood from a shunted region returns unoxygenated to the right side of the heart.

Shunting is normal in certain lung areas. For instance, in an *anatomic shunt,* 2% to 5% of the right ventricular output entering the bronchial, pleural, or thebesian veins bypasses the pulmonary capillaries.

Abnormal shunting may result from a congenital or acquired lung disorder, such as atelectasis, mucus plugs, and lung consolidation. The most common cause of hypoxemia, such shunting may lead to severe arterial oxygen desaturation. During shunting, carbon dioxide may continue to diffuse from the blood into functional alveoli and then leave the body dur-

---

Calculating DO_2

To calculate oxygen delivery (DO_2) in arterial and mixed venous blood, use the following equation:

$$DO_2 = CO \times O_2 \text{ content} \times 10$$

In this equation, CO stands for cardiac output, expressed in liters/minute; O_2 content is the total amount of oxygen in the blood (arterial or mixed venous); and 10 is the standard conversion factor.

The following examples show how the equation works to determine arterial and mixed venous oxygen delivery.

Arterial oxygen delivery (DaO_2)

CO is 5 liters/minute and CaO_2 (normal arterial oxygen content) is 19.8 ml O_2/dl blood.

$$DaO_2 = 5 \times 19.8 \times 10 = 990 \text{ ml } O_2/\text{minute}$$

Mixed venous oxygen delivery ($D\bar{v}O_2$)

CO is 5 liters/minute and $C\bar{v}O_2$ (normal mixed venous oxygen content) is 15.19 ml O_2/dl blood.

$$D\bar{v}O_2 = 5 \times 15.19 \times 10 = 760 \text{ ml } O_2/\text{minute}$$

---

ing exhalation. (The total amount of shunted blood from anatomic and intrapulmonary shunts is called the *physiologic shunt.*)

Dead-space ventilation

When perfusion is reduced in relation to ventilation, *dead-space ventilation* occurs, causing an above-normal $\dot{V}/\dot{Q}$ ratio. Carbon dioxide from dead-space areas accumulates in the blood, and little or none is exhaled. Dead-space ventilation increases with such conditions as hypovolemia, hypotension, pulmonary embolism, and cardiac arrest.

Silent units

When both ventilation and perfusion decrease, silent lung units may form to compensate for the $\dot{V}/\dot{Q}$ imbalance. Silent units divert blood flow to better-ventilated lung areas.

Recognizing common respiratory patterns

Use this chart as a guide when assessing your patient's respiratory rate, rhythm, and depth.

PATTERN	CHARACTERISTICS
Eupnea	Normal respiratory rate and rhythm. For adults and teenagers, 12 to 20 breaths/minute; for children ages 2 to 12, 20 to 30 breaths/minute; for neonates, 30 to 50 breaths/minute. Occasionally, deep breaths at a rate of 2 or 3 per minute.
Tachypnea	Increased respiratory rate, as seen with fever. Respiratory rate increases about 4 breaths/minute for every degree Fahrenheit above normal.
Bradypnea	Slower but regular respirations. Can occur when the brain's respiratory control center is affected by an opiate, a tumor, alcohol, a metabolic disorder, or respiratory decompensation. This pattern is normal during sleep.
Apnea	Absence of breathing; may occur periodically.
Hyperpnea	Deeper, faster respirations.
Cheyne-Stokes respirations	Respirations gradually become faster and deeper than normal, then slower, over a 30- to 170-second period. Periods of apnea for 20 to 60 seconds.
Biot's respirations	Faster and deeper respirations than normal, with abrupt pauses. Each breath has same depth. May occur with spinal meningitis or other central nervous system conditions.
Kussmaul's respirations	Faster and deeper respirations without pauses; in adults, over 20 breaths/minute. Breathing usually sounds labored, with deep breaths that resemble sighs. May accompany or result from renal failure or metabolic acidosis.
Apneustic breathing	Prolonged gasping inspiration, followed by extremely short, inefficient expiration. May accompany or result from lesions in the brain's respiratory center.

Pulse oximetry

A noninvasive procedure, pulse oximetry measures SaO_2 by determining the amount of hemoglobin that's carrying oxygen within the arterial bed. A sensor containing a photodetector and light sources is placed on the finger, toe, nose, hand, or forehead. The photodetector measures the relative absorption of red and infrared light within the arterial bed and then relays this data to a monitor, which displays the SaO_2 value with each heartbeat and shows the pulse rate measured at the sensor site. An arterial oxygen saturation measurement provided by a pulse oximeter is commonly referred to as SpO_2.

Some monitors also display a waveform, called a plethysmogram, and a pulse amplitude bar. Because blood volume changes constantly, the plethysmogram shows variations in the

Ventilation-perfusion spectrum

When ventilation (the movement of air in the alveoli) and perfusion (the movement of blood around the alveoli) are equal, the gas exchange between blood and alveoli operates at full efficiency. Two reflexes try to adjust ventilation to perfusion, or perfusion to ventilation; these reflexes keep the normal ventilation-perfusion ($\dot{V}/\dot{Q}$) ratio at 0.8 (ventilation = 4 liters/minute, perfusion = 5 liters/minute). As these illustrations show, the $\dot{V}/\dot{Q}$ ratio increases with conditions that cause dead-space ventilation and decreases with shunting.

Dead-space ventilation (high $\dot{V}/\dot{Q}$)

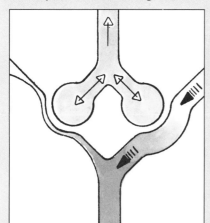

Normal range ($\dot{V}/\dot{Q}$ = 0.8)

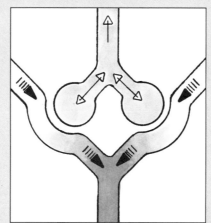

Shunting (low $\dot{V}/\dot{Q}$)

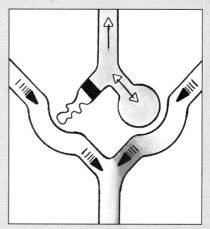

amount of light absorbed by the arterial bed during systole or diastole. (Motion or weak pulse signals may cause the plethysmogram to deviate from its normal appearance, rendering pulse oximetry measurements unreliable.)

Because pulse oximetry detects hypoxemia early, this technique is indicated whenever hypoxemia is a risk — for example, in patients receiving anesthesia or opioid drugs, those with sleep apnea syndrome or cardiopulmonary disease, and neonatal and pediatric patients. Its rapid detection of SpO₂ changes allows you to gauge the effect of interventions on your patient's oxygenation status. If the SpO₂ value worsens, you may need to change or discontinue an intervention. (See *Relying on pulse oximetry,* page 120.)

Pulse oximetry also may prove useful during diagnostic and outpatient procedures and for long-term, short-term, or spot-check monitoring.

Pulse oximetry has no contraindications. However, because it requires adequate arterial pulsations, it won't work if the patient lacks an arterial pulse, or may be unreliable if his pulse is weak. The only potential complication is altered skin integrity from improper sensor application and use. (See *Choosing the right pulse oximetry sensor,* page 121.)

Equipment

Pulse oximetry requires a pulse oximeter and a sensor of the appropriate type and size. (See *Performing pulse oximetry,* pages 124 and 125.) Two types of sensors can be used. A *transmission sensor,* the most common type, has the light sources and photodetector directly opposite one another. It's usually positioned on the patient's finger, toe, nose, or hand. In a *reflectance sensor,* the light sources are adjacent to the photodetector. This type of

(Text continues on page 122.)

Relying on pulse oximetry

Pulse oximetry provides ongoing assessment data that can prove crucial when caring for the patient with respiratory compromise. The oxygen saturation (SpO_2) value obtained with this technique helps you detect hypoxemia immediately, such as from fever, activities of daily living, airway clearance measures, and mechanical ventilator adjustments. Based on oximetry values, you can take measures to increase your patient's SpO_2 value, such as administering prescribed antipyretics or antianxiety drugs, suctioning, providing rest periods, giving more oxygen, or changing ventilator settings.

Consider, for example, the case of Donald Markham, age 77, who has just been placed in your care.

Initial care
Mr. Markham's chief complaint is dyspnea on exertion. He has a long history of chronic obstructive pulmonary disease and chronic anxiety. On admission, his body temperature measured 99.3° F (37.4° C); pulse, 140 beats/minute; respirations, irregular at 32 breaths/minute; and blood pressure, 150/100 mm Hg. Auscultation revealed inspiratory and expiratory rhonchi. Arterial blood gas (ABG) analysis revealed the following:
- pH: 7.38
- PaO_2: 51.7 mm Hg
- $PaCO_2$: 54 mm Hg
- HCO_3^-: 33.8 mEq/liter
- SaO_2: 88.6%.

Based on Mr. Markham's history and physical examination findings, the doctor diagnosed pneumonia, intubated him, and then began mechanical ventilation. He ordered an aminophylline drip, ampicillin, methylprednisolone, cimetidine, and metaproterenol. To treat the patient's anxiety, he prescribed lorazepam I.V. p.r.n.

After 6 days of nasoendotracheal intubation, with little progress in weaning from the ventilator, Mr. Markham underwent a tracheotomy.

Care on your unit
Because Mr. Markham requires minute-to-minute monitoring, which ABG analysis can't provide, you begin pulse oximetry to monitor his SaO_2 values continuously. As ordered, you administer oxygen (0.35 of inspired oxygen [FIO_2]) through a T piece fitted onto the tracheostomy tube.

Over the next 7 days, Mr. Markham is weaned to the T piece. His SaO_2 value ranges from 85% to 97%, falling 2% to 4% during tracheal suctioning and tracheostomy care. On four occasions while moving from his bed to the chair and back again, his SaO_2 value measures from 90% to 96%, 89% to 92%, 91% to 92%, and 90% to 94%.

On the fourth occasion, several minutes after Mr. Markham returns to bed, the pulse oximetry network alarm sounds at the nurses' station. Noting his SaO_2 value of 80%, you rush to his room, where you find him unconscious. You start resuscitation measures immediately.

The health care team determines that Mr. Markham has suffered a hypoxic event and initiates cardiac monitoring, which reveals occasional premature ventricular contractions. Manual ventilation (FIO_2 of 1.0) rapidly improves Mr. Markham's level of consciousness. Within 5 minutes, he's fully alert and responsive. The cardiac monitor now shows a normal sinus rhythm, and pulse oximetry reveals normal SaO_2 values. The doctor orders mechanical ventilation to support adequate oxygenation.

Throughout the next day, Mr. Markham's SaO_2 values fall to 85% to 90% whenever he becomes agitated or feverish. However, they improve to 92% to 97% after you administer lorazepam I.V. or acetaminophen rectally. Once you begin weaning him to the T piece, you note that his SaO_2 value drops significantly on two occasions (from 96% to 91% and from 97% to 90%). Each time, you return him to the ventilator briefly. Because pulse oximetry detects hypoxemia so rapidly, you're able to avert further compromise.

Choosing the right pulse oximetry sensor

Selecting the correct sensor can promote accurate pulse oximetry results. Keep in mind that weight limits for sensors overlap, which will allow you to use a sensor appropriate for the patient's size. You could use the pediatric sensor for a small adult, for example.

After you've chosen the appropriate sensor, position it correctly. Place the pediatric and adult adhesive sensors and the finger-clip sensor for adults on the index, middle, or ring finger. You can also place the infant, pediatric, and adult adhesive sensors on a toe, but don't put the finger-clip sensor there. Also, avoid the toe if your patient has compromised circulation in the lower extremities.

Place the neonatal sensor on either a neonate's foot or hand or on an adult's finger. Put the nasal sensor on the cartilaginous portion of the nose, just below the bridge.

Adhesive neonatal sensor
Less than 3 kg (6.6 lb) or more than 40 kg (88 lb)

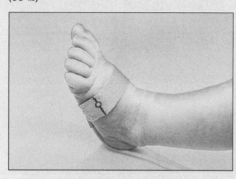

Adhesive infant sensor
1 to 20 kg (2.2 to 44 lb)

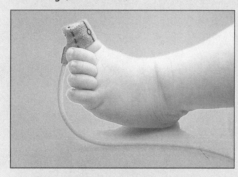

Adhesive pediatric sensor
10 to 50 kg (22 to 110 lb)

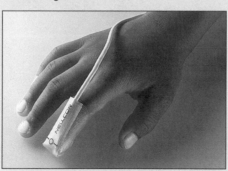

Adhesive adult sensor
More than 30 kg (66 lb)

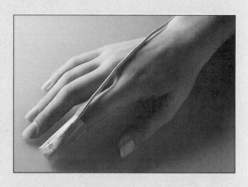

Adhesive adult nasal sensor
More than 50 kg (110 lb)

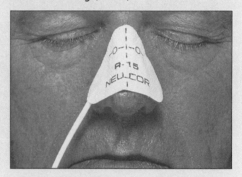

Finger-clip sensor
More than 40 kg (88 lb)

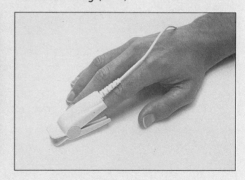

sensor is placed on a flat surface, such as the forehead or temple.

The choice of sensor also depends on the expected duration of monitoring, the patient's activity level and weight, and infection concerns. An adhesive sensor, designed for single-patient use, is appropriate for either short- or long-term SaO_2 monitoring. For a highly active patient, an adhesive sensor provides a stabilizing, "second-skin" fit. Its light sources and photodetector are more likely to remain securely positioned, allowing it to move with the patient and provide more reliable readings. A sterile adhesive sensor is preferred for the patient with an increased risk for infection, such as a neonate or an immunosuppressed patient.

A reusable sensor may be indicated for short-term or SpO_2 spot-check monitoring. However, on a highly active patient, it may become dislodged or produce unreliable readings. A reusable sensor isn't sterile and thus is a poor choice for a patient with an infection or for one with an increased risk for infection. Between patients, clean a reusable sensor with a 70% alcohol solution or other cleaning agent, as recommended by the manufacturer.

Preparation

Explain the monitoring technique to the patient. Tell him that the monitor will painlessly measure the amount of oxygen in his body on an ongoing basis. Mention how long monitoring will last. Inform him where the sensor will be placed or, if possible, have him choose the site. Instruct him to avoid moving the sensor site excessively to ensure reliable readings, and tell him to report any discomfort at the site. Caution him and his family not to alter the alarm settings or volume.

Following the manufacturer's recommendations, choose a sensor appropriate for the selected monitoring site, patient's weight and activity level, expected duration of monitoring, and any infection-control concerns. Check the patient's pulse and capillary refill proximal to the sensor site because impaired circulation may cause unreliable readings. To prevent circulatory compromise, avoid placing the sensor on an extremity with an arterial or I.V. line, a blood pressure cuff, or an arteriovenous shunt.

If you're using a fingertip sensor, remember that skin oils and nail polish can interfere with sensor readings. Therefore, if necessary, clean the sensor site to remove excessive oils or polish. Then let the site air-dry.

Procedure

• Wash your hands. Next, apply the sensor according to the manufacturer's instructions. Some sensors have markings that help you properly align the light sources and photodetector. If you're using a transmission sensor, make sure these markings align directly across the arterial bed. Misalignment may cause an inaccurate reading — or none at all.
• Assess whether the sensor fits properly. Make sure the adhesive isn't so tight that it impedes blood flow to the site. Don't use additional tape to secure the sensor unless the manufacturer directs you to do so.
• Connect the sensor to the pulse oximeter and turn on the monitor.
• Make sure the alarm settings are appropriate for your patient and consistent with hospital policy or doctor's orders. Check alarm volume and adjust it, if necessary. If the oximeter you're using has an audible beep tone that varies with SpO_2 value, adjust the tone so you can hear variations.
• Some manufacturers provide networking systems that relay bedside pulse oximetry data and alarms to a central station. If your unit has such a system, make sure all connections for the network are intact, and check the central monitor to verify that it's receiving information about your patient. Also confirm that the audible alarms at the central station are turned on.

Interpretation of findings

Normal SpO_2 for a healthy adult ranges from 95% to 100%. When the value falls below 90% (corresponding to a PaO_2 of approximately 60 mm Hg on a normal oxyhemoglobin dissociation curve), even minute PaO_2 changes may cause significant desaturation and a rapid decline in oxygen content. (However, newborn nurseries and neonatal intensive care units commonly accept lower SpO_2 levels.) Be sure to compare ongoing readings with baseline values to help evaluate whether your patient's oxygenation status is getting better or worse.

Nursing considerations

• If your patient has poor perfusion — for example, from peripheral vascular disease, vasoconstrictive drugs, hypotension, hypovolemia, or hypothermia — consider using a sensor that measures a more centrally perfused site, such as the nose.

• To reduce the effect of venous pulsations, don't apply the sensor too tightly. Also, don't place the sensor distal to a tourniquet or an occlusive dressing. Ideally, the sensor should be positioned at heart level.

• Consider using a telemetry system if pulse oximeter alarms aren't loud enough for the nursing staff to hear.

• Change the sensor site at least as frequently as the manufacturer recommends, and document all site changes.

• Document and report any signs of impaired skin integrity at the sensor site.

• Be aware that abnormal SpO_2 values may result from technical problems, such as excessive motion at the sensor site, as well as such clinical conditions as venous pulsations. (See *What affects pulse oximetry readings?* page 126.) To avoid technical problems, keep the sensor site clean and dry, instruct the patient to avoid moving the sensor, and minimize outside light.

• Be aware that injection of intravascular dyes, such as methylene blue, may cause false-low SpO_2 readings for several minutes after injection. Be sure to assess the patient for signs of an anaphylactic response to the dye.

• Keep in mind that pulse oximetry can't determine the occurrence or degree of hyperoxemia. When hyperoxemia is a concern, especially with premature infants, supplement oximetry readings with periodic arterial blood gas (ABG) measurements to detect hyperoxemia. (See *Interpreting ABG values,* page 127.)

• If your patient has mild to moderate anemia, periodically obtain hemoglobin values to help evaluate total oxygen content. His SpO_2 values may seem adequate, but reduced hemoglobin levels may compromise total oxygen content.

When hemoglobin values fall below 5 g/dl, the oximeter may fail to provide SpO_2 values.

• Document SpO_2 values according to your patient's needs and your hospital's policy. For example, for a patient without respiratory compromise or related interventions, document SpO_2 values at least as often as you document routine vital signs. If your patient has a labile respiratory status requiring more intensive support and management, document SpO_2 values more frequently, including before and after any change in treatment.

• Keep in mind that pulse oximetry and ABG analysis may yield different SpO_2 values. That's because oximetry measures oxygen saturation directly, whereas the ABG value is calculated from measured PaO_2. If an unexplained shift in the oxyhemoglobin dissociation curve occurs, the ABG value may not represent the patient's true SaO_2 value.

• If your patient has confirmed or suspected carbon monoxide poisoning and requires complete oxygenation assessment, expect the doctor to order carboxyhemoglobin levels and SaO_2 analysis as measured by a laboratory co-oximeter. This technique directly measures the percentage of oxyhemoglobin relative to several hemoglobin species in the blood (including carboxyhemoglobin), yielding a fractional oxygen saturation value. For this patient, SaO_2 values derived through an ABG analysis won't be accurate because they're calculated from measured PaO_2, which usually remains normal or elevated with carbon monoxide poisoning.

• Usually, pulse oximetry is discontinued when the patient's oxygenation status remains stable for approximately 24 hours and he no longer runs the risk of hypoxemia and altered oxygen transport. However, a patient who's been receiving narcotic analgesics may require pulse oximetry for up to 24 hours after the narcotic is withdrawn to ensure SaO_2 stability. The decision to discontinue monitoring depends on the patient's specific needs and the discretion of the health care team. Usually, monitoring is reinstated if the patient shows signs of respiratory compromise or a risk for compromise.

(Text continues on page 126.)

Performing pulse oximetry

For pulse oximetry, you may use one of two types of sensors. A *transmission sensor* works by placing the light sources (light-emitting diodes [LEDs]) and photodetector in direct opposition to one another over an arterial bed. It's usually positioned on the patient's finger, toe, nose, or hand. A *reflectance sensor* positions the LEDs and photodetector next to one another on a flat surface, such as the forehead or temple.

First, select a sensor site that the manufacturer recommends. Check the strength of the patient's pulse and the adequacy of capillary refill at the proposed site. If the patient has poor peripheral perfusion, consider using a nasal or reflectance sensor (these primarily monitor central rather than peripheral blood flow). Also, avoid placing a sensor in a poorly perfused area or on an extremity with a blood pressure cuff, an arterial or intravenous line, or a pressure dressing.

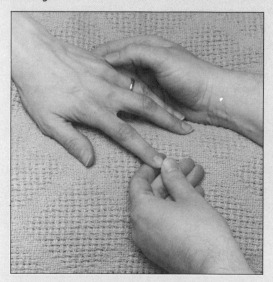

If you're placing the sensor on the patient's finger, remove any nail polish, which could block light transmission and interfere with reliable readings. And although skin preparation isn't necessary, you may want to remove oil from the patient's skin with an alcohol wipe before applying a reflectance sensor.

Next, apply the sensor according to the manufacturer's instructions. Properly align the LEDs and photodetector as indicated by the markings on the sensor. If you're placing a sensor on the patient's finger, position the patient's hand at heart level to eliminate venous pulsations and to promote accurate readings.

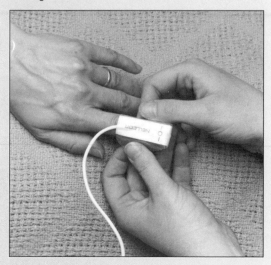

Connect the sensor to the extension cable.

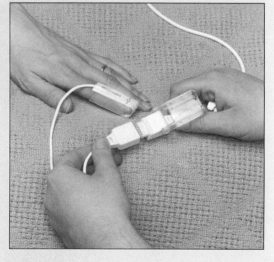

Switch on the power. A self-test display should flash on the monitor. After a few seconds, an SpO_2 value and pulse rate will appear on the screen. Note this initial information as well as the pulse amplitude and any status messages.

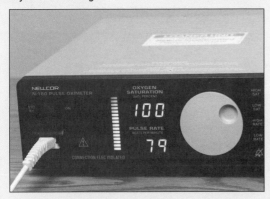

Depending on the type of oximeter, you may hear a beep with each heartbeat. Typically, the beep rises in pitch as SpO_2 increases and falls as SpO_2 decreases. To adjust the beep's volume, turn the control knob clockwise to increase the volume and counterclockwise to decrease it.

Even if your system has preset alarm limits, you'll need to check the high- and low-limit alarms. The high limit for SpO_2 is 100% for adults and 95% for neonates; the low limit is 85% for adults and 80% for neonates. The high pulse limit is 140 beats/minute for adults and 200 beats/minute for neonates; the low limit is 50 beats/minute for adults and 100 beats/minute for neonates.

If necessary, adjust the alarm limits according to the hospital's policy, the patient's condition, or the doctor's order. On the model shown here, you would press the appropriate alarm limit button and simultaneously adjust the control knob.

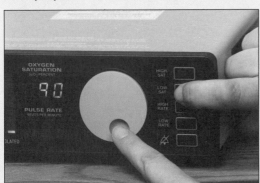

Next, set the averaging mode according to the patient's activity level. Press the high and low rate buttons simultaneously as you turn the control knob. Continue turning the control knob until the desired mode number appears in the display.

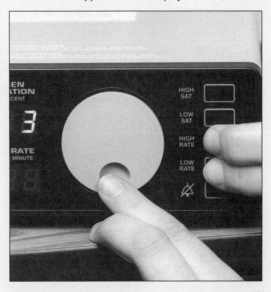

For inactive patients you'll usually select mode 1, which averages readings over 5 to 7 seconds to produce the SpO_2 value. For sleep studies, choose mode 2, which averages readings over 2 to 3 seconds. For active patients, select mode 3, which averages readings over 10 to 15 seconds. Whichever mode is ordered, document the patient's SpO_2 values as often as required by the patient's condition or your hospital's policy. In most cases, you'll document the measurements whenever you take vital signs or whenever the patient's clinical status changes.

To silence the alarm, press the button labeled AU-DIO ALARM OFF. This will silence the audible alarm for 60 seconds; however, the visual alarm will continue to flash as long as the alarm situation exists. Although the audible alarm will reset after 60 seconds, make sure that you've turned the alarms back on before leaving the patient's bedside.

What affects pulse oximetry readings?

If your patient is being monitored by pulse oximetry, be sure to maintain a continuous display of the oxygen saturation (SpO_2) value. Here are some factors that commonly affect pulse oximetry readings—and measures you can take to prevent or correct false readings.

Poor skin contact
To prevent this problem, apply an adhesive sensor with fresh adhesive.

Movement
If the patient is moving the finger or toe to which the sensor is attached, the pulse oximeter may identify the motion as arterial pulsations, causing an inaccurate SpO_2 value. To minimize motion artifact, use an adhesive sensor or stabilize the sensor by immobilizing the monitor site.

You can also try connecting the oximeter to an electrocardiograph (ECG). The ECG will tell the sensor to work only when blood pulsation results from heart contractions (called ECG synchronization).

Low perfusion
Only small amounts of blood may flow through the finger's arterial bed if the patient has poor perfusion (such as from peripheral vascular disease or vasoconstrictive drugs). That means the oximeter won't identify the arterial pulse and may not

display an SpO_2 value. To prevent this problem, use a nasal sensor or place a reflectance sensor on the patient's forehead.

Venous pulsation
Normally nonpulsatile, venous blood may pulsate from right ventricular heart failure, a tight sensor, or any tourniquet-like effect. Because the oximeter looks for pulsating blood, it will detect both pulsating venous blood and pulsating arterial blood, producing a false SpO_2 value. Usually, you can avoid this problem simply by making sure the sensor isn't too tight.

Outside light
The SpO_2 value may be inaccurate if the photodetector senses large amounts of outside light (such as direct sunlight, procedure lamps, or bilirubin lights in the nursery). You can easily correct this by covering the sensor with a sheet or towel.

Anemia
Always double-check the patient's hemoglobin level. Even if he's anemic with a hemoglobin value of 5 g/dl, his SpO_2 value may seem normal because the hemoglobin that's available to carry oxygen is fully saturated. Yet he may have insufficient oxygen to meet his metabolic needs. To correct this problem, be prepared to administer red blood cells or whole blood.

Transcutaneous oxygen and carbon dioxide monitoring

Used primarily in neonates, transcutaneous oxygen ($TcPO_2$) and carbon dioxide ($TcPCO_2$) monitoring evaluate the adequacy of gas exchange. These two noninvasive techniques may be done alone or in combination. An electrode or a sensor containing a transducer system,

heating device, and temperature probe is applied to the skin with an adhesive ring. Partial pressure sensing devices measure oxygen and carbon dioxide diffusion through the skin from capillaries directly beneath the surface. This procedure supplements the established methods of observing skin color and obtaining periodic ABG values to detect hypoxemia and hyperoxemia. However, obtaining periodic ABG values is the most accurate method of evaluating gas exchange.

In $TcPO_2$ monitoring, the electrode is heated to a constant temperature above skin

Interpreting ABG values

Arterial blood gas (ABG) values provide crucial information about the efficiency of your patient's gas exchange and acid-base balance. You can also use ABG values to monitor the effects of respiratory interventions.

Although ABG measurement requires blood sampling, an invasive procedure that sometimes causes pain (especially for patients without an arterial line), the information it provides allows more thorough assessment of gas exchange. Here are normal ABG values:

• Blood pH: 7.35 to 7.45
• Partial pressure of oxygen in arterial blood (Pao_2): 80 to 100 mm Hg (decreases with age)
• Partial pressure of carbon dioxide in arterial blood ($Paco_2$): 35 to 45 mm Hg
• Bicarbonate (HCO_3^-): 22 to 26 mEq/liter
• Arterial oxygen saturation (Sao_2): 95% to 100%.

Evaluating acid-base balance

To interpret ABG results, start by evaluating acid-base balance. Suspect *alkalosis* as the primary or initiating disorder if the pH exceeds 7.45. Suspect *acidosis* if the pH is below 7.35. With normal pH, ABG values may be normal if a patient has compensated for his problem. For example, kidneys can compensate by retaining HCO_3^- if the lungs can't eliminate enough carbon dioxide.

To determine the specific type of alkalosis or acidosis, analyze the $Paco_2$ and HCO_3^- values. If the former is abnormal but the latter normal, suspect acute respiratory alkalosis or acidosis without metabolic compensation by the kidneys. If the HCO_3^- value is abnormal but the $Paco_2$ value is normal, suspect metabolic alkalosis or acidosis.

A borderline high or low pH combined with an abnormal $Paco_2$ or HCO_3^- value indicates whether or not the acid-base disorder is compensated (pH has returned to normal.) With compensated respiratory acidosis, pH is borderline low, $Paco_2$ is high, and HCO_3^- is high.

Assessing oxygenation status

To assess your patient's oxygenation status, check the Pao_2 and Sao_2. Note the fraction of inspired oxygen he was receiving when the blood sample was drawn. Decreased Pao_2 and Sao_2 values may indicate hypoxemia.

Be sure to track serial ABG measurements, noting whether any significant changes followed medical or nursing interventions.

---

temperature—usually 109° to 111° F (43° to 44° C). Normally, skin Po_2 is near zero, although it may be higher in premature infants. Heating the electrode causes the lipid matrix of the stratum corneum epidermidis, the skin's outermost layer, to melt, enhancing capillary blood flow and promoting oxygen diffusion through the tissue under the electrode or sensor. Chemically reduced, diffused oxygen provides a current proportional to the Po_2 level at the oxygen-permeable membrane on the sensor surface. Because skin heating increases metabolism, this method may slightly underestimate Po_2.

Typically, carbon dioxide in unheated skin is approximately equal to carbon dioxide in venous blood. In $TcPco_2$ monitoring, the heated sensor causes carbon dioxide to diffuse from capillaries across a carbon dioxide–permeable membrane on the sensor. Carbon dioxide then reacts with an electrolyte solution, allowing $TcPco_2$ measurement. Because heating increases metabolism, $TcPco_2$ values may somewhat overestimate $Paco_2$. (See *How transcutaneous monitoring works,* page 128.)

Equipment

This procedure requires a $TcPo_2$ monitor, a $TcPco_2$ monitor, or a combination $TcPo_2$–$TcPco_2$ monitor; an electrode or a sensor; a contact medium or water; and an adhesive ring. If the sensor requires maintenance, you

How transcutaneous monitoring works

In transcutaneous oxygen and carbon dioxide monitoring, a heated electrode is placed on the skin, where it melts the lipid matrix of the stratum corneum epidermidis. This dramatically enhances capillary blood flow and increases oxygen and carbon dioxide diffusion through the tissue beneath the electrode. The monitor measures the amount of diffused oxygen or carbon dioxide.

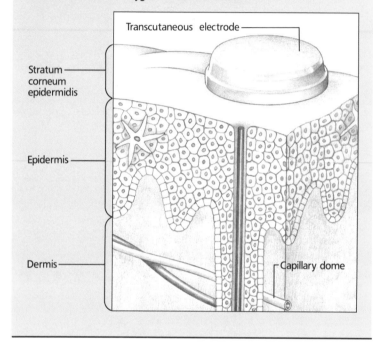

Transcutaneous electrode

Stratum corneum epidermidis

Epidermis

Dermis

Capillary dome

and costophrenic margin. If you're caring for a neonate or an infant with patent ductus arteriosus, choose a $TcPO_2$ sensor site carefully because right-to-left blood shunting may occur. A sensor placed on the right upper chest region will reflect the higher, preductal PaO_2, whereas a sensor placed on the abdomen or thigh usually will reflect the lower, postductal PaO_2. In some cases, you may place two $TcPO_2$ sensors on the infant with right-to-left shunting to monitor both preductal and postductal values, which can provide valuable data about intracardiac shunting.

Procedure
• Set up the monitor and calibrate it as required, following the manufacturer's instructions.
• Wash your hands. Using an alcohol sponge, clean the electrode or sensor application site to remove skin oils and ensure good contact. Let the skin air-dry.
• Attach the double-sided adhesive ring to the electrode or sensor. As the manufacturer directs, moisten the site with a drop of water or a special contact gel to enhance contact.
• Place the electrode or sensor on the skin site, making sure the adhesive ring is tight and free from air gaps.
• Set the alarm switches and electrode or sensor temperature according to the manufacturer's instructions or hospital policy.

may need additional equipment, as specified by the manufacturer.

Preparation
Explain the monitoring procedure to the patient. If you're caring for an infant, explain the procedure to the parents. Provide emotional support to the parents, as needed, and answer any questions.

Choose a site for electrode placement. The transcutaneous electrode can be placed on any flat site—preferably one with good capillary blood flow, few fatty deposits, and no bony prominences. In a neonate, the upper chest, abdomen, and inner thigh are common monitoring sites; you should avoid the extremities

Interpretation of findings
After you apply a $TcPO_2$ sensor, the patient's $TcPO_2$ value should fall rapidly because ambient air has a higher oxygen concentration than the skin surface. Once vessels at the sensor site dilate from heat (roughly 10 to 20 minutes), the value should rise accordingly. Normal $TcPO_2$ values range from 50 to 90 mm Hg.

After you apply a $TcPCO_2$ sensor, the patient's $TcPCO_2$ value should rise because ambient air has a lower carbon dioxide concentration than the skin surface. After 10 to 20 minutes, the value may drop slightly. Normal $TcPCO_2$ values range from 35 to 45 mm Hg.

Although $TcPO_2$ values estimate PaO_2 fairly accurately, they're most accurate with PaO_2

values below 80 mm Hg. This is one reason why $TcPO_2$ monitoring is generally recommended only for neonates.

With adequate blood flow to the sensor site and maximal diffusion across the skin, $TcPO_2$ values help establish the PaO_2 trend. However, if circumstances aren't ideal, $TcPO_2$ values may underestimate PaO_2 values. For example, poor perfusion (such as from hypotension, hypovolemia, or hypothermia) may decrease blood flow to the sensor even with adequate sensor temperature. Vasoconstrictive drugs and extensive edema may also impair blood flow. Variations in skin thickness may contribute to altered oxygen diffusion from the capillaries, possibly affecting the $TcPO_2$ value. Generally, the thicker the skin, the wider the variance between $TcPO_2$ and PaO_2 values — another reason why this form of monitoring is preferred for neonates and elderly people, who have thinner skin.

Falling $TcPO_2$ values that vary widely from PaO_2 values call for further investigation. For example, $TcPO_2$ may decrease from ineffective respiration, poor circulation, or a combination of the two. To ensure proper assessment and intervention, you should assess the patient closely for signs and symptoms of circulatory and respiratory impairment.

Because carbon dioxide diffuses more easily than oxygen, $TcPCO_2$ values correlate more closely with $PaCO_2$ values. Typically, $TcPCO_2$ values are less sensitive to changes in blood flow to the skin. Also, gestational age (in neonates and infants), body temperature, decreased blood flow, and vasoactive drugs are less likely to cause inaccurate or unreliable $TcPCO_2$ values.

Nursing considerations
• Carefully monitor and rotate the sensor site every 2 to 4 hours to prevent skin irritation or burns. (A very premature infant may require more frequent site changes.) Ensure appropriate temperature limits.
• Stay alert for burns and blisters from the electrode and skin reactions to the adhesive ring. Frequently assess the patient's skin integrity and tolerance for monitoring. Document and report any changes in skin integrity, and intervene appropriately.
• Although slight erythema may occur at the sensor site, it should subside shortly after sensor removal. If erythema does occur, explain the cause to the patient or his parents and reassure them that the redness probably will disappear within a few hours.
• Make sure the sensor isn't occluded or covered by any source, because pressure on the sensor may interfere with blood flow to the sensor site and cause pressure necrosis and burns.
• Once the sensor reaches equilibrium, expect a delayed response time (30 to 80 seconds) before the monitor responds to PaO_2 or $PaCO_2$ changes. Keep this in mind if you're sampling blood for ABG analysis, because monitor values may differ from ABG values if respiratory changes or activity occurs during this interval. Always note the transcutaneous value when drawing a blood sample for ABG analysis to determine how closely the values are tracking one another.
• A sudden change in transcutaneous values unrelated to a change in patient status may mean the sensor has become partially or fully detached from the skin. If this happens, recalibrate the monitor and reapply the sensor as instructed by the manufacturer.
• Be aware that $TcPO_2$ and $TcPCO_2$ values may change with nursing interventions. Carefully assess your patient's tolerance for care procedures, such as suctioning and chest physiotherapy, and modify these interventions as needed to prevent or minimize respiratory compromise.
• Expect transcutaneous values to vary with patient oxygenation changes caused by activity, such as crying, feeding, and exercise. Be prepared to obtain a blood sample for ABG analysis and to start resuscitation if you suspect a change in transcutaneous values that may reflect patient compromise.
• Be sure to obtain periodic ABG values, because transcutaneous monitoring doesn't assess pH and may not always reflect actual PaO_2 and $PaCO_2$ values.
• Document $TcPO_2$ and $TcPCO_2$ values at least

How ETCO₂ monitoring works

The optical portion of an end-tidal carbon dioxide (ETCO$_2$) monitor contains an infrared light source, a sample chamber, a special carbon dioxide (CO$_2$) filter, and a photodetector. The infrared light passes through the sample chamber and is absorbed in varying amounts, depending on the amount of CO$_2$ the patient has just exhaled. The photodetector measures the CO$_2$ content and then relays this information to the microprocessor in the monitor, which displays the CO$_2$ value and waveform.

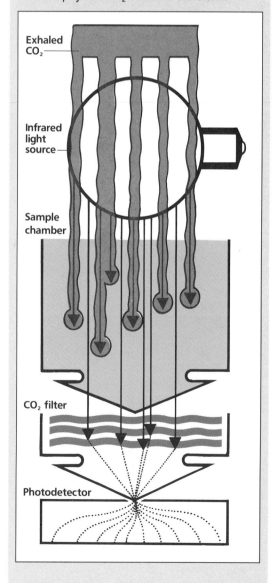

Exhaled CO$_2$

Infrared light source

Sample chamber

CO$_2$ filter

Photodetector

as often as vital signs and before and after respiratory interventions. Also document all sensor site changes.
• Usually, transcutaneous monitoring ends when the patient regains a stable cardiopulmonary status and no longer needs mechanical ventilation and oxygen therapy. After monitoring ends, assess your patient's respirations for comfort and regularity. Consider resuming monitoring if cardiorespiratory compromise recurs.

End-tidal carbon dioxide monitoring

End-tidal carbon dioxide (ETCO$_2$) monitoring determines the carbon dioxide (CO$_2$) concentration in exhaled gas. In this technique, a photodetector measures the amount of infrared light absorbed by airway gas during inspiration and expiration. (Light absorption increases along with the CO$_2$ concentration.) A monitor converts this data to a CO$_2$ value and a corresponding waveform, or capnogram, if capnography is used. (See *How ETCO$_2$ monitoring works.*)

ETCO$_2$ monitoring provides information about the patient's pulmonary, cardiac, and metabolic status that aids patient management and helps prevent clinical compromise. This technique has become a standard care measure during anesthesia administration and mechanical ventilation. For a patient with a stable acid-base balance, it may be used to aid weaning from mechanical ventilation. It also reduces the need for frequent ABG measurements, especially when combined with pulse oximetry.

Other uses for ETCO$_2$ monitoring include assessing resuscitation efforts and identifying the return of spontaneous circulation. Because no CO$_2$ is exhaled when breathing stops, this technique also detects apnea.

When used during endotracheal (ET) intubation, ETCO$_2$ monitoring can avert neurologic injury and even death by confirming correct ET tube placement and detecting accidental esophageal intubation, since CO$_2$ is not normally produced by the stomach. Ongoing $ETCO_2$ monitoring throughout intubation also can prove valuable because an ET tube may become dislodged during manipulation or patient movement or transport. $ETCO_2$ monitoring has no contraindications.

Equipment

Required equipment includes a mainstream or sidestream CO_2 monitor, a CO_2 sensor, and an airway adapter. The sensor, which contains an infrared light source and a photodetector, is positioned at one of two sites in the monitoring setup. With a mainstream monitor, it's positioned directly at the patient's airway with an airway adapter, between the ET tube and the breathing circuit tubing. With a sidestream monitor, the airway adapter is positioned at the airway (whether or not the patient is intubated) to allow aspiration of gas from the patient's airway back to the sensor, which lies either within or close to the monitor.

Some CO_2 detection devices provide semiquantitative indications of CO_2 concentrations, supplying an approximate range rather than a specific value for $ETCO_2$. Other devices simply indicate whether CO_2 is present during exhalation. (See *Colorimetric $ETCO_2$ detection*.)

Preparation

If the patient requires ET intubation, an $ETCO_2$ detector or monitor is usually applied immediately after the tube is inserted. If he doesn't require intubation or is already intubated and alert, explain the purpose and expected duration of monitoring. Tell an intubated patient that the monitor will painlessly measure the amount of CO_2 he exhales. Inform a nonintubated patient that the monitor will track his CO_2 concentration to make sure his breathing is effective.

To prepare the equipment, choose the right size airway adapter for your patient, as recommended by the manufacturer. For example, a neonatal adapter may have a much smaller dead space, making it appropriate for a smaller patient.

Colorimetric $ETCO_2$ detection

A recent innovation in end-tidal carbon dioxide ($ETCO_2$) monitoring, colorimetric $ETCO_2$ detection uses a disposable device that changes color to signal the presence of carbon dioxide in the airway. On exhalation, a color change from purple to yellow or tan reveals the approximate $ETCO_2$ concentration. Color changes may occur for up to 2 hours of monitoring.

Colorimetric $ETCO_2$ detectors are commonly available in code carts, intubation kits, and emergency transport vehicles. They can be used for any intubated patient, especially if electronic $ETCO_2$ monitoring is unavailable.

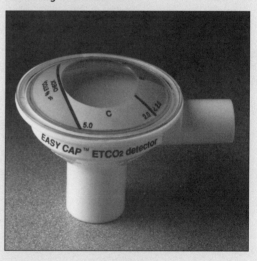

If the monitor you're using isn't self-calibrating, calibrate it as the manufacturer directs. If you're using a sidestream CO_2 monitor, be sure to replace the water trap between patients, if directed. (The trap allows humidity from exhaled gases to be condensed into an attached container.) Newer sidestream models don't require water traps.

Procedure

• Wash your hands. After turning on the monitor and calibrating it (if necessary), position the airway adapter and sensor as the manufacturer directs. For an intubated patient, position the adapter directly on the ET tube. For a nonintubated patient, place the adapter at or near the patient's airway. (An oxygen-delivery cannula may have a sample port through which gas can be aspirated for monitoring.)

• Turn on all alarms and adjust alarm settings as appropriate for your patient. Make sure the alarm volume is loud enough to hear.

• Document the initial $ETCO_2$ value and all ventilator settings. Describe the waveform, if one appears on your monitor. If the monitor has a printer, you may want to print out a sample waveform and include it in the patient's medical record.

Interpretation of findings

With adequate alveolar ventilation and blood flow to the lungs, normal $ETCO_2$ values should approximate $PaCO_2$ values. However, with significantly reduced pulmonary blood flow (as from cardiac arrest), $ETCO_2$ will drop below $PaCO_2$ — or may even measure zero.

Normal $ETCO_2$ values range from 35 to 45 mm Hg. They're usually 2 to 5 mm Hg less than a $PaCO_2$ value obtained by ABG measurement. This differential between arterial and $ETCO_2$ values is called the a-$ADCO_2$ value. This normal variance assumes that your patient has a normal $\dot{V}/\dot{Q}$ ratio and that you're sampling the gas correctly.

Decreased $ETCO_2$

The a-$ADCO_2$ value may exceed 5 mm Hg, especially if dead-space conditions are present or if you're not sampling the gas correctly. Dead-space conditions occur when lung perfusion decreases relative to ventilation, as in hypotension, hypovolemia, pulmonary embolism, and cardiac arrest. Because decreased perfusion impairs CO_2 transport, the $ETCO_2$ value will drop below normal and the waveform will show decreased $ETCO_2$ in both the real-time and trend modes. If $ETCO_2$ decreases exponentially within a few breaths, suspect a catastrophic cardiopulmonary event.

A sudden $ETCO_2$ drop to or near zero also signals a potentially catastrophic loss of ventilation. Usually, this results from esophageal intubation, disconnection of airway from ventilator, complete ET tube obstruction, or total ventilator malfunction. Assess the patient immediately to determine if ventilation is impaired; then take appropriate steps to restore an airway and support ventilation. Once you've evaluated the patient for ventilatory failure, check the CO_2 monitor to rule out a blocked sample tube.

A gradual drop in $ETCO_2$ may signal decreasing CO_2 production, increased CO_2 removal caused by hyperventilation, or diminishing pulmonary perfusion. Causes of decreased CO_2 production include hypothermia and sedation. Increased CO_2 removal may result from inappropriate ventilator settings. (However, this condition may be desirable when managing a patient with neurologic dysfunction.) Diminishing pulmonary perfusion may reflect blood loss, which may necessitate volume replacement.

A common abnormal waveform shows sustained low $ETCO_2$ without an alveolar plateau. An absent or abnormal alveolar plateau usually indicates incomplete exhalation. This condition may be caused by lung secretions, bronchospasm, or a partially kinked ET tube. Incomplete exhalation causes a rounded CO_2 waveform. Without an alveolar plateau, the $ETCO_2$ value doesn't reliably estimate $PaCO_2$. When the above conditions are corrected, such as by suctioning, administering bronchodilators, or eliminating kinks in the tube, the $ETCO_2$ value and CO_2 waveform usually return to normal.

A low $ETCO_2$ value and a rounded CO_2 waveform also may result from improper gas sampling. For instance, the airway adapter may be placed too far from the patient's airway; exhaled gas then mixes with fresh gas flow from the ventilator, diluting $ETCO_2$. To correct this problem, move the airway adapter closer to the patient's airway or adjust fresh gas flow rates.

$ETCO_2$ dilution is more likely with a sidestream aspirating system that samples large amounts of exhaled gas per minute. This can be a particular problem when monitoring infants, who normally have lower tidal volumes. When caring for a smaller patient, try to obtain one of the newer sidestream CO_2 monitors that samples smaller gas volumes.

Increased ETCO$_2$
A gradual increase in ETCO$_2$ may result from hypoventilation, increasing CO_2 production, or partial airway obstruction. During hypoventilation, CO_2 accumulates in the blood and the patient may exhale more of it than usual. Such factors as increased body temperature and pain also may increase CO_2 production. Partial airway obstruction may increase ETCO$_2$ by compromising ventilation.

A sudden rise in ETCO$_2$ may stem from an acute increase in the amount of CO_2 in blood perfusing the lungs — for example, from sodium bicarbonate administration or tourniquet release. However, such a rise usually is transient.

Occasionally, the waveform shows a cleft near the end of exhalation in the normally smooth alveolar plateau. Most common in patients undergoing neuromuscular blockade, this represents partial recovery from the blockade. Administering additional neuromuscular blocking agents should provide a fuller state of blockade and eliminate the cleft.

Evaluating spontaneous respirations
ETCO$_2$ monitoring may help distinguish spontaneous respirations from mechanical-ventilator respirations. Ineffective spontaneous respirations may cause below-normal ETCO$_2$ values and a rounded waveform. Spontaneous respirations that more closely resemble a normal waveform, including the alveolar plateau, may more accurately indicate the patient's readiness to be weaned. You may see a rounded waveform with below normal ETCO$_2$ values when monitoring a nonintubated patient. In this case, you should observe trends.

Nursing considerations
• Wear gloves when handling the airway adapter to prevent cross-contamination. Make sure the adapter is changed with every breath-

ing circuit and ET tube change.
• Place the adapter as close to the ET tube as possible to avoid contaminating exhaled gases with fresh gas flow from the ventilator. If you're using a heat and moisture exchanger, you may be able to position the airway adapter between the exchanger and breathing circuit.
• If your patient's ETCO$_2$ values and PaCO$_2$ values differ, assess him for factors that can influence ETCO$_2$ — especially when the a-ADCO$_2$ value is above normal.
• Interpreting the a-ADCO$_2$ value correctly will provide useful information about your patient's status. For example, an increased a-ADCO$_2$ value may mean your patient has worsening dead-space disease — especially if his VT remains constant.
• Remember that ETCO$_2$ monitoring doesn't replace ABG measurements because it doesn't assess oxygenation or blood pH. Supplementing ETCO$_2$ monitoring with pulse oximetry may provide more complete information.
• If the CO_2 waveform is available, assess it for height, frequency, rhythm, baseline, and shape to help evaluate gas exchange. Be sure you know how to recognize a normal waveform and can identify abnormal waveforms and their possible causes. If a printer is available, record and document any abnormal waveforms in the patient's medical record. (See *CO$_2$ waveform*, page 134.)
• In a nonintubated patient, use ETCO$_2$ values to establish trends. Be aware that in this patient, exhaled gas is more likely to mix with ambient air and exhaled CO_2 may be diluted by fresh gas flow from the nasal cannula.
• ETCO$_2$ monitoring commonly is discontinued when the patient has been weaned effectively from mechanical ventilation or when he's no longer at risk for respiratory compromise. Carefully assess your patient's tolerance for weaning. After extubation, continuous ETCO$_2$ monitoring may detect the need for reintubation.
• Document ETCO$_2$ values at least as often as vital signs, whenever significant changes in waveform or patient status occur, and before

CO₂ waveform

The carbon dioxide (CO_2) waveform, or capnogram, produced in end-tidal carbon dioxide ($ETCO_2$) monitoring reflects the course of CO_2 elimination during exhalation. A normal capnogram (shown below) consists of several segments, which reflect the various stages of exhalation and inhalation.

Normally, any gas eliminated from the airway during *early exhalation* is dead-space gas, which hasn't undergone exchange at the alveolocapillary membrane. Measurements taken during this period contain no CO_2.

As exhalation continues, *CO_2 concentration rises* sharply and rapidly. The sensor now de-

tects gas that has undergone exchange, producing measurable quantities of CO_2.

The final stages of alveolar emptying occur during late exhalation. During the *alveolar plateau* phase, CO_2 concentration rises more gradually because alveolar emptying is more constant.

The point at which the $ETCO_2$ value is derived is the *end of exhalation*, when CO_2 concentration peaks. Unless an alveolar plateau is present, this value doesn't accurately estimate alveolar CO_2. During inhalation, the *CO_2 concentration declines* sharply to zero.

mm Hg

Alveolar plateau

Rise of CO_2 concentration

Early exhalation of dead-space gas

End of exhalation

Decline of CO_2 concentration

and after weaning, respiratory, and other interventions. Periodically obtain samples for ABG analysis as the patient's condition dictates, and document the corresponding $ETCO_2$ value.

Mixed venous oxygen saturation monitoring

An invasive procedure, mixed venous oxygen saturation ($S\bar{v}O_2$) monitoring reveals the balance between oxygen supply and demand. A special fiber-optic catheter placed in the pulmonary ar-

tery continuously measures the oxygen saturation of hemoglobin in mixed venous blood. The resulting $S\bar{v}O_2$ value represents oxygen reserve—the amount of oxygen available during periods of increased oxygen demand.

$S\bar{v}O_2$ values also provide important information about the interactive aspects of oxygenation, including oxygen content, oxygen delivery, and oxygen demand. If any of these factors are compromised, oxygenation can be affected, especially if compensatory mechanisms fail. For example, if oxygen content is lower than normal, cardiac output can increase to sustain oxygen delivery and oxygen demand increases.

Potential complications of this technique include pneumothorax, pulmonary artery perforation, air emboli, thrombosis, infection, and cardiac arrhythmias.

For a resting adult, normal oxygen delivery to the tissues is approximately 1,000 ml/minute; normal oxygen consumption, roughly 250 ml/minute. The tissues normally extract about 25% of the available oxygen, leaving 75% in reserve. Thus, $S\bar{v}O_2$ normally measures approximately 75%, although it may range from 60% to 80%.

When oxygen needs increase, oxygen consumption rises; a 1.8° F (1° C) rise in body temperature may increase oxygen consumption up to 10%. To compensate, cardiac output normally rises. However, in a critically ill patient, oxygen delivery may be impaired, preventing a compensatory increase in cardiac output. For example, if the hemoglobin or SaO_2 value decreases, arterial oxygen content may drop. With any of these factors, oxygen delivery may be compromised and the tissues may extract a greater percentage of available oxygen, lowering the $S\bar{v}O_2$ value.

Many conditions increase tissue oxygen needs, including hyperthermia, shivering, burns, head injuries, seizures, pain, exercise, infection, chest trauma, and dyspnea. Recovery from anesthesia and certain nursing interventions, such as weighing and chest physiotherapy, also may increase oxygen needs.

Oxygen consumption may diminish in a patient receiving anesthetics, analgesics, sedatives, or neuromuscular blockers. Sepsis and conditions that increase hemoglobin-oxygen binding also may reduce oxygen consumption by reducing oxygen extraction by the tissues.

Equipment
To perform continuous $S\bar{v}O_2$ monitoring, you'll need a kit that contains a flow-directed, thermodilution pulmonary artery (PA) catheter with fiber-optic filaments, an optical module, and a computerized oximeter. The catheter continuously emits light into pulmonary blood, which reflects light relative to the oxyhemoglobin content. The optical module determines how much light has been reflected and then relays this information to the $S\bar{v}O_2$ monitor,

which converts it to an $S\bar{v}O_2$ value and waveform. The monitor may also display cardiac output and other hemodynamic values.

You may also need a strip recorder for documenting the $S\bar{v}O_2$ measurements. A printer, an optional piece of equipment, lets you record the graphic display.

Preparation
Before the procedure, make sure that the patient or guardian is fully informed and signs a consent form. For information on setting up the monitoring system, see *Continuous $S\bar{v}O_2$ monitoring*, pages 136 to 139.

Procedure
• For directions on how to proceed with monitoring, see *Continuous $S\bar{v}O_2$ monitoring*, pages 136 to 139.
• Document the initial $S\bar{v}O_2$ value; then continue to document values hourly or more frequently if they vary significantly.
• Also document the $S\bar{v}O_2$ value before and after any intervention intended to improve oxygen delivery or decrease oxygen demand. You may want to attach selected strips from the recorder to the patient's medical record.

Interpretation of findings
An $S\bar{v}O_2$ value from 60% to 80% usually indicates sufficient oxygen delivery to meet oxygen demands. Compare serial readings to the patient's baseline value.

If the $S\bar{v}O_2$ value is below 60% or varies more than 10% from the patient's baseline, reassess the patient and the monitoring system. A below-normal value reflects increased oxygen needs, impaired oxygen delivery, or both. A value of 50% or lower suggests marginal oxygen delivery.

A value above 80% may signal increased oxygen delivery, reduced oxygen needs, or complications associated with the PA catheter. Each condition warrants further assessment. Be sure to assess the $S\bar{v}O_2$ waveform, which may help evaluate your patient's response to therapy. (See *Understanding $S\bar{v}O_2$ waveform variations*, page 140.)

(Text continues on page 140.)

Continuous $S\bar{v}O_2$ monitoring

To perform continuous mixed venous oxygen saturation ($S\bar{v}O_2$) monitoring, you'll need to obtain a kit that contains a flow-directed, thermodilution pulmonary artery catheter with fiber-optic filaments (to be inserted by the doctor). You'll need an optical module and a computerized oximeter. You may also need a strip recorder for documenting the $S\bar{v}O_2$ measurements. A printer, an optional piece of equipment, lets you record the graphic display.

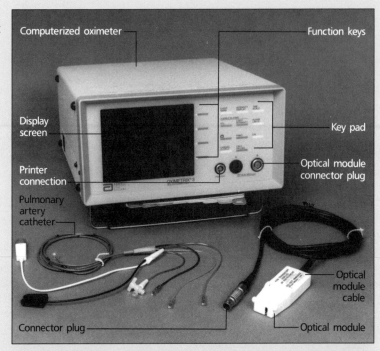

Computerized oximeter

Function keys

Display screen

Key pad

Printer connection

Optical module connector plug

Pulmonary artery catheter

Optical module cable

Connector plug

Optical module

Turning on the oximeter
To begin, connect the optical module cable to the oximeter by aligning the red dot on the connector plug at the end of the cable with the red mark on the oximeter. Then push in the plug until it locks in place.

Turn on the oximeter by flipping the power switch to a forward position. On the display screen, you should see a version number in the upper left corner, the current date and time under the version number, and the mode $S\bar{v}O_2$.

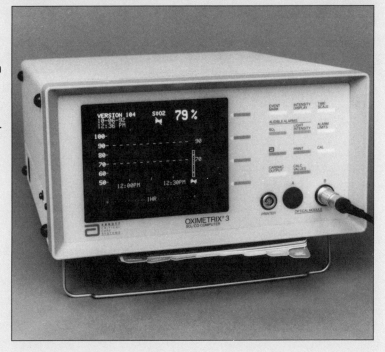

Continuous S⊽O₂ monitoring (continued)

Preparing the catheter and optical module

Inspect the pulmonary artery catheter package for any rips or tears. Then remove the outer wrapping from the package while leaving the inner wrapping over the catheter intact.

Peel back the lift tab on the inner wrapping (as shown near right). Place the optical module in the specially designed recess in the tray.

With the optical module still in the tray, open the module's lid by pulling it straight out in the direction of the arrow and then lifting. A LOW LIGHT message will appear on the display screen when you open the lid. Next, slide the optical connector, located at the distal end of the pulmonary artery catheter, into the optical module (as shown far right). Make sure that the word TOP on the connector faces up. Then close the lid.

Next, check that the black optical reference is in position by verifying that the catheter tip is in the reference.

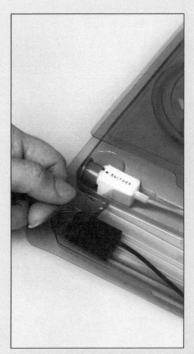
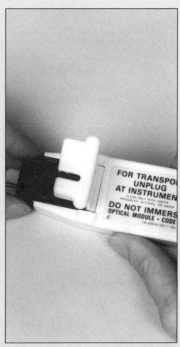

Calibrating the monitor before catheter insertion

Before the doctor inserts the pulmonary artery catheter, calibrate the equipment so that it's ready to function. First, press the key labeled CAL. The display screen should list the calibration options. Then, with the catheter still in the package, select the preinsertion function by pressing the function key next to the block labeled P.

The message shown at right should then appear on the display screen. To initiate calibration, press the function key next to the block labeled Y. Expect the screen to display only the letters CAL and the monitoring mode (S⊽O₂) for up to 1 minute. When the system completes the calibration, the screen will display the message CAL OK in the upper right corner. If the message CAL FAIL appears, repeat the calibration steps.

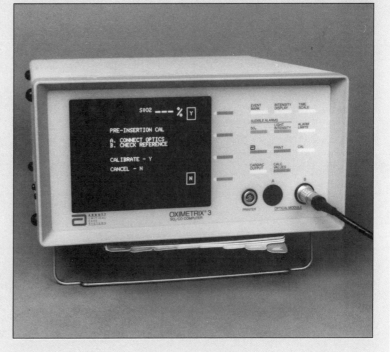

(continued)

Continuous S̄vO₂ monitoring *(continued)*

Calibrating the monitor after catheter insertion

You may need to calibrate the monitor once the catheter is in place—for example, if calibration wasn't done before insertion, if the catheter disconnects from the optical module, if the fiber-optic filaments sustain damage, if you suspect an incorrect reading, or if a catheter has been in place for an extended period.

Before doing so, make sure that the patient's SaO₂ level is relatively stable. Also, set the intensity of the signal display so that it's within normal limits. Then press the CAL key.

Next, press the function key next to the block labeled I (as shown). This selects in vivo calibration.

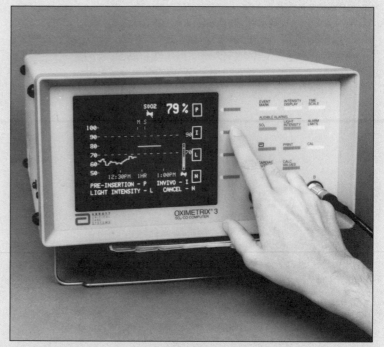

Drawing blood

Press the function key next to the block labeled Y, as shown, to continue with in vivo calibration. In response, the oximeter will store the preceding 5 seconds of oxygen saturation data, and the display screen will signal DRAW BLOOD for 12 seconds.

When this message appears, clear the distal lumen of the pulmonary artery line, draw a blood sample, and send it to the laboratory for S̄vO₂ analysis. The screen will display the in vivo calibration process and exhibit the stored oxygen saturation values in the upper left corner.

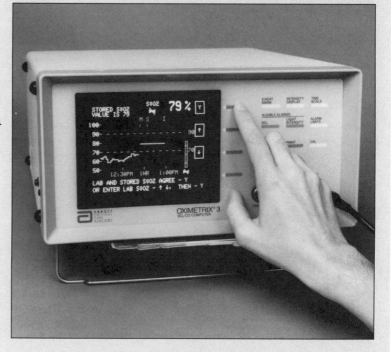

Continuous S̄vO₂ monitoring (continued)

Comparing values and adjusting equipment

After you receive the laboratory's S̄vO₂ results, compare them with the stored value that appears in the upper left corner of the display screen. Is the new value within 4 saturation units of the stored value? If not, enter the laboratory value by manipulating the function keys next to the blocks showing the up and down arrows.

Once you've entered the correct saturation number – or if the laboratory value was within 4 saturation units of the value displayed by the computer – press the key next to the block labeled Y.

After calibration, adjust the rest of the equipment. Begin by calibrating the light intensity. First, press the CAL key. Next, press the function key beside the block labeled L for light intensity (as shown). When the next screen display appears, press the function key next to the block labeled Y to confirm that you want to proceed. The computer will then begin calibration, after which the screen will display the letter L and the light intensity signal should center in the vertical intensity bar on the screen.

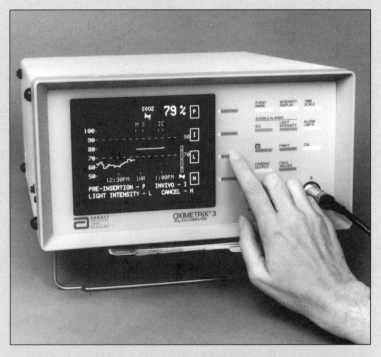

Setting alarm limits

To set the alarm limits, first press the ALARM LIMITS key.

Then adjust the alarm limits as necessary by manipulating the function keys next to the blocks labeled with an up or down arrow (as shown).

After you've set the appropriate limits, again press the ALARM LIMITS key. The on-screen display should return to the monitoring mode.

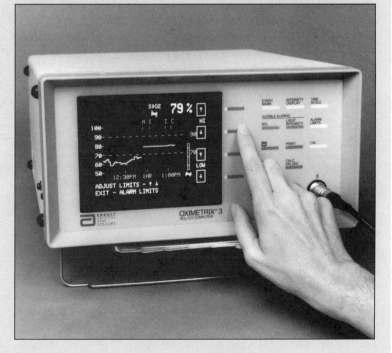

Understanding SⱱO₂ waveform variations

The first illustration is a normal mixed venous oxygen saturation (S$\bar{\text{v}}$O₂) waveform. The second depicts variations that may occur when a patient is suctioned, turned, and weighed. The third waveform shows the variations produced when positive end-expiratory pressure (PEEP) is initiated or the fraction of inspired oxygen (FIO₂) is decreased.

Normal S$\bar{\text{v}}$O₂ waveform

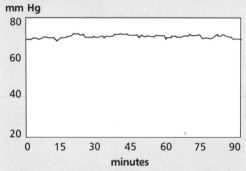

S$\bar{\text{v}}$O₂ with patient activities

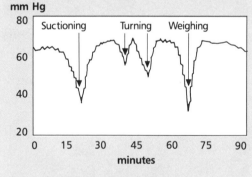

S$\bar{\text{v}}$O₂ with PEEP and FIO₂ changes

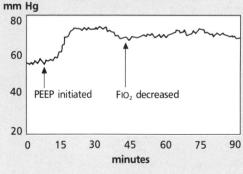

Nursing considerations

• Document and report any S$\bar{\text{v}}$O₂ value below 60%, above 80%, or more than 10% above or below the baseline value over a period of 3 minutes. Be sure to check for trends in S$\bar{\text{v}}$O₂ values. (See *Detecting S$\bar{\text{v}}$O₂ trends*.)

• If your patient has abnormal S$\bar{\text{v}}$O₂ values, try to identify the cause and intervene appropriately to improve his respiratory and hemodynamic status. For example, you may need to correct anemia or hypoxemia, enhance cardiac output, or decrease oxygen demands.

If S$\bar{\text{v}}$O₂ values fall below 60% or are more than 10% below baseline, carefully assess the patient for increased oxygen demands, reduced oxygen delivery, or both. Reduced oxygen delivery may result from decreased hemoglobin values (as with anemia and hemorrhage), decreased SaO₂ (as with hypoxia, suctioning, respiratory failure, airway obstruction, and impaired oxygen diffusion), or reduced cardiac output (as with cardiogenic shock, hypotension, hypovolemia, vasoconstriction, arrhythmias, acidosis, and sepsis). As appropriate, adjust nursing interventions to avoid further increasing the patient's oxygen demands or reducing his oxygen delivery. For example, excessive positive end-expiratory pressure (PEEP) therapy may reduce oxygen delivery by decreasing blood return to the heart. Reducing PEEP to a more tolerable level may improve blood flow to the heart, improving oxygen delivery.

If the patient's S$\bar{\text{v}}$O₂ values exceed 80%, assess him for causes of increased oxygen delivery or reduced oxygen needs, and reevaluate interventions. Increased oxygen delivery may stem from a rise in SaO₂ (such as from a high fraction of inspired oxygen) or increased cardiac output (such as from fluid or positive inotropic therapy or intra-aortic balloon pump support). Hemoglobin values may increase after administration of blood products. Vasoconstriction, sepsis, sedation, chemical paralysis, and hypothermia also may reduce oxygen needs.

• Take steps to avoid technical problems that can cause abnormal values. For example, make sure all connections between the fiber-optic PA catheter and the monitor are secure and verify that the catheter is patent and not kinked. If the $S\bar{v}O_2$ waveform appears damped or erratic, aspirate blood from the catheter to check its patency. If you're unable to aspirate blood, the line may be clotted; notify the doctor so the catheter can be replaced. If the pulmonary artery waveform is altered, suspect wedging of the catheter against the vessel wall. Try to unwedge it by flushing the line, repositioning the patient, or asking him to cough. Notify the doctor immediately if you can't correct catheter wedging.

• To minimize the risk of infection, change the sterile dressing every 24 hours, or more often if it becomes loose or soiled. Carefully inspect the site and document its appearance with each dressing change. Immediately report any signs or symptoms of infection.

• Change I.V. tubing every 24 hours, or as specified by hospital policy. Document the dates and times of tubing changes.

• Usually, $S\bar{v}O_2$ monitoring is discontinued when the patient's oxygenation and hemodynamic status stabilize or if complications (such as infection from catheterization) occur. Carefully follow your hospital's policy when assisting with catheter removal. Apply pressure and a pressure dressing to minimize bleeding from the insertion site.

Bedside pulmonary function monitoring

Pulmonary function tests (PFTs) help assess the integrity and function of the airways, pulmonary vasculature, and pulmonary interstitium. Besides detecting lung disease and abnormal lung function, they help reveal the type of impairment (obstructive or restrictive) and its extent, analyze disease progression, and evaluate the effects of therapy. PFTs also can identify patients at risk for respiratory compromise.

Although comprehensive PFTs usually are

Detecting $S\bar{v}O_2$ trends

Changes in mixed venous oxygen saturation ($S\bar{v}O_2$) values may precede obvious deterioration in a patient's clinical status. Therefore, detecting $S\bar{v}O_2$ trends allows earlier intervention and management.

For instance, don't assume that an $S\bar{v}O_2$ value between 60% and 80% is always normal. In some cases, it may suggest a dangerous trend. To detect trends, be sure to compare each new $S\bar{v}O_2$ value to the patient's baseline $S\bar{v}O_2$ and to evaluate successive values for changes over time.

Consider the patient whose baseline $S\bar{v}O_2$ is 79%. His latest $S\bar{v}O_2$ value is 68%. Although this falls within the normal range, you should consider a value of 68% a possible sign of decreased oxygen delivery, increased oxygen demand, or both. This downward trend may provide an early clue that he's less able to compensate for changes in his oxygenation.

---

performed in a pulmonary function laboratory, simpler bedside procedures now are available to monitor changes in the acutely ill patient. Bedside monitoring may include such measurements as VT, MV, vital capacity (VC), maximal voluntary ventilation (MVV), maximal inspiratory and expiratory pressures (MIP, MEP), forced vital capacity (FVC), forced expiratory volume (FEV), forced expiratory flow (FEF), and peak expiratory flow (PEF).

Bedside monitoring supplements other assessment procedures, such as ABG analysis, chest X-rays, physical examination, and complete PFTs. Results help guide nursing care and medical management. The need for specific information, the type of equipment available, and the patient's ability to participate in testing determine which measurements are taken.

Equipment
Equipment depends on the specific test. For example, PEF measurement requires a peak-flow meter; MIP and MEP measurements require a pressure manometer; and VT, MV, VC,

MVV, and expiratory flow rate measurements require a spirometer. (See *Devices used in bedside monitoring.*)

A spirometer measures the volume of inhaled and exhaled air. As the patient breathes, a spirogram — a tracing of changes in lung volume — may be recorded.

For some tests, additional equipment may include a mouthpiece, an airway adapter, and a noseclip. You may also need a pulse oximeter to determine the oxygen saturation of the patient's blood before or during testing.

Preparation

Explain to the patient the purpose of pulmonary function monitoring, and tell him how he's expected to participate. Because patient cooperation, motivation, and effort can significantly affect test results, make sure he isn't too fatigued or sedated to follow directions. Have him refrain from smoking, eating heavy meals, and drinking beverages before testing to avoid interference with maximal breathing effort. Complete any bronchial hygiene procedures, including postural drainage and suctioning, before testing starts. Withhold bronchodilators, unless the doctor orders otherwise.

If the patient is on a mechanical ventilator, position him in Fowler's or semi-Fowler's position. Otherwise, have him sit or stand, as the test requires. Make sure he's comfortable.

Gather all equipment. Obtain a flow sheet for immediate recording of measurements. If your patient is prone to oxygen desaturation, measure his SaO_2 value with a pulse oximeter before testing; if indicated, hyperoxygenate him.

Procedure

As indicated by the specific test, follow the appropriate procedure for measuring lung volumes or capacities.

Tidal volume

V_T usually is measured with a spirometer.
• If the patient is on a mechanical ventilator, disconnect the ventilator. Then wait about 30 to 60 seconds to reestablish his normal respiratory pattern before measuring V_T. To determine if he's becoming hypoxemic during testing, use a pulse oximeter.
• Attach the mouthpiece to the spirometer. Place a noseclip on the patient, and have him verify that he can't pass air through his nose. Then place the mouthpiece in his mouth.
• Ask the patient to breathe normally. After 10 breaths, note the volume on the spirometer. Divide this volume by 10 to obtain an average V_T. Reconnect the patient to the ventilator when measurements are complete.

Minute volume

MV is the product of respiratory frequency and V_T.
• Follow the procedure for measuring V_T. Then multiply V_T by the respiratory rate per minute to obtain the patient's MV.

Vital capacity

Representing the greatest possible breathing capacity, VC is the amount of air that can be exhaled after maximum inspiratory effort. (VC is often measured in a patient with tachypnea because an increased respiratory rate commonly results from reduced oxygen reserve.)
• Attach the mouthpiece to the spirometer and instruct the patient to inhale as deeply as possible. Then insert the mouthpiece so his lips are sealed tightly around it. This helps prevent air leakage and ensures an accurate digital readout or spirogram recording.
• Press the button on the spirometer to reset the dial to zero. Ask the patient to exhale completely. Then read the measurement on the spirometer.
• Let the patient rest briefly. Then repeat the procedure twice to obtain three measurements.

Maximal voluntary ventilation

Also called maximal breathing capacity, MVV refers to the total volume of air that can be exchanged in 1 minute with the patient's maximum voluntary effort. MVV reflects overall respiratory efficiency, including respiratory muscle status, lung compliance, airway resistance, and neurologic coordination.
• Attach the mouthpiece to the spirometer. Ask the patient to breathe into the spirometer

Devices used in bedside monitoring

These illustrations show two common devices you'll use to perform bedside tests—the Wright spirometer and the inspiratory pressure manometer. Both are being used on a patient with a tracheostomy tube.

Wright spirometer

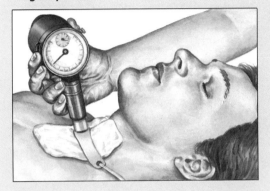

Inspiratory pressure manometer

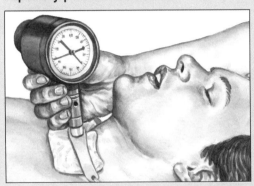

as deeply and rapidly as possible over a specified period—usually 10, 12, or 15 seconds.
• Multiply the expired volume measurement by a factor of 6, 5, or 4, respectively, to obtain MVV.

Maximal inspiratory pressure
Representing maximal alveolar pressure during inspiration, MIP reflects inspiratory muscle strength and diaphragm function and helps assess a patient's readiness for weaning from mechanical ventilation. MIP also is called peak inspiratory pressure, negative inspiratory force, negative inspiratory effort, or peak inspiratory force.
• Make sure the airway is free of secretions. If the patient is on a ventilator, disconnect it.
• Attach the inspiratory force meter or pressure manometer to the mouthpiece or airway adapter.
• Apply a noseclip to the patient, and have him verify that he can't pass air through his nose.
• Instruct the patient to exhale.
• With your thumb or fingertip, occlude the airway by covering the safety port on the inspiratory force meter or pressure manometer.

• Ask the patient to breathe as deeply as possible as you block his airway. As he does so, note the value on the pressure manometer.

Maximal expiratory pressure
Commonly used to determine respiratory muscle strength in patients with neuromuscular problems, MEP measurement also evaluates coughing ability.
• Connect the pressure manometer to the mouthpiece; then place the mouthpiece in the patient's mouth.
• Put a noseclip on the patient, and have him verify that he can't pass air through his nose.
• Ask the patient to inhale as deeply as possible. Occlude the airway by closing the safety port or valve on the pressure gauge with your thumb or fingertip.
• Instruct the patient to exhale as deeply as possible as you block his airway. Note the value on the manometer; MEP is the maximal pressure produced for 2 or 3 seconds.

Expiratory flow (forced vital capacity, forced expiratory volume, and forced expiratory flow)

Expiratory flow consists of three parameters — FVC (the amount of air exhaled forcefully and quickly after maximal inspiration), FEV (the amount of air exhaled in the first, second, or third second of an FVC maneuver), and FEF (the average flow rate during the middle of an FVC maneuver). All three measurements can be derived from the same bedside spirometry procedure, using a spirometer that produces a graphic reading.
• Attach the mouthpiece to the spirometer, and place the noseclip on the patient.
• Place the mouthpiece in the patient's mouth. Ask him to inhale deeply, then exhale forcefully, quickly and completely.
• Read the measurement on the spirometer. This measurement is the FVC. To obtain the FEF, average the flow rate obtained over the course of the FVC procedure.
• Observe the recording on the spirometer to obtain the amount of FVC exhaled in 1, 2, or 3 seconds. This is the FEV.
• Let the patient rest briefly, and repeat the procedure three times to make sure your measurements are accurate.

Peak expiratory flow

PEF represents the highest flow attained during an FVC maneuver. Sometimes called maximal expiratory flow rate, this measurement helps determine the extent of obstructive disease or bronchospasm. When done before or after bronchodilator administration or respiratory therapy, it helps gauge therapeutic effectiveness.
• Attach the mouthpiece to the peak-flow meter.
• Have the patient sit up. Then instruct him to inhale as deeply as possible. Insert the mouthpiece and have him seal his lips tightly around it.
• Instruct the patient to exhale forcefully into the flow meter in one short, sharp blast.
• Note the PEF reading on the dial, recorded in liters per second or minute.

Interpretation of findings

For any PFT, an above-normal or below-normal value may indicate the need for additional testing. Be sure to consider the patient's age, weight, and diagnosis when interpreting bedside PFT results. Also analyze findings in conjunction with ABG results. Consider PFT results to be suspect if the patient grows fatigued or short of breath during testing. These results may not reflect the patient's true expiratory potential.

Evaluate serial measurements to help determine disease progression. As indicated, compare bedside measurements with comprehensive PFT measurements (if available) for a more complete evaluation of the patient's condition.

VT values. Normal VT is 10 to 15 ml/kg of body weight. Causes of decreased VT include restrictive lung disease, ventilatory muscle fatigue, and central nervous system (CNS) depression. Causes of increased VT include hypoxemia and CNS stimulation.

MV values. Normal MV is 5 to 10 liters. An increased value reflects excessive CO_2 production, such as from increased oxygen needs. MV results may also help assess whether a mechanically ventilated patient is ready for weaning. For example, if $PaCO_2$ remains stable at approximately 40 mm Hg and MV is below 10 liters, the patient has a good chance for successful weaning.

VC values. Normal VC is based on predicted values obtained from nomograms. A VC may be compromised by acute and chronic lung diseases, conditions that reduce the intrathoracic space, neuromuscular disease, and chest or abdominal surgery. In a normal adult, a VC below 10 ml/kg reflects an inability to sustain spontaneous ventilation for prolonged periods. A VC above 10 ml/kg may signal the patient's readiness to be weaned from a mechanical ventilator.

MVV values. Normal MVV is 170 liters/minute. MVV decreases with moderate to severe lung obstruction. With restrictive disease, it may be normal or slightly decreased. Because

MVV measurement depends heavily on the patient's efforts, its application may be limited. It's most useful in evaluating patients with neuromuscular disorders and assessing a surgical patient's postoperative pulmonary risk.

MIP values. Normal MIP is at least -80 cm H_2O. MIP may decrease with neuromuscular disorders. A value more negative than -25 cm H_2O may indicate readiness to be weaned from a mechanical ventilator; a less negative value means a continued need for mechanical ventilation.

MEP values. Normal MEP ranges from $+80$ to $+100$ cm H_2O. An effective cough requires MEP of at least $+40$ cm H_2O. MEP may decrease with neuromuscular disease.

Expiratory flow. When interpreting this value, compare it to predictive nomograms. Consider any value below 80% abnormal. Expiratory flow commonly decreases with obstructive disease and sometimes with restrictive disease. Usually, patients who respond to treatment, such as bronchodilator therapy, show an improving expiratory flow value. Repeated measurements help determine therapeutic effectiveness. If values don't improve, the disease is considered irreversible and bronchodilators may be discontinued or contraindicated.

PEF values. Normal PEF measures approximately 400 to 700 liters/minute or 10 liters/second. Decreased PEF signals interference with airflow, such as from obstructive lung disease.

Nursing considerations

• Try to schedule bedside testing during a quiet time when both you and the patient are free from distractions.
• If the patient is likely to develop hypoxemia or difficulty breathing during measurement, provide oxygen before and after the test.
• For single-breath maneuvers, expect to repeat the test three times and record the highest value. Between measurements, have the patient rest and return him to the ventilator, if indicated.

• For serial testing, have the patient use the same position each time because variations in positioning may cause an inconsistent performance and unreliable results. Document the position along with test results.
• Take measures to prevent infection — a crucial concern with bedside pulmonary function equipment. Use disposable components whenever possible. Follow hospital policy on handling used equipment.
• Document measurements on the patient's medical record, noting mechanical ventilator settings, bronchodilator administration, and patient positioning. Compare new values with previous results, including baseline measurements, and report significant variations to the doctor.
• Bedside PFTs usually are discontinued once the patient becomes stable or has been successfully weaned from a mechanical ventilator.
• Before the patient is discharged, provide appropriate teaching. If his condition warrants, teach him how to obtain PFT measurements at home to help assess disease progress and identify any need for more aggressive intervention.

Apnea monitoring

Commonly used at the bedside, apnea monitoring provides an early warning of impending apneic episodes, documents the incidence and degree of apnea, and assesses the effectiveness of interventions.

In adults, apnea is defined as an absence of breathing lasting 10 seconds or longer. Apnea occurs in two distinct types: central and obstructive. Mixed apnea — a combination of central and obstructive apnea — also may occur.

In *central apnea,* the patient has no central respiratory output and therefore no respiratory effort. Central apnea is related to abnormal CNS functions that aren't fully understood.

In *obstructive apnea,* central respiratory output occurs but pharyngeal closure prevents airflow. Obstructive apnea may result from collapse of the compliant pharyngeal muscles, altered airway configuration caused by positioning, failure of smaller airways to remain patent, anatomic airway narrowing from fat or tissue edema, chronic inflammation caused by snoring, or increased upper airway resistance secondary to swelling or obstruction.

Many people normally experience brief periods of apnea during sleep. In *sleep apnea syndrome (SAS),* multiple episodes of obstructive or mixed apnea occur, accompanied by loud, repetitive snoring and daytime somnolence. Although definitions of SAS vary, the term usually refers to 30 or more periods of apnea per 7 hours of sleep or more than 5 such episodes per hour. SAS may cause problems ranging from mild to serious, including insomnia, daytime hypersomnolence, personality changes, cognitive dysfunction, arrhythmias, and laboratory test abnormalities (such as polycythemia, hypercapnia, and hypoxemia).

Among preterm infants, apneic episodes commonly are accompanied by bradycardia. Infantile apnea may result from an immature respiratory control center, respiratory center depression, failure of peripheral chemoreceptors to override hypoxemic depression of the respiratory center, reflex responses of the posterior pharynx and lungs, or airway obstruction related to positioning.

Equipment
Apnea monitoring usually requires a thoracic impedance monitor unit and chest electrodes. The monitor detects changes in thoracic impedance, which increases during inspiration and decreases during expiration. A respiratory amplifier displays the respiratory rate. Some monitors also display a respiratory waveform, whose amplitude reflects respiratory depth.

Preparation
Explain the monitoring procedure to the patient and his family. Tell them you'll be using a device to monitor the patient's breathing. Explain how the device is applied and describe the information the monitor will display. Warn them never to change the alarm settings or turn off the monitor.

Procedure
• Plug the power cable into a grounded electrical outlet. Wash your hands. Next, clean the patient's chest and abdomen at the sites where electrodes will be placed. Dry the skin thoroughly.
• Place electrodes on the chest and abdomen, as the manufacturer directs. Attach the lead wires to the electrodes. Be sure to target areas where chest wall movement is greatest to help detect an adequate signal.
• Turn on the monitor. Set the high and low respiratory rate alarms and adjust the apnea time period. Make sure the alarm volume is audible and the printer (if available) is loaded with paper.
• Observe the respiratory rate, waveform, and heart rate displayed on the monitor. Document these in the patient's medical record at least as often as you record routine vital signs. Report and document the presence and degree of any apneic episodes, including their time, frequency, and duration. Also document any associated bradycardia or other findings.

Interpretation of findings
Normally, respirations are regular and rhythmic, without prolonged interruption. Therefore, consider frequent apnea a significant finding, especially when accompanied by other symptoms. The patient may need additional evaluation, including complete polysomnography assessment.

Apnea duration and frequency may relate to such treatments as drug therapy, continuous positive airway pressure, or surgery. As interventions change, note any improvement or deterioration in the patient's respiratory rate and pattern.

Nursing considerations
• When an apnea alarm sounds, first assess the patient, checking for bradycardia and other arrhythmias, cyanosis, and airway obstruction. Be prepared to ventilate and oxygenate the patient if he remains unresponsive to stimulation. Carefully assess airway adequacy and intervene as necessary to maintain patency.

• After correcting apnea, evaluate the patient for the underlying cause by thoroughly assessing his respiratory, neurologic, and metabolic status. If you suspect sepsis, obtain cultures and administer antibiotics, as ordered. Specific therapy aims to treat the underlying cause of apnea.

• If your patient has obstructive apnea, stay alert for airway obstruction during apnea monitoring. The chest wall may continue to move even though the airway is obstructed. Because the apnea monitor can't distinguish between effective and ineffective ventilation, a patient with unstable respiratory status may require additional monitoring, such as pulse oximetry and capnography.

• If artifact or poor signal quality triggers the apnea alarm, reassess the position and integrity of chest electrodes. If necessary, reposition or replace electrodes to enhance signal quality. Also replace any loose electrodes. Remove electrodes carefully, particularly if the patient has an actual or potential skin integrity impairment.

• If ordered, use airway thermistors and $ETCO_2$ monitoring devices to detect apnea. Airway thermistors produce varied electrical resistance in response to normal temperature changes that occur during inspiration and expiration (the air is cooler on inspiration than expiration). $ETCO_2$ monitoring devices detect apnea by measuring airway CO_2 levels, which are absent when breathing ceases.

• Before discharge, teach the patient and his family how to use an apnea monitor at home, if indicated.

• Apnea monitoring usually is discontinued after testing has been completed or when apneic episodes decrease in frequency and duration to a clinically acceptable level. It also may be discontinued if the doctor orders an alternate form of respiratory monitoring, such as $ETCO_2$ monitoring.

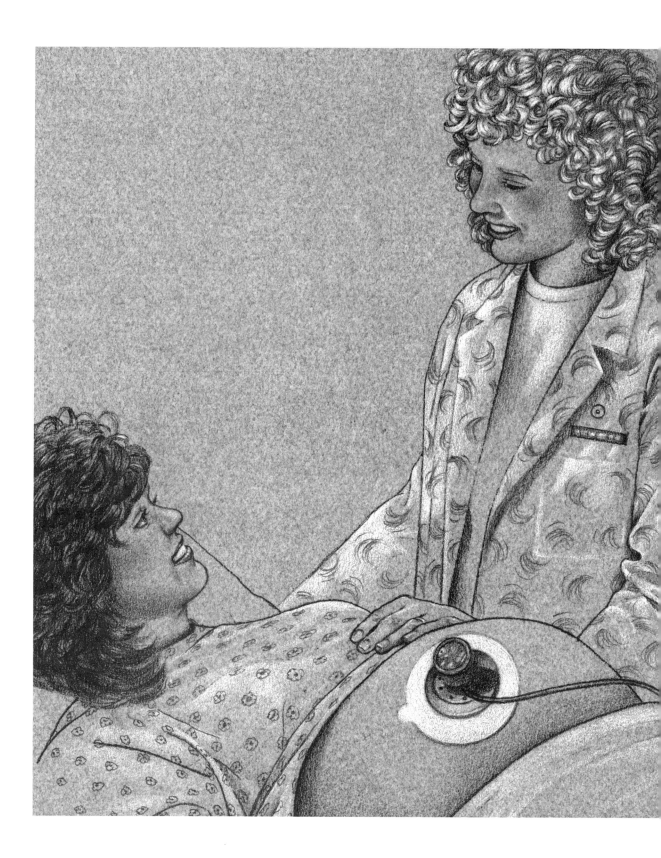

CHAPTER

Monitoring fetal status

Fetal well-being during labor and delivery depends on a complex physiologic balance between the mother and fetus. By carefully monitoring fetal status and the mother's uterine function, you can identify potential threats to fetal well-being before serious complications occur.

This chapter describes the concepts and techniques involved in assessing the fetal heart rate (FHR) using external and internal electronic fetal monitoring (EFM). To help you understand the dynamics of fetal monitoring, the chapter reviews the physiology of labor. Then it describes the equipment, preparation, and procedures used in both forms of EFM; explains how to interpret fetal monitor strips; and describes related nursing considerations.

Physiology of labor

During normal labor, the mother's regular rhythmic contractions cause cervical dilation and effacement, eventually leading to fetal descent through the pelvis. (See *Cervical effacement and dilation*.) The cardinal movements of labor, a series of positional changes, propel the fetus through the pelvis during the first and second stages of labor. (See *Cardinal movements of labor*, pages 152 and 153.)

Mild contractions occurring 5 to 20 minutes apart and lasting 30 to 40 seconds signal the start of the first stage of labor. This stage can last as long as 8 hours. As labor progresses, contractions typically increase in frequency, intensity, and duration. By the end of the first stage, approaching complete cervical dilation, contractions occur every 2 minutes and last 60 to 90 seconds. During the second stage, which culminates in delivery, contractions space out to every 3 to 4 minutes but still last 60 to 90 seconds. The patient may push with each contraction.

Although each contraction affects the fetus, a healthy fetus with normal oxygen reserves can tolerate normal contractions. However, certain factors can impair oxygen transport from mother to fetus and carbon dioxide removal from the fetal circulation. For example, maternal hypotension or hypertension, uterine hypertonus (minimal or absent resting tone of the uterus), and umbilical cord compression can lead to fetal hypoxia and eventually acidosis if not reversed or controlled. These conditions can be identified from the FHR pattern.

Maternal hypotension may impair blood flow to the uterus by reducing blood return to the heart. During labor, hypotension can result from a dorsal recumbent position. In this position, the uterus compresses the great vessels, especially the aorta and inferior vena cava. This reduces blood return to the heart, which leads to decreased cardiac output. As a result, the uterus receives less blood and placental perfusion diminishes.

In contrast, pregnancy-induced hypertension and chronic maternal hypertension increase vascular resistance, which may directly reduce blood flow to the uterus.

Uterine hypertonus directly increases intrauterine pressure, thereby reducing the uterine blood flow and jeopardizing the fetal blood supply and oxygenation. Causes of uterine hypertonus include uterine distention, multiple gestation, polyhydramnios, and oxytocin hyperstimulation.

In nearly 5% of labors, the umbilical cord is wrapped around the fetus's neck or another body part. Such cord compression may temporarily reduce blood flow and oxygen supply to the fetus.

Performing electronic fetal monitoring

When used properly, EFM is probably the most reliable method currently in use for assessing fetal status. External EFM is performed routinely at most hospitals. Internal EFM, a far more invasive and more complex procedure, is generally used only when external EFM yields inconclusive results, or when the health care team needs more information about the condition of the fetus or its mother. Several high-risk factors may warrant continuous EFM (see *Indications for electronic fetal monitoring*, page 154).

Although the indications and techniques for external and internal EFM differ, both forms of monitoring have the same goal: to detect potentially dangerous abnormalities early. To perform EFM reliably, you need to know how to set up and use the equipment, interpret a fetal monitor strip, and intervene quickly and appropriately if necessary.

External EFM

A noninvasive procedure, external (indirect) EFM uses two devices strapped to the patient's abdomen. One device evaluates the FHR; the other detects uterine contractions. In high-risk pregnancies, external EFM provides critical in-

Cervical effacement and dilation

As labor begins and uterine contractions intensify, the cervix effaces and dilates. Effacement — progressive thinning and shortening of the vaginal portion of the cervix — is measured as a percentage from 0% to 100%. Dilation — progressive enlargement of the cervical os — is measured from 0 to 10 cm. A primigravid patient usually experiences effacement first, then dilation, as shown below. A multigravid patient experiences both simultaneously.

Before labor

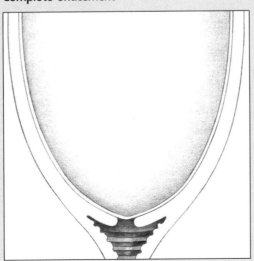

Early effacement

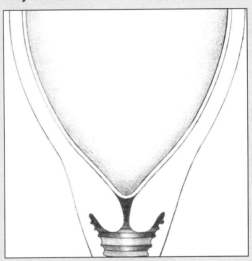

Complete effacement

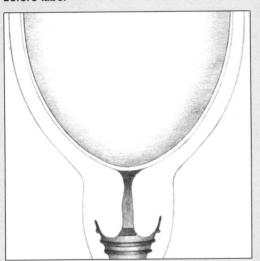

Complete dilation

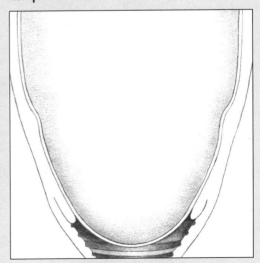

Cardinal movements of labor

During labor, the fetus progresses through a series of positional changes as it passes through the pelvis: engagement, descent, flexion, internal rotation, extension, external rotation (restitution and shoulder rotation), and expulsion. These illustrations show the fetus in each position; each inset shows the fetal presenting part at the corresponding stage.

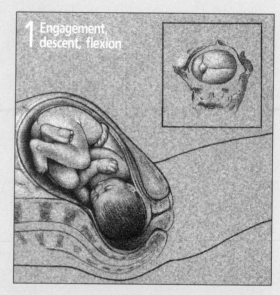

1 Engagement, descent, flexion

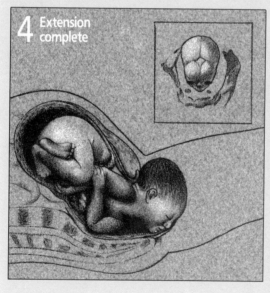

4 Extension complete

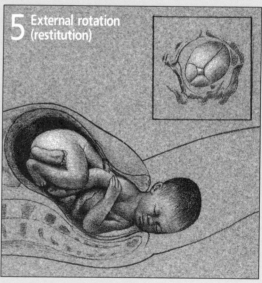

5 External rotation (restitution)

formation about fetal status during the antenatal period. The more advanced external EFM devices can monitor twins simultaneously.

Indications for external EFM include high-risk pregnancy and oxytocin-induced labor. However, many labor and delivery units use external EFM for all patients. EFM also is used for the nonstress test and the nipple stimulation contraction stress test (used to assess fetal well-being during the antenatal period).

External EFM has certain disadvantages. For instance, it may be difficult to perform on

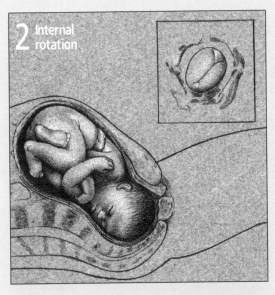

2 Internal rotation

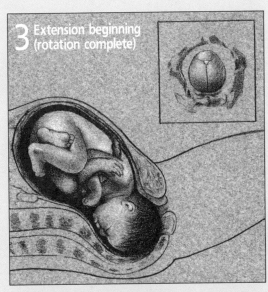

3 Extension beginning (rotation complete)

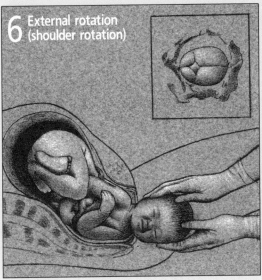

6 External rotation (shoulder rotation)

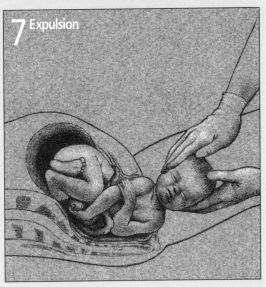

7 Expulsion

patients or patients with polyhydram-
ind on hyperactive or premature fetuses.
ionitoring belts may be uncomfortable
iually must be adjusted when the patient
es position. Also, the patient can't move
much during monitoring because the belt cables are hooked to the monitor.

The monitor may make counting errors
when the FHR falls below 60 beats/minute.
Conversely, with an accelerated FHR
(200 beats/minute or faster), the monitor

Indications for electronic fetal monitoring

For many patients, electronic fetal monitoring (EFM) offers advantages over other monitoring methods, such as fetal heart rate auscultation and uterine palpation. The following high-risk maternal and fetal factors typically call for continuous EFM.

Maternal factors
Preexisting factors
• Cardiac disease
• Diabetes
• Hypertension
• Pregnancy-induced hypertension
• Previous stillbirth
• Renal disease

Pregnancy factors
• Amnionitis
• Hydramnios or oligohydramnios
• Postterm labor
• Premature rupture of the membranes
• Preterm labor
• Third-trimester bleeding

Labor factors
• Failure of labor to progress
• Induction or augmentation of labor
• Multiple gestation (more than one fetus)
• Regional anesthesia

Fetal factors
• Abnormal heart rate on auscultation
• Intrauterine growth retardation
• Meconium staining
• Rh disease

derstand the factors that can affect the uteroplacental unit. In addition, you must know how to identify FHR tracings that indicate fetal hypoxia.

Internal EFM

Also called direct fetal monitoring, this sterile, invasive procedure uses a spiral electrode and an intrauterine catheter to evaluate fetal status during labor. By providing an electrocardiogram (ECG) of the FHR, internal EFM assesses fetal response to uterine contractions more accurately than does external EFM. It precisely measures intrauterine pressure, tracks labor progress, and allows evaluation of short- and long-term FHR variability.

Internal EFM is indicated whenever direct, beat-to-beat FHR monitoring is required. Specific indications include maternal diabetes or hypertension, fetal postmaturity, suspected intrauterine growth retardation, and meconium-stained fluid. However, internal EFM is performed only if the amniotic sac has ruptured, the cervix is dilated at least 2 cm, and the presenting part of the fetus is at least at the −1 station. (See *Understanding fetal station.*)

Contraindications for internal EFM include maternal blood dyscrasias, suspected fetal immune deficiency, placenta previa, face presentation or uncertainty about the presenting part, and cervical or vaginal herpetic lesions.

Maternal complications of internal EFM may include uterine perforation and intrauterine infection. Fetal complications may include abscess, hematoma, and infection.

Equipment
External EFM
This technnique uses an ultrasound transducer and a pressure-sensitive tocotransducer. The ultrasound transducer transmits high-frequency sound waves through soft tissues to the fetal heart. The waves rebound from the heart through the abdominal wall, where the transducer receives them. The transducer then relays the sound waves to a fetal monitor, which translates them into both a signal and a tracing on the monitor strip.

counts only half the beats. Also, a high incidence of artifact with external EFM may render tracings illegible or inaccurate.

Although external EFM provides valuable information, you shouldn't rely solely on this technology. Check EFM results by auscultating the FHR, particularly if you know of any potential interfering factors. Also, keep in mind that to perform external EFM properly and interpret the results successfully, you need to un-

PHYSIOLOGY

Understanding fetal station

Fetal station refers to the relationship of the fetal presenting part to the maternal ischial spine. Fetal station is measured in centimeters, from − 5 to + 5. When the largest diameter of the presenting part is level with the ischial spine, the fetus is at station 0. Numbers from 1 to 5 reflect how many centimeters the presenting part of the fetus is above or below the ischial spine.

A presenting part above the ischial spine is designated from − 1 to − 5. A presenting part below this point is classified from + 1 to + 5. Successful vaginal delivery requires progressive fetal descent from a minus station to 0 and then to a plus station during labor.

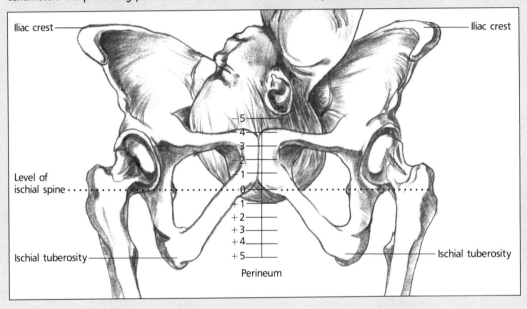

The pressure-sensitive tocotransducer monitors labor by responding to pressure exerted by uterine contractions and simultaneously recording their duration and frequency. The monitoring apparatus traces FHR and uterine contraction data onto the same printout paper.

Internal EFM
A spiral electrode is the most commonly used device for internal EFM. Shaped like a corkscrew, the electrode is attached to the presenting fetal part (usually the scalp). It detects the fetal heartbeat and then transmits it to the monitor, which converts the signals to a fetal ECG waveform.

A pressure-sensitive catheter, called an Intran catheter, though not as widely used as the tocotransducer, is the most accurate method of determining the true intensity of contractions. It's particularly helpful in dysfunctional labor and in preventing or rapidly determining the need for a cesarean section. The potential for infection or uterine perforation associated with this device is high, however.

Preparation
Before external or internal EFM, make sure that the patient is fully informed about the procedure, and obtain a signed consent form. You'll then need to prepare both the patient and the monitoring equipment.

External EFM

Describe the entire procedure to the patient and her partner, if present, and explain how the equipment works. Reassure them that the monitoring device won't harm the fetus.

Ask the patient to empty her bladder. Provide privacy and wash your hands. Then help her into a semi-Fowler or left lateral position, and expose her abdomen. *Don't let her lie supine* because pressure from the gravid uterus on the inferior vena cava may cause maternal hypotension, leading to decreased uterine perfusion and possible fetal hypoxia.

Explain to the patient and her partner how to use the monitor's printout to time and prepare for contractions. Explain that the distance from one dark vertical line to the next on the printout grid represents 1 minute. By knowing how often contractions are occurring, the patient's partner can prepare the patient for the onset of new contractions and can guide and slow her breathing as each contraction subsides.

Gather the necessary equipment, including an electronic fetal monitor, an ultrasound transducer, and a tocotransducer. Also obtain ultrasound conduction gel, two abdominal belts, and graph paper. Because fetal monitor features vary in type and complexity, you should review the operator's manual before proceeding.

If the monitor has two paper speeds, select the slower speed (typically 3 cm/minute) to ensure an easy-to-read tracing. At higher speeds — for example, 1 cm/minute — the printed tracings are more condensed, making results harder to decipher and interpret accurately.

Internal EFM

Describe the procedure to the patient and her partner, if present, and explain how the equipment works. Tell the patient that a doctor or specially trained nurse will perform a vaginal examination to identify the position of the fetus.

Gather the necessary equipment. Besides an electronic fetal monitor, you'll need a spiral electrode and a drive tube, a disposable leg plate pad or reusable leg plate with Velcro belt, conduction gel, antiseptic solution, hypoallergenic tape, two pairs of sterile gloves, an Intran catheter connection cable and pressure-sensitive catheter, graph paper, and an operator's manual. Be sure to review the operator's manual before using the equipment.

If the monitor has two paper speeds, set it at 3 cm/minute to ensure a readable tracing. A tracing at 1 cm/minute is more condensed and harder to interpret accurately.

Connect the Intran cable to the uterine activity outlet on the monitor. Wash your hands and open the sterile equipment, maintaining aseptic technique.

Procedure

The procedures for external and internal EFM differ significantly. Make sure that you're familiar with each.

External EFM

• Palpate the patient's abdomen to locate the fundus, the area of greatest muscle density in the uterus, where contractions occur. (See *Palpating uterine contractions.*)

• Using Leopold's maneuvers, palpate the fetal back, where fetal heart tones are most audible. (See *Performing Leopold's maneuvers,* pages 158 and 159.)

• Plug the tocotransducer cable into the uterine activity jack, and plug the ultrasound transducer cable into the phono-ultrasound jack. Attach the abdominal belts to the tocotransducer and to the ultrasound transducer.

• Secure the transducer over the site where the fetal heartbeat is loudest, and secure the tocotransducer over the fundus. (See *Applying an external electronic fetal monitor,* page 160.)

• Apply conduction gel to the ultrasound transducer crystals to promote an airtight seal and ensure optimal sound-wave transmission.

• Adjust the pen set tracer controls so that the baseline values on the monitor strip read between 5 and 15 mm Hg. This prevents triggering the alarm that indicates the tracer has dropped below the paper's margins. The proper setting varies among tocotransducers.

• Label the printout paper with the patient's hospital number or name and birthdate, the date, maternal vital signs and position, the pa-

Palpating uterine contractions

To palpate your patient's uterine contractions, locate the fundus by finding the area of greatest muscle density in the uterus. Then place the palmar surface of your fingers there and palpate lightly.

When palpating contractions, note that each contraction has three phases: increment (building up) phase, acme (peak) phase, and decrement (letting down) phase. Palpate during several contractions, determining the frequency, duration, and intensity of each one. You'll feel the uterine tightening and abdominal lifting that accompany each contraction.

To assess the frequency of contractions, time the period from the beginning of one contraction to the beginning of the next. To evaluate duration, time the period from the onset of uterine tightening to its relaxation.

While the uterus is tightened, determine the intensity of the contraction by pressing your fingertips into the fundus. During mild contractions, the fundus indents easily and feels like a chin. In moderate contractions, it doesn't indent as easily and feels more pointed, like the tip of a nose. With strong contractions, the fundus is firm, resists indenting, and feels like a forehead.

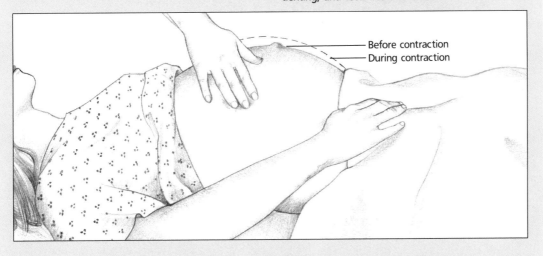

Before contraction
During contraction

per speed, and the number on the monitor strip. This helps ensure accurate, consecutive monitoring records. If the patient vomits, changes position, or is restless or agitated, document this on both her flow sheet and the monitor's printout paper. If she receives any drugs, has a vaginal examination, or has her blood pressure taken, indicate this on both as well.

• Make a mental note of the baseline FHR. Normally, FHR ranges from 120 to 160 beats/minute.

• Assess periodic accelerations or decelerations from the baseline FHR. Then compare FHR patterns with uterine contraction patterns. Note the timing of a deceleration relative to the onset of a uterine contraction, and the timing of the lowest level of a deceleration relative to the peak of a contraction. Also note the range of deceleration. These data can help you distinguish fetal distress from benign head compression.

• Move the ultrasound transducer and the tocotransducer to accommodate any changes in maternal or fetal position. Readjust both devices periodically, and assess the patient's skin for reddened areas caused by pressure from the abdominal belt. Also, document her skin condition.

• Clean the ultrasound transducer periodically

Performing Leopold's maneuvers

You can determine fetal position by performing Leopold's maneuvers. First ask the patient to empty her bladder; then assist her to a supine position and expose her abdomen. Perform the four maneuvers in the order described here.

First maneuver
Facing the patient, warm your hands and place them on her abdomen to determine fetal position in the uterine fundus. Curl your fingers around the fundus. With the fetus in vertex position, you'll feel the buttocks—irregularly shaped and firm. With the fetus in breech position, you'll feel the head—hard, round, and movable.

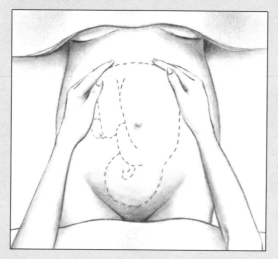

Second maneuver
Move your hands down the sides of the abdomen and apply gentle pressure. If the fetus lies in vertex position, you'll feel a smooth, hard surface on one side—the fetus's back. On the other side, you'll feel lumps and knobs—the knees, hands, feet, and elbows. If the fetus lies in breech position, you may not feel the back at all.

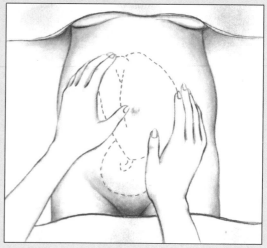

with a damp cloth to remove any dried conduction gel, which can interfere with ultrasound transmission and readings. Apply fresh gel as necessary.
• Handle equipment carefully to avoid dropping or banging transducers. Clean and store transducers according to department policy or the operating manual.
• Clean or discard abdominal belts before the next patient's use, according to department policy.

Internal EFM
Label the printout paper with the patient's hospital number or name and birthdate, the date, the paper speed, and the number on the monitor strip.

Monitoring uterine contractions. Follow these steps to monitor contractions.
• Assist the patient into the lithotomy position for a vaginal examination. The doctor puts on sterile gloves. *Note:* You may do this procedure if you're specially trained.
• Attach the connection cable to the appropriate outlet on the monitor marked UA (uterine activity). Connect the cable to the Intran catheter. Next, zero the catheter with a gauge provided on the distal end of the catheter. This will help determine the resting tone of the

Third maneuver

Spread apart the thumb and fingers of your hand, and place them just above the symphysis pubis. Then bring your fingers together. If the fetus lies in vertex position and hasn't descended, you'll feel the head. If the fetus lies in vertex position and has descended, you'll feel a less distinct mass.

Fourth maneuver

Use this maneuver in late pregnancy. Place your hands on both sides of the lower abdomen. Apply gentle pressure with your fingers as you slide your hands downward toward the symphysis pubis. If the head presents, one hand's descent will be stopped by the cephalic prominence; the other hand will be unobstructed.

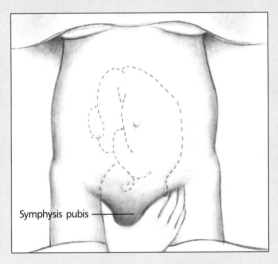

Symphysis pubis

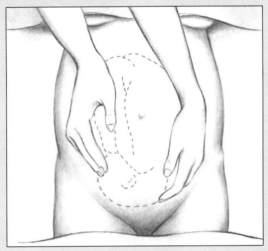

uterus, usually 5 to 15 mm Hg.

• Cover the patient's perineum with a sterile drape, if hospital policy so dictates. Then clean the perineum with antiseptic solution, according to hospital policy. Using aseptic technique, the doctor inserts the catheter into the uterine cavity while performing a vaginal examination. The catheter is advanced to the black line on the catheter and secured with hypoallergenic tape along the inner thigh.

• Observe the monitoring strip to verify proper placement of the catheter guide and to ensure a clear tracing. Periodically evaluate the monitoring strip to determine the exact amount of pressure exerted with each contraction. Note all such data on the monitoring strip and on the patient's care record.

• The Intran catheter is usually removed during the second stage of labor or at the doctor's discretion. Dispose of the catheter, and clean and store the cable according to hospital policy. (See *Applying an internal electronic fetal monitor,* page 161.)

Monitoring FHR. Follow these steps to monitor FHR.

• Apply conduction gel to the leg plate. Then secure the leg plate to the patient's inner thigh with Velcro straps or 2″ tape. Connect the leg

(Text continues on page 162.)

Applying an external electronic fetal monitor

External electronic fetal monitoring evaluates the fetal heart rate (FHR) using ultrasound and detects uterine contractions with a tocotransducer. To apply an external electronic fetal monitor, follow these steps.

Ultrasound transducer

Position the ultrasound transducer over the fetus's heart and tighten the abdominal belt. Verify the location by the tracing on the fetal heart monitor strip.

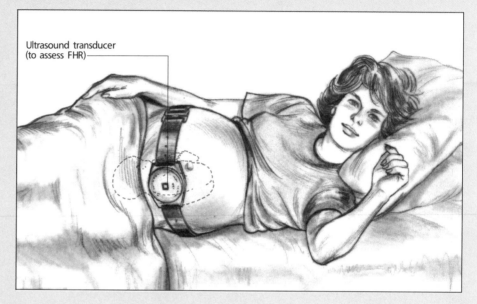

Ultrasound transducer (to assess FHR)

Tocotransducer

Place the tocotransducer over the uterine fundus where it contracts, either midline or slightly to one side. Place your hand on the fundus, and palpate for a contraction to verify proper placement. Secure the tocotransducer with its abdominal belt.

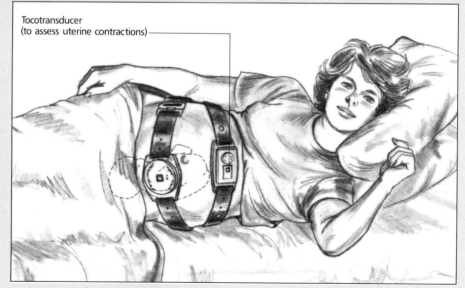

Tocotransducer (to assess uterine contractions)

Applying an internal electronic fetal monitor

During internal electronic fetal monitoring, a spiral electrode monitors the fetal heart rate (FHR) and an internal catheter monitors uterine contractions.

Monitoring FHR

The spiral electrode is inserted after a vaginal examination that determines the position of the fetus. As shown at right, the electrode is attached to the presenting fetal part, usually the scalp or buttocks.

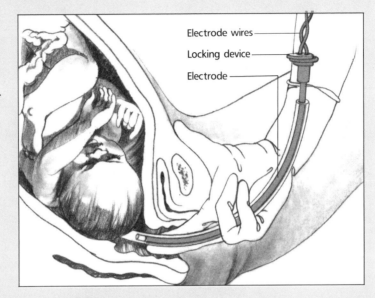

Electrode wires
Locking device
Electrode

Monitoring uterine contractions

The intrauterine catheter is inserted up to a premarked level on the tubing and then connected to a monitor that interprets uterine contraction pressures.

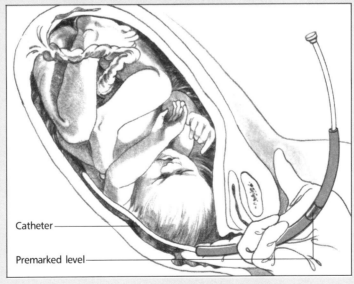

Catheter
Premarked level

plate cable to the ECG outlet on the monitor.
• Tell the patient she'll have a vaginal examination to identify the fetal presenting part (usually the scalp or buttocks) and determine its level of descent, and to apply the electrode. Explain that this examination ensures against attaching the electrode to fetal suture lines, fontanels, face, or genitalia. The spiral electrode will be placed in a drive tube and advanced through the vagina to the fetal presenting part. To secure the electrode, mild pressure will be applied and the drive tube turned clockwise 360 degrees.
• After the electrode is in place and the drive tube has been removed, connect the color-coded electrode wires to the corresponding color-coded leg plate posts.
• Turn on the recorder. Note the time on the printout paper.
• Assist the patient to a comfortable position, and evaluate the strip to verify proper placement and a clear FHR tracing.

Monitoring the patient. Begin by noting the frequency, duration, and intensity of uterine contractions. Normal intrauterine pressure ranges from 8 to 12 mm Hg. (See *Reading a fetal monitor strip.*) Then follow these steps.
• Check the baseline FHR. Assess periodic accelerations or decelerations from the baseline FHR.
• Compare the FHR pattern with the uterine contraction pattern. Note the interval between the onset of an FHR deceleration and the onset of a uterine contraction; the interval between the lowest level of an FHR deceleration and the peak of a uterine contraction; and the range of FHR deceleration.
• Check for FHR variability, which is a measure of fetal oxygen reserve and neurologic integrity and stability.

Interpretation of findings
Use the baseline FHR—the starting point for all fetal assessments—as a reference point for all subsequent readings. To obtain the baseline FHR, observe the FHR tracing for 5 to 10 minutes when the patient isn't in labor, when the fetus isn't moving, between uterine contractions, when no fetal stimulation is taking place

(for example, from vaginal examination or electrode application), or during the interval between periodic changes (transient accelerations or decelerations). The tracing should register 120 to 160 beats/minute.

Variations from the baseline FHR include bradycardia, tachycardia, and increased or decreased variability. Other FHR deviations are called *periodic changes* and *nonperiodic changes*. Notify the doctor immediately if the FHR changes significantly from the baseline, especially during or immediately after a contraction. Usually, signs of fetal distress immediately follow a contraction. (See *Identifying baseline FHR irregularities,* pages 164 to 166.)

Baseline tachycardia
In this irregular heart rate, the FHR remains above 160 beats/minute for at least 10 minutes. Fetal tachycardia may result from maternal or fetal fever, chronic fetal hypoxia and acidosis, fetal hypovolemia, or a maternal metabolic disorder (such as hyperthyroidism). Certain drugs used by the mother, including parasympathetic agents (for example, atropine and scopolamine) and beta-adrenergics (for example, ritodrine and terbutaline) can also cause baseline tachycardia.

Baseline bradycardia
Defined as an FHR below 120 beats/minute for at least 10 minutes, baseline bradycardia may be benign if the FHR shows normal beat-to-beat variability with no late decelerations. However, when accompanied by late decelerations and minimal or absent variability, baseline bradycardia is an ominous sign of advanced fetal distress from hypoxia and acidosis. Congenital heart block, a rare defect, produces baseline bradycardia of 60 to 80 beats/minute; a fetus with heart block must be delivered in a hospital where cardiac surgery can be performed.

Variability
The most important indicator in assessing fetal well-being, variability results from interaction of the sympathetic nervous system, which speeds up the FHR, and the parasympathetic nervous system, which slows down the FHR.

Reading a fetal monitor strip

Presented in two parallel recordings, the fetal monitor strip records the fetal heart rate (FHR) in beats per minute in the top recording and uterine activity in millimeters of mercury (mm Hg) in the bottom recording. You can obtain information about fetal status and labor progress by reading the strips horizontally and vertically.

Reading horizontally on the FHR or uterine activity strip, note that each small block represents 10 seconds. Six consecutive small blocks, separated by a dark vertical line, represent 1 minute. Reading vertically on the FHR strip, note that each block represents an amplitude of 10 beats/minute. Reading vertically on the uterine activity strip, you'll see that each block represents 5 mm Hg of pressure.

Assess the baseline FHR—the resting heart rate—between uterine contractions when fetal movement diminishes. Normally between 120 and 160 beats/minute, the baseline FHR pattern serves as a reference for subsequent FHR tracings produced during contractions.

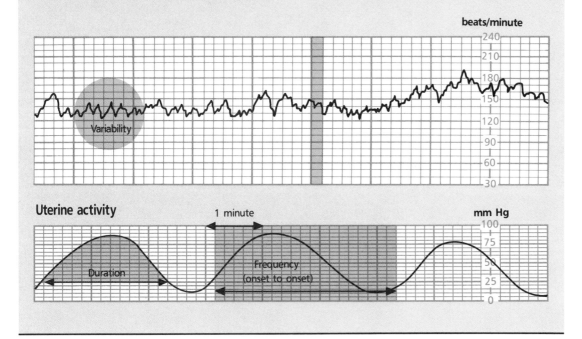

Variability has two components—long-term and short-term. *Long-term variability* refers to the larger periodic and rhythmic deviations above and below the baseline FHR. Normal long-term variability ranges from 5 to 20 beats/minute in rhythmic fluctuations of three to five times per minute.

Short-term variability refers to differences in successive heartbeats, as measured by the R-R interval of the QRS complex on the ECG waveform. It represents actual beat-to-beat FHR fluctuations and the balance between the sympathetic and parasympathetic nervous systems. Short-term variability is classified as present or absent. Normal short-term variability, 2 to 3 beats/minute, is considered the most reliable single indicator of fetal well-being.

Periodic changes
Caused by uterine contractions and fetal movements, periodic changes include transient accelerations or decelerations from the baseline FHR. They represent normal rhythmic fluctua-

(Text continues on page 166.)

Identifying baseline FHR irregularities

IRREGULARITY	POSSIBLE CAUSES	CLINICAL SIGNIFICANCE	NURSING INTERVENTIONS
Baseline tachycardia beats/minute 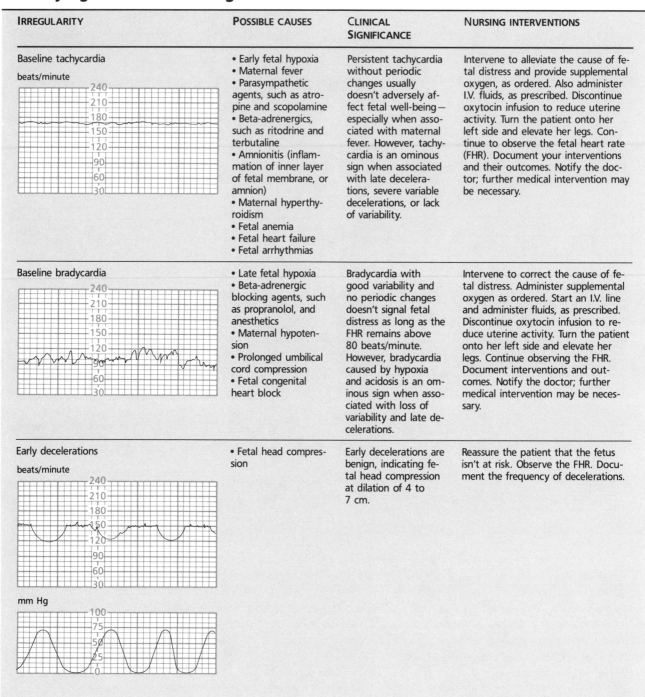	• Early fetal hypoxia • Maternal fever • Parasympathetic agents, such as atropine and scopolamine • Beta-adrenergics, such as ritodrine and terbutaline • Amnionitis (inflammation of inner layer of fetal membrane, or amnion) • Maternal hyperthyroidism • Fetal anemia • Fetal heart failure • Fetal arrhythmias	Persistent tachycardia without periodic changes usually doesn't adversely affect fetal well-being—especially when associated with maternal fever. However, tachycardia is an ominous sign when associated with late decelerations, severe variable decelerations, or lack of variability.	Intervene to alleviate the cause of fetal distress and provide supplemental oxygen, as ordered. Also administer I.V. fluids, as prescribed. Discontinue oxytocin infusion to reduce uterine activity. Turn the patient onto her left side and elevate her legs. Continue to observe the fetal heart rate (FHR). Document your interventions and their outcomes. Notify the doctor; further medical intervention may be necessary.
Baseline bradycardia 240 210 180 150 120 90 60 30	• Late fetal hypoxia • Beta-adrenergic blocking agents, such as propranolol, and anesthetics • Maternal hypotension • Prolonged umbilical cord compression • Fetal congenital heart block	Bradycardia with good variability and no periodic changes doesn't signal fetal distress as long as the FHR remains above 80 beats/minute. However, bradycardia caused by hypoxia and acidosis is an ominous sign when associated with loss of variability and late decelerations.	Intervene to correct the cause of fetal distress. Administer supplemental oxygen as ordered. Start an I.V. line and administer fluids, as prescribed. Discontinue oxytocin infusion to reduce uterine activity. Turn the patient onto her left side and elevate her legs. Continue observing the FHR. Document interventions and outcomes. Notify the doctor; further medical intervention may be necessary.
Early decelerations beats/minute 240 210 180 150 120 90 60 30 mm Hg 100 75 50 25 0	• Fetal head compression	Early decelerations are benign, indicating fetal head compression at dilation of 4 to 7 cm.	Reassure the patient that the fetus isn't at risk. Observe the FHR. Document the frequency of decelerations.

Identifying baseline FHR irregularities *(continued)*

IRREGULARITY	POSSIBLE CAUSES	CLINICAL SIGNIFICANCE	NURSING INTERVENTIONS
Late decelerations 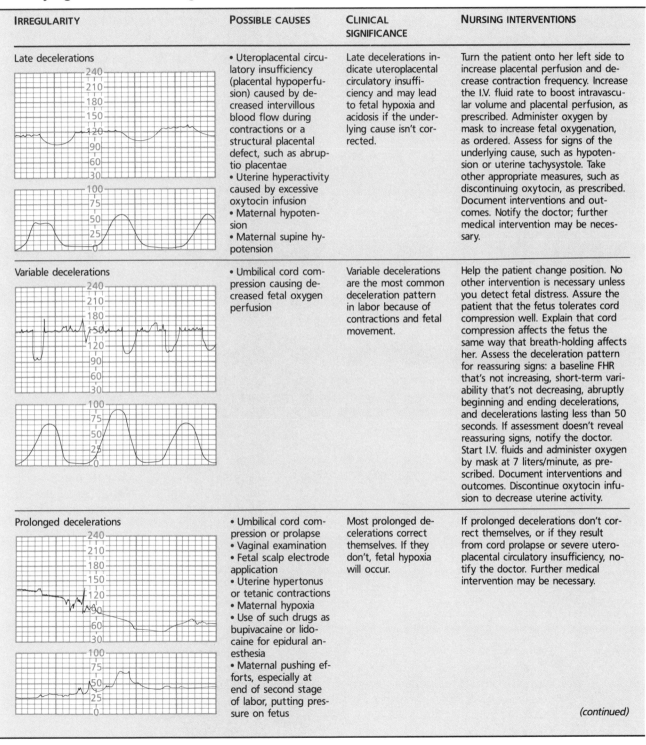	• Uteroplacental circulatory insufficiency (placental hypoperfusion) caused by decreased intervillous blood flow during contractions or a structural placental defect, such as abruptio placentae • Uterine hyperactivity caused by excessive oxytocin infusion • Maternal hypotension • Maternal supine hypotension	Late decelerations indicate uteroplacental circulatory insufficiency and may lead to fetal hypoxia and acidosis if the underlying cause isn't corrected.	Turn the patient onto her left side to increase placental perfusion and decrease contraction frequency. Increase the I.V. fluid rate to boost intravascular volume and placental perfusion, as prescribed. Administer oxygen by mask to increase fetal oxygenation, as ordered. Assess for signs of the underlying cause, such as hypotension or uterine tachysystole. Take other appropriate measures, such as discontinuing oxytocin, as prescribed. Document interventions and outcomes. Notify the doctor; further medical intervention may be necessary.
Variable decelerations	• Umbilical cord compression causing decreased fetal oxygen perfusion	Variable decelerations are the most common deceleration pattern in labor because of contractions and fetal movement.	Help the patient change position. No other intervention is necessary unless you detect fetal distress. Assure the patient that the fetus tolerates cord compression well. Explain that cord compression affects the fetus the same way that breath-holding affects her. Assess the deceleration pattern for reassuring signs: a baseline FHR that's not increasing, short-term variability that's not decreasing, abruptly beginning and ending decelerations, and decelerations lasting less than 50 seconds. If assessment doesn't reveal reassuring signs, notify the doctor. Start I.V. fluids and administer oxygen by mask at 7 liters/minute, as prescribed. Document interventions and outcomes. Discontinue oxytocin infusion to decrease uterine activity.
Prolonged decelerations	• Umbilical cord compression or prolapse • Vaginal examination • Fetal scalp electrode application • Uterine hypertonus or tetanic contractions • Maternal hypoxia • Use of such drugs as bupivacaine or lidocaine for epidural anesthesia • Maternal pushing efforts, especially at end of second stage of labor, putting pressure on fetus	Most prolonged decelerations correct themselves. If they don't, fetal hypoxia will occur.	If prolonged decelerations don't correct themselves, or if they result from cord prolapse or severe uteroplacental circulatory insufficiency, notify the doctor. Further medical intervention may be necessary.

(continued)

Identifying baseline FHR irregularities (continued)

IRREGULARITY	POSSIBLE CAUSES	CLINICAL SIGNIFICANCE	NURSING INTERVENTIONS
Mixed patterns	• Same as for early, late, variable, and prolonged decelerations	Same as for early, late, variable, and prolonged decelerations.	Turn the patient onto her left side or place her in Trendelenburg's position, with legs elevated. Administer oxygen by mask, as ordered. Discontinue oxytocin infusion to reduce uterine activity. Increase the I.V. infusion rate to boost perfusion of intervillous placental spaces. Continue to observe the FHR. Document interventions and outcomes. Notify the doctor; further medical intervention may be necessary.

tions from the fetal resting pulse. Accelerations that are uniform in shape and timing usually signal fetal well-being and adequate oxygen reserve. Accelerations may also stem from partial umbilical cord compression.

Periodic decelerations from a normal baseline FHR are classified as early, late, or variable, depending on when they occur and on their waveform shape.

Early decelerations. Signaling fetal head compression, early decelerations have a uniform shape and appear as mirror images of contractions on the waveform. Reflecting an intact vagal response to increased intracranial pressure, these benign variations have no pathologic significance. Fetal head compression may result from uterine contractions, vaginal examinations, fundal pressure, or internal electrode placement.

Late decelerations. These patterns begin at or after the peak of a uterine contraction. The waveform resembles that of an early deceleration: Descent and return are smooth and gradual, and no accelerations appear. Late decelerations are usually accompanied by loss of variability with a rising baseline FHR or tachycardia. Usually repetitive, they typically occur with

each contraction; however, in some cases, they occur only with stronger contractions.

Late decelerations are caused by uteroplacental circulatory insufficiency, which leads to inadequate oxygen exchange and fetal hypoxia and acidosis. Factors that contribute to late decelerations include advanced maternal age, maternal supine hypotension, chronic maternal hypotension, pregnancy-induced hypertension, maternal cardiac disease, maternal diabetes, maternal anemia, fetal postmaturity, intrauterine growth retardation, placenta previa, abruptio placentae, conduction anesthetics, and uterine hyperstimulation from oxytocin augmentation or induction.

Late decelerations are a sign of a potentially difficult or dangerous pregnancy and warrant immediate interventions. If interventions fail, cesarean delivery or another medical intervention may be necessary.

Variable decelerations. The most common pattern during labor, variable decelerations can occur at any time during the uterine contracting phase. Characterized by irregular waveform shape, they vary in depth, duration, and timing.

Essentially benign, variable decelerations can be mild, moderate, or severe. They result from umbilical cord compression, as occurs from a supine maternal position; wrapping of the cord around the fetus's neck, leg, arm, or other body part; or a short, knotted, or prolapsed cord.

A reassuring variable pattern has an abrupt onset and end. The baseline FHR doesn't increase and short-term variability doesn't decrease.

A nonreassuring variable pattern includes signs of hypoxemia. Variability increases initially but the baseline FHR remains within normal limits. Eventually, however, the FHR accelerates to a baseline tachycardia as the fetus tries to compensate for the growing oxygen deficit. Hypoxia becomes more evident as variability decreases. The variable decelerations may take on a more rounded shape, and the onset and end grow smoother, indicating adverse effects on the central nervous system.

Although common, variable decelerations shouldn't be ignored because fetal reserves vary considerably. One fetus may tolerate severe variable decelerations, whereas another may be unable to cope with even mild variable decelerations. Most variable decelerations can be corrected by changing maternal position. If they persist, further intervention may be necessary.

Nonperiodic changes

Prolonged decelerations, variable decelerations between contractions, and spontaneous accelerations may occur at any time during labor and aren't always associated with contractions. Sinusoidal and pseudosinusoidal patterns — two unusual FHR patterns — are also considered nonperiodic changes.

Prolonged decelerations. Generally isolated incidents linked with sudden vagal stimulation, prolonged decelerations vary in shape and may occur at any time during labor. Typically, they last from 2 to 10 minutes.

Causes of prolonged decelerations include umbilical cord compression or prolapse, vaginal examination, fetal scalp electrode application, uterine hypertonus, tetanic contractions, maternal hypoxia, or use of such drugs as bupivacaine or lidocaine for epidural anesthesia. Especially at the end of the second stage of labor,

the mother's pushing efforts may put pressure on the fetus, causing prolonged decelerations.

When the cause is removed or corrected, prolonged decelerations typically correct themselves within 10 minutes, giving the fetus time to recover. However, if prolonged decelerations result from cord prolapse or severe uteroplacental circulatory insufficiency, cesarean delivery or another medical intervention will probably be necessary.

Spontaneous accelerations. These changes are accompanied by fetal movement, although the mother may not always feel it. A "spike" on the uterine activity monitor strip recorded 1 to 3 seconds before a spontaneous acceleration may signal fetal movement. These spikes may be recurring and indicate an adequate fetal oxygen reserve.

Mixed patterns. Combinations of early, late, and variable decelerations may occur.

Sinusoidal pattern. A rare but potentially ominous FHR pattern, a sinusoidal pattern usually results from fetal anemia, a fetal-maternal bleed, or Rh isoimmunization.

A sinusoidal pattern produces a highly distinctive waveform pattern that's smooth and undulating, with no short-term variability and with a cycle frequency of 4 to 8 beats/minute. Don't confuse a true sinusoidal pattern with a pseudosinusoidal pattern, characterized by an irregular waveform pattern and short-term variability. A pseudosinusoidal pattern requires no medical intervention, but a sinusoidal pattern requires immediate delivery by cesarean section.

Nursing considerations

• Make sure that the patient and her partner understand the purpose of EFM, and allow time for their questions.
• Apply monitoring belts snugly to ensure accurate monitoring, but make sure that they're not so tight that they're uncomfortable.
• Interpret the FHR and uterine contractions at regular intervals. Guidelines of the Association of Women's Health, Obstetric, and Neonatal Nurses specify that high-risk patients need

Sampling fetal scalp blood

If the health care team suspects fetal hypoxia, a fetal scalp blood sampling test may be performed to evaluate fetal acid-base status.

Before fetal scalp blood sampling can be performed, the patient's cervix must be dilated 2 to 3 cm and her membranes must have ruptured. The fetal presenting part should be reasonably immobile. The doctor or a nurse-midwife inserts an endoscopic tube equipped with a light source into the patient's cervix. As shown in the illustration below, a blade device cuts the fetus's scalp to obtain a blood sample. A pH test is then performed in the hospital laboratory.

Indications

Fetal scalp blood sampling is performed when fetal monitoring reveals a periodic pattern of repetitive late decelerations or repetitive moderate to severe variable decelerations, or a pattern of persistent tachycardia or bradycardia with absent or minimal variability. The results of fetal scalp blood sampling can determine the need for emergency cesarean delivery.

Implications of findings

A normal pH (7.25 to 7.35) requires no further intervention. When the test reveals an abnormal pH (7.20 to 7.24), it should be repeated in 20 minutes. An emergency cesarean delivery should be performed when the pH test reveals acidosis (a reading less than 7.20).

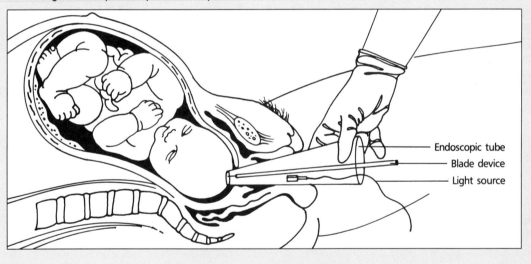

Endoscopic tube
Blade device
Light source

continuous FHR monitoring, whereas low-risk patients should have the FHR auscultated every 30 minutes after a contraction during the first stage and every 15 minutes after a contraction during the second stage. Many obstetricians request continuous external EFM for all patients because high-risk patients may be hard to identify.

First determine the baseline FHR within 10 beats/minute; then assess the degree of baseline variability. Note the presence or absence of short-term or long-term variability. Identify periodic FHR changes, such as decelerations (early, late, variable, or mixed) or nonperiodic changes such as a sinusoidal pattern.

• Keep in mind that acute fetal distress can result from any change in the baseline FHR that causes fetal compromise. If necessary, take steps to counteract FHR changes. First, turn the patient onto her left side or have her assume Trendelenburg's position. Elevate her legs to redistribute the weight on the contracting uterus and alleviate pressure from the umbilical cord. Correct supine hypertension by removing uterine pressure from the vena cava to ease venous return and from the aorta or common iliac arteries to decrease arterial pressure in the pelvis and legs.

Other steps to eliminate FHR changes include increasing the I.V. fluid infusion rate to enhance perfusion of the placental intervillous spaces and carefully regulating or discontinuing oxytocin infusion, as ordered, to reduce uterine activity (which increases perfusion of placental intervillous spaces and enhances oxygen–carbon dioxide transfer across the placenta). You may also administer oxygen by nonrebreather mask at 7 to 8 liters/minute, as ordered, to increase the maternal-fetal oxygen gradient. If fetal hypoxia has occurred, administer I.V. glucose, as ordered. Be sure to notify the doctor, who may perform fetal scalp blood sampling or other medical interventions. (See *Sampling fetal scalp blood.*)
• Prepare for delivery. If vaginal delivery isn't imminent (within 30 minutes) and fetal distress patterns don't improve, cesarean delivery will be necessary.

Documentation
• Document all activity related to monitoring. (A fetal monitoring strip becomes part of the patient's permanent record, so it's considered a legal document.) Be sure to document the type of monitoring your patient receives and all interventions. Identify the monitoring strip with the patient's name, her doctor's name, your name, and the date and time. Also note the paper speed.
• Record the patient's vital signs at regular intervals. Note her pushing efforts and record any change in her position. Document any I.V. line insertion and any changes in the I.V. solution or infusion rate. Note the use of oxytocin, regional anesthetics, or other medications.
• After a vaginal examination, document cervical dilation and effacement as well as fetal station, presentation, and position. Also document membrane rupture, including the time it oc-

curred and whether it was spontaneous or artificial. Note the amount, color, and odor of the fluid. If internal EFM was used, document electrode placement.

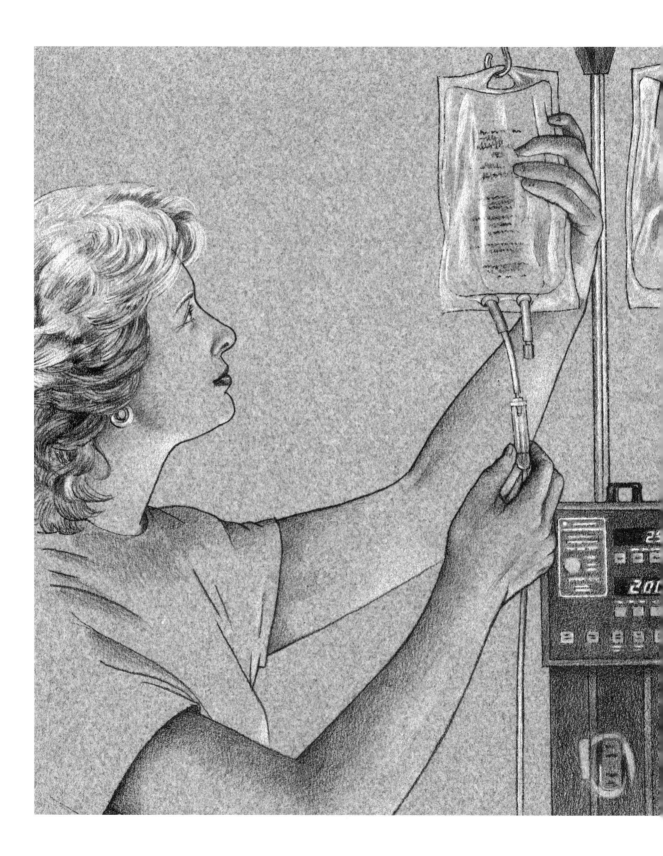

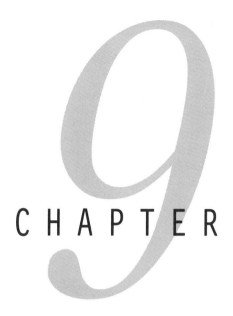

CHAPTER 9

Monitoring fluid and electrolyte balance

Whether you work in a hospital, an extended care facility, or some other setting, maintaining fluid and electrolyte balance in your patient is a primary goal. To accomplish this goal, you must know how to monitor for both actual and potential fluid and electrolyte disturbances.

Many problems — illness, injury, surgery, and even some treatments, for instance — can disrupt a patient's fluid and electrolyte balance. Yet the changes that herald such disruptions may be quite subtle. To identify these changes before serious problems occur, you need keen observational skills and expertise in measuring and recording intake and output. You must also know which laboratory studies to monitor — and what abnormal results could mean.

This chapter begins by describing the physiology of fluids and electrolytes, including the body's fluid compartments and the mechanisms that regulate fluid and electrolyte balance. It then explains how to ensure your

How body fluids are distributed

Within the body, fluid exists in two major compartments, which are separated by capillary walls and cell membranes. Two-thirds of the fluid (40% of total body weight) exists within the cells: the intracellular fluid (ICF). One-third of it (20% of total body weight) lies outside the cells: the extracellular fluid (ECF).

The ECF, in turn, has two major compartments: interstitial fluid (15% of total body weight), which bathes the cells; and intravascular fluid, or plasma (5% of total body weight), the blood's liquid component.

 Intracellular fluid

 Interstitial fluid

■ Plasma

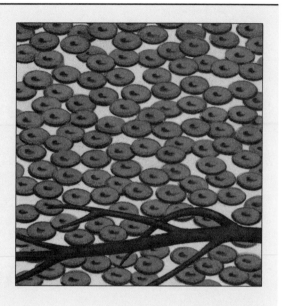

patient's fluid and electrolyte balance by monitoring intake and output, I.V. fluid therapy, and blood and urine studies. The chapter also explains how to use the vascular intermittent access system to evaluate a patient's electrolyte status and how to monitor intra-abdominal pressure to help assess fluid balance.

Physiology

Water, the essential component of body fluid, accounts for approximately 60% of total body weight in the normal adult. Body water transports gases and nutrients, helps regulate temperature, transports wastes to excretion sites, and helps maintain cell shape.

Solutes include electrolytes and various nonionized substances. Electrolytes, such as sodium, potassium, calcium, and chloride, are essential to maintaining the body's fluid and acid-base balance. They also conduct the elec-

trical current needed to maintain homeostasis. Nonionized substances include glucose, creatinine, and urea.

Fluid compartments

Two-thirds of body water is *intracellular*, remaining within cells. The other third is *extracellular*, remaining outside cells. Intracellular fluid (ICF) totals about 25 liters and accounts for 40% of total body weight. Extracellular fluid (ECF) totals roughly 15 liters and accounts for 20% of total body weight. (See *How body fluids are distributed*.)

ECF is subdivided into interstitial, intravascular, and transcellular fluid. *Interstitial* fluid, which surrounds cells, makes up 80% of the total ECF. *Intravascular* fluid consists of plasma, the liquid component of blood. It accounts for about 20% of the total ECF. *Transcellular* fluid, found in such spaces as the cerebrospinal column, GI tract, and peritoneal cavity, makes up only a minute portion of the total ECF. Consisting of epithelial cell secretions, transcellular fluid differs from interstitial and intravascular fluid in ionic composition.

Body composition affects total body water. Unlike skeletal tissue, adipose (fat) tissue contains little water. Consequently, an obese person may have only half the total body water of a lean person. Likewise, the typical woman, with more fat cells than the typical man, has a somewhat lower percentage of total body fluid. Elderly people have less total body fluid because body fluid diminishes with age while the number of fat cells increases. These differences have important nursing implications: Fluid and electrolyte replacement dosages that are appropriate for a lean man may be excessive for an obese, female, or elderly patient.

Electrolytes

These chemical compounds dissociate in solution into electrically charged particles called ions. *Cations* form a positive charge, whereas *anions* form a negative charge. The electrical charge conducts the electrical current required for normal cell function.

Electrolytes exist within both ECF and ICF. Although the various electrolytes differ in concentration, their totals balance to achieve a neutral electrical charge. (*Concentration* refers to the number of dissolved particles or solutes in a liter of fluid.)

Most electrolytes help maintain acid-base balance by interacting with hydrogen ions. The major electrolytes also have specialized functions that contribute to metabolism and fluid and electrolyte balance. (See *Understanding electrolytes,* page 174.)

Sodium and chloride are the major electrolytes in ECF. Sodium concentration determines osmolality and ECF volume. (*Osmolality* refers to the total number of osmotically active particles in a volume of solution.) Sodium also contributes to nerve and muscle cell activation. Chloride helps maintain osmotic pressure and is needed for hydrochloric acid production by gastric mucosal cells.

Other electrolytes found in ECF include calcium and bicarbonate. Calcium helps maintain cell permeability and is required for nerve impulse transmission, muscle contraction, blood coagulation, and bone and tooth formation. Bi-

carbonate helps regulate acid-base balance.

In ICF, potassium and phosphate are the most abundant electrolytes. Potassium helps regulate cell excitability and plays an essential role in nerve impulse conduction. It also affects resting membrane potential, contributes to muscle contraction and myocardial membrane responsiveness, and controls ICF osmolality and energy metabolism. Phosphate, also essential for energy metabolism, combines with calcium to form a key component for bones and teeth. Magnesium, another electrolyte in ICF, takes part in the cellular enzyme system.

Electrolytes contribute to homeostasis through these various functions, both specifically and in relation to other electrolytes. An imbalance of one electrolyte commonly affects several others. Electrolytes are also affected by fluid intake and output, acid-base balance, hormone secretion, and normal cell functioning.

Fluid and solute movement

Fluid and solutes constantly move between fluid compartments by passing through the semipermeable cell membrane. Movement occurs through one of four mechanisms: diffusion, osmosis, capillary filtration, or active transport.

Most solutes move by *diffusion.* In this passive process, the solute moves from an area of high concentration to one of lower concentration. Eventually, such movement leads to equal solute distribution in fluid.

Osmosis occurs when two areas with different concentrations are separated by a membrane that allows water but not solutes to pass. Water moves passively across such a membrane, from an area of low solute concentration to one of higher solute concentration, until solute concentrations on both sides are equal. Volume on one side of the membrane increases as more water enters to dilute the concentration; volume on the other side decreases.

Water moves by osmosis between ECF and ICF according to the osmolarity of these compartments. (*Osmolarity* refers to the concentration of a solute in a volume of solution.) Normally, ECF and ICF have equal osmotic pressures. If ECF osmolarity increases, water shifts

Understanding electrolytes

Electrolytes help regulate water distribution, govern acid-base balance, and transmit nerve impulses. They also contribute to energy generation and blood clotting. This table summarizes the functions of the body's major electrolytes. The illustration shows electrolyte distribution in and around the cell.

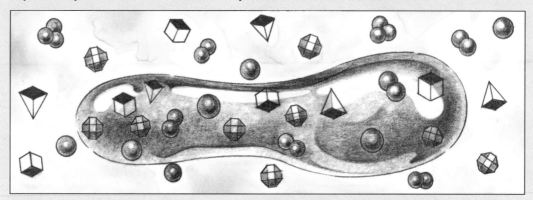

Potassium (K⁺)

- The dominant cation in intracellular fluid (ICF)
- Regulates cell excitability (unlike most other ions, K^+ can permeate cell membranes, thereby affecting the cell's electrical status)
- Helps to control energy metabolism and ICF osmolarity and, consequently, ICF osmotic pressure

Magnesium (Mg⁺⁺)

- A leading ICF cation
- Contributes to many enzymatic and metabolic processes, particularly protein synthesis
- Modifies nerve impulse transmission and skeletal muscle response (unbalanced magnesium concentrations dramatically affect neuromuscular processes)

Phosphate (HPO₄⁻⁻)

- The major ICF anion
- Promotes energy storage as well as carbohydrate, protein, and fat metabolism
- Acts as a hydrogen buffer

Sodium (Na⁺)

- The main extracellular fluid (ECF) cation
- Helps govern normal ECF osmolarity (for example,

a shift in Na^+ concentrations triggers a fluid volume change to restore normal solute and water ratios)
- Helps maintain acid-base balance
- Activates nerve and muscle cells
- Influences water distribution (with chloride)

Chloride (Cl⁻)

- The main ECF anion
- Helps maintain normal ECF osmolarity
- Affects body pH
- Plays a vital role in maintaining acid-base balance (combines with hydrogen ions to produce hydrochloric acid)

Calcium (Ca⁺⁺)

- A major cation in teeth and bones, found in fairly equal concentrations in ICF and ECF
- Also found in cell membranes, where it helps cells adhere to one another and maintain their shape
- Within cells, acts as an enzyme activator (for example, muscle cells must have Ca^{++} for contraction)
- Aids coagulation
- Affects cell membrane permeability and firing level

by osmosis from ICF to ECF. Conversely, if ICF osmolarity increases, water shifts from ECF to ICF.

Filtration occurs when water and dissolved substances move through a semipermeable membrane from an area of high pressure to one of lower pressure. In body fluids, hydrostatic (capillary) pressure resulting from the heart's pumping action aids filtration. When blood pressure inside the capillary exceeds pressure outside the capillary, water and solutes are forced out through pores in capillary walls and into the interstitial fluid.

In *active transport,* physiologic pumps move substances against a concentration gradient — a process that requires adenosine triphosphate for energy. The sodium-potassium pump, for instance, moves sodium ions from ICF, an area of greater concentration, to ECF, where concentration is lower. The reverse occurs with potassium, so greater amounts of potassium remain in ICF. Active transport of sodium, potassium, chloride, sugars, and amino acids also requires a carrier substance, which provides specific attachment sites for the solute.

Fluid balance and regulation

Fluid balance refers to a total body water content that remains relatively constant, with consistent distribution among the main fluid compartments. This balance depends on both water and electrolytes. In fact, fluid balance and electrolyte balance are so interdependent that a change in one alters the other.

To maintain normal fluid volume and concentration, fluid gains must equal fluid losses. Each day, the body gains and loses an average of 2,600 ml of fluid. Fluid gains come from ingestion of fluids and solids and oxidative metabolism. Fluid losses occur through urine and fecal excretion and evaporation through the lungs and skin. (See *Fluid gains and losses.*)

Fluid and electrolyte balance depend on homeostatic mechanisms that strive to keep fluid volume and composition within normal ranges. This balancing act involves several organs and hormones. The kidneys, the primary organs responsible for regulating body fluid, normally filter about 170 liters of plasma and excrete just 1.5 liters daily. In response to aldo-

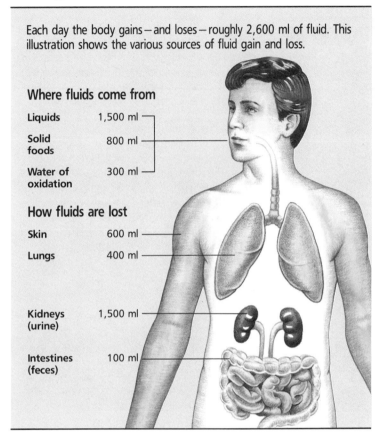

Fluid gains and losses

Each day the body gains — and loses — roughly 2,600 ml of fluid. This illustration shows the various sources of fluid gain and loss.

Where fluids come from

Liquids	1,500 ml
Solid foods	800 ml
Water of oxidation	300 ml

How fluids are lost

Skin	600 ml
Lungs	400 ml
Kidneys (urine)	1,500 ml
Intestines (feces)	100 ml

sterone and antidiuretic hormone (ADH), the kidneys selectively conserve or excrete water and electrolytes according to the body's needs, helping to regulate ECF volume, serum pH, osmolality, and electrolyte content.

Other organs that contribute to fluid and electrolyte balance include the heart and lungs and the pituitary, adrenal, and parathyroid glands. The heart provides the pumping action that circulates blood through vessels and organs, including the kidneys; without adequate perfusion, the kidneys couldn't provide the filtration so crucial to fluid and electrolyte regulation. The lungs serve as a source of insensible water loss, removing approximately 300 ml of water daily via exhalation.

The posterior pituitary gland releases ADH in response to increased serum osmolarity. Cir-

Recognizing fluid volume deficit and excess

Too much or too little fluid volume can have serious consequences. To ensure prompt detection and correction of an imbalance, make sure you're familiar with common assessment findings and the appropriate interventions.

Fluid volume deficit
Fluid volume deficit reflects loss of water and electrolytes from the extracellular fluid (ECF) compartment. Three types of fluid volume deficits exist. A *hypertonic deficit* occurs when the ECF loses proportionately more water than sodium or when its sodium content increases. In contrast, a *hypotonic deficit* occurs when the ECF loses proportionately more sodium than water. An *isotonic deficit* reflects a proportionate loss of sodium and water from the ECF.

Assessment findings
The patient with a fluid volume deficit may complain of thirst, fatigue, and urine output changes. He may experience vomiting or diarrhea, abdominal pain, and difficulty concentrating. Physical findings include a systolic blood pressure decrease of 10 mm Hg or more when the patient moves from a supine to a standing position. You may also note a subnormal temperature, elevated pulse and respiratory rates, and a weak pulse.

Other findings include dry mucous membranes, poor skin turgor, sunken eyes, pinched facial expression, flat neck veins when supine, slow hand-vein filling, cold extremities, and increased tongue furrows (wrinkles). With a severe fluid volume deficit, stupor or coma may occur. A weight loss of 2% suggests a mild fluid volume deficit; 5%, a moderate deficit; 8% or more, a severe deficit.

Interventions
• Assess the patient's vital signs and level of consciousness (LOC) at least every 4 hours or as necessary.
• Check for signs and symptoms of dehydration: decreased skin turgor, dry oral mucous membranes, and thirst.
• Monitor serum electrolyte levels and check urine specific gravity every 8 hours.
• Weigh the patient daily at the same time, on the same scale, while he's wearing the same type of clothing.
• Maintain accurate intake and output records. Record intake and output every 8 hours, and report and correct an imbalance.
• Encourage adequate fluid intake. To promote compliance with increased intake, determine the patient's fluid likes and dislikes.
• If the patient experiences diarrhea, notify the doctor.
• If indicated, initiate parenteral fluid administration.
• Teach the patient how to recognize fluid volume deficit.

Fluid volume excess
Fluid volume excess reflects an increased accumulation of water and electrolytes in the ECF.

Assessment findings
The patient with fluid volume excess may complain of lethargy, shortness of breath, acute weight gain, and a bloated sensation. He may be experiencing ankle and eyelid edema, anorexia, nausea, vomiting, or abdominal cramps. Suspect fluid volume ex-

culating in the plasma to the kidneys, ADH triggers increased water reabsorption by the renal tubules, eventually restoring normal osmolarity. The pituitary gland also stores and releases corticotropin, which affects aldosterone production and release. A mineralocorticoid secreted by the adrenal gland, aldosterone pro-

motes sodium and water reabsorption in the distal tubule. This leads to increased ECF volume, which in turn enhances blood volume. Aldosterone also causes renal excretion of potassium. The parathyroid glands regulate the balance of calcium and phosphate, important electrolytes, by secreting parathyroid hormone.

cess if the patient has seizures and you detect an altered LOC.

During the physical examination, check for edema, distended neck veins, ascites, pleural effusion, and crackles. Other findings may include engorged peripheral veins; slow hand-vein emptying; a full, bounding pulse; an increase in blood pressure; and polyuria.

Note whether the patient is receiving corticosteroids, chlorpropamide, vasopressin, phenylbutazone, or guanethidine. All of these drugs can cause a fluid volume excess.

A weight gain of 2% indicates a mild fluid volume excess; 5%, a moderate excess; 8% or more, a severe excess.

Interventions
• Assess the patient's vital signs and LOC at least every 4 hours or as necessary.
• Check for ankle or sacral edema.
• Monitor serum electrolyte levels and check urine specific gravity every 8 hours.
• Weigh the patient daily at the same time, on the same scale, while he's wearing the same type of clothing.
• Maintain accurate intake and output records. Record intake and output every 8 hours, and notify the doctor if an imbalance occurs.
• Maintain dietary sodium restrictions, if indicated. Teach the patient about his prescribed diet, advising him of the sodium content of various foods.
• Maintain fluid restrictions, as indicated. Teach the patient about fluid restrictions and the signs and symptoms of fluid retention.
• Evaluate the effectiveness of diuretics and watch for any adverse reactions.

Monitoring intake and output

The cornerstone of assessing fluid and electrolyte balance, intake and output monitoring is indicated for any patient with an actual or potential fluid or electrolyte imbalance. Accurate intake and output records are mandatory for patients with burns, renal failure, an electrolyte imbalance, congestive heart failure, or severe vomiting or diarrhea; for those who've had surgery recently; and for those receiving diuretics or corticosteroids. They're also important for patients with nasogastric (NG) tubes or drainage collection devices and for those receiving I.V. therapy.

Procedure
• On the patient's intake and output record, note the date and time you initiated monitoring, and document appropriate patient information.
• Identify, measure, and record all fluid gained or lost as separate entries on the intake and output record, along with the time of day. Record amounts in cubic centimeters (cc) or milliliters (ml).
• If required, record 8-hour summaries with 24-hour totals. Depending on the patient's condition, you may also need to document hourly intake and output.

Interpretation of findings
Normally, the patient's intake and output record should show a balance between the amount of fluid he takes in and the amount he loses. Suspect a fluid volume deficit (hypovolemia) if his output exceeds his intake; suspect a fluid volume excess (hypervolemia) if his intake exceeds his output. However, if he's receiving fluid replacement therapy to treat hypovolemia, his intake *should* exceed his output. (See *Recognizing fluid volume deficit and excess.*)

Nursing considerations
• Make sure not to overlook any source of fluid gain or loss when recording your patient's intake and output. Such an error could delay detection and treatment of a fluid imbalance. (See *Avoiding common mistakes in intake and output monitoring,* pages 178 and 179.)
• When recording intake, include all fluids entering the body, including beverages, fluids contained in solid foods taken by mouth, and foods that are liquid at room temperature, such as flavored gelatin, custard, and ice

Avoiding common mistakes in intake and output monitoring

Measuring fluid intake and output accurately can pose a challenge unless you're aware of potential sources of error—and take steps to prevent them. This chart lists common mistakes caregivers make when measuring and recording intake and output and describes measures you can take to prevent them.

MISTAKE	PREVENTIVE MEASURES
Discarding body fluids without measuring them	• Make sure all staff members know which patients require intake and output measurement. For instance, verify that the card file contains a list of these patients' names, and post a list of the names in a convenient area for quick reference. • Supply an adequate patient report to all personnel. • Attach a "Measure intake and output" sign to the patient's bed.
Failing to elicit the patient's cooperation	• Make sure the patient and his family understand the importance of monitoring intake and output. • Teach the patient and his family how to help caregivers maintain an accurate record of intake and output.
Incorrectly measuring small amounts of oral fluids	• Use an appropriate device to measure small amounts of oral fluids. • Keep small, calibrated paper cups at the patient's bedside to more easily measure oral fluids.
Ascribing inconsistent volumes to fluid containers	• Designate a specific volume for each container used to measure fluids, and make sure all staff members record the same volume consistently. • Keep a bedside record that lists the designated volumes for each container.
Overestimating fluid intake from iced beverages	• Be aware that iced beverages have a lower fluid volume than uniced beverages (from fluid displacement by ice). • Record intake from ice chips as roughly half the volume of the ice chips; an ounce of ice chips equals roughly 15 ml of water. • Keep ice in beverages to a minimum to promote more accurate intake measurement.
Inaccurately estimating fluids ingested from meal trays	• Don't assume the patient drank the entire contents of an empty fluid container. Instead, ask him if he drank all the fluid himself or gave some to another person.
Underestimating fluid intake from parenteral fluid	• Keep in mind that parenteral fluid bottles are overfilled. A 1,000-ml bottle may contain 1,100 ml of fluid; a 100-ml bottle, 150 ml. • Run excess fluid through tubing during setup, or record actual volume infused.
Failing to estimate fluid lost through perspiration	• Record the amount of clothing and bed linens saturated with perspiration. Be aware that each necessary bed change represents at least 1 liter of fluid lost. • If required, estimate perspiration as 1, 2, 3, or 4 (with 1 representing barely visible sweating and 4 representing profuse sweating).
Failing to record vomitus	• Don't record uncaught vomitus as a lost specimen. Instead, estimate and document the amount of fluid lost in vomitus.
Failing to record fluid lost through urinary incontinence	• Estimate the amount of urine lost through incontinence by assessing the amount of clothing and bed linens saturated with urine.
Failing to record fluid lost in liquid stools	• Encourage the patient to use a bedpan, or place a measuring device over the toilet to allow direct measurement. • Estimate the amount of fluid lost in liquid stools through fecal incontinence.

Avoiding common mistakes in intake and output monitoring *(continued)*

MISTAKE	PREVENTIVE MEASURES
Failing to estimate fluid lost in wound exudate	• Measure and document the amount of drainage on a dressing by measuring the width of the stained area and determining dressing thickness. • If necessary, weigh the dressing before applying and after removing it to estimate fluid loss. • If the patient has a fistula, apply a stoma bag to catch and measure drainage.
Failing to assess urinary catheter patency if urine drainage decreases	• Don't assume that decreased drainage from an indwelling urinary catheter results from reduced urine formation. If drainage decreases, first determine if the catheter is patent.
Inaccurately measuring small amounts of urine	• Obtain an appropriate measuring device for frequent checks of urine output. (An error as small as 10 ml could have important consequences when dealing with small amounts of urine.) • Use a collecting device calibrated to measure small amounts of urine.
Failing to record intake and output from irrigation	• Add the amount of irrigating solution infused to the intake column, and add the amount of fluid withdrawn during irrigation to the output column. Alternatively, you may compare the amount of irrigating solution to the amount of fluid withdrawn during irrigation. If the amount added exceeds the amount removed, record the excess in the intake column. If the amount removed exceeds the amount added, record the excess in the output column.

cream. Intake also should include GI instillations, bladder irrigations, and I.V. fluids.

• When recording output, include all fluid that leaves the patient's body, including urine, loose stools, vomitus, aspirated fluids, and drainage from surgical drains, NG tubes, and chest tubes. Also estimate and record output from other sources, such as insensible losses from the lungs and skin.

• Measure — don't estimate — intake and output.

• When recording intake and output, enlist the patient's help, if possible, to ensure the most accurate records.

• For a small child, weigh diapers, if appropriate.

• Review intake and output during each shift, and notify the doctor if amounts differ significantly over a 24-hour period. To identify trends, review daily totals for several consecutive days.

• Document your findings in the appropriate location; describe any fluid restrictions and the patient's compliance with them.

Monitoring I.V. fluids

Administer prescribed I.V. fluids to meet a patient's daily nutritional needs, to replace abnormal fluid losses, or to correct electrolyte imbalances. Patients receiving I.V. fluids require careful monitoring for fluid imbalances.

Balanced I.V. solutions, used to treat and correct specific electrolyte imbalances, resemble plasma in fluid and electrolyte content. After adequate renal function has been established, the patient may receive Ringer's or lactated Ringer's solution. The latter is especially useful in treating mild acidosis.

Therapeutic solutions, usually infused through a subclavian catheter, are indicated when oral intake is contraindicated for a prolonged period. Hypertonic solutions, used in parenteral nutrition, contain 20% to 50% glucose in 500 ml of water (depending on the patient's needs) or 5% to 8% amino acids in 500 ml of water. These solutions, which supply roughly 440 calories and 4 g of nitrogen/liter, replace lost GI fluids and electrolytes volume for volume.

Colloids draw fluid into the bloodstream by increasing intravascular osmotic pressure. They remain in the vascular space for several days, provided that the capillary endothelium is normal. (Colloids are not considered true I.V. fluid solutions because they contain undissolved proteins or starch molecules that are uniformly distributed.) Colloids include albumin, plasma protein fraction, dextran, and hetastarch. (See *Guide to colloids*.)

Procedure

Administer the correct solutions at the prescribed rate and volume.

Nursing considerations

• Be sure you know how the prescribed I.V. fluid therapy will affect the patient's fluid and electrolyte balance.
• Consider the patient's normal electrolyte requirements when providing I.V. fluids. The sodium requirement is 1 to 2 mEq/kg/day; potassium, 0.5 to 1 mEq/kg/day; and chloride, 1 to 2 mEq/kg/day, for instance. Are the solutions being infused providing these electrolytes? Also consider how long the patient has been receiving I.V. fluids and whether his electrolyte requirements are being supplemented by oral intake.
• Carefully assess the I.V. insertion site for signs of infiltration, phlebitis, local infection, and catheter occlusion. These complications may alter the rate and volume of fluid administration, leading to fluid imbalance.

Monitoring blood and urine tests

The results of certain blood and urine tests can provide valuable information about your patient's fluid and electrolyte status — especially if you correlate them with his history and physical findings. Blood tests that help assess fluid and electrolyte status include serum sodium, potassium, chloride, calcium, phosphate, magnesium, glucose, protein, and creatinine levels; serum osmolality; blood urea nitrogen

(BUN) levels; BUN-creatinine ratio; and hematocrit. Urine tests include routine urinalysis and sodium, chloride, potassium, calcium, and magnesium levels.

These test results are commonly part of the patient's preadmission laboratory studies. However, if your patient is at risk for or has a fluid or electrolyte imbalance, you should obtain and monitor test results repeatedly.

Procedure

• Usually, a laboratory technician obtains venous blood samples. Be sure to provide guidance, as needed, to prevent misleading or invalid test results. For instance, if your patient is receiving I.V. fluids, make sure blood samples are taken from the opposite arm or an area below the I.V. insertion site. Also, be aware that hemolysis of the blood sample may occur if the skin is too wet from the antiseptic, if the tourniquet remains on too long, if a large amount of blood is withdrawn through a small-gauge needle, or if the sample is shaken vigorously. Hemolysis may affect serum potassium, magnesium, and phosphate levels; a too-tight tourniquet may cause a false-high serum potassium value.
• The doctor may order a single urine specimen or a 24-hour urine specimen. Collect all urine specimens in a clean container to avoid contamination, which could cause false results. You may collect single specimens at any time, although the first morning voiding is preferred because it's more concentrated. To avoid changes in a single specimen kept longer than 1 hour, refrigerate the specimen.

Interpretation of findings

Make sure you're familiar with normal and abnormal laboratory values as well as the implications of abnormal results. (For normal blood and urine values, see *Laboratory tests used to monitor fluid and electrolyte balance*, pages 182 to 185.)

Nursing considerations

• Tell the laboratory technician if your patient has a clotting disorder or is receiving anticoagulant therapy. After the sample is withdrawn,

(Text continues on page 185.)

Guide to colloids

You may need to administer colloids to a patient with a fluid volume deficit. This chart provides essential information about major colloids.

COLLOID	CONTENTS	USES	NURSING IMPLICATIONS
plasma protein fraction (Plasmanate): 5% solution of human plasma proteins mixed in 0.9% sodium chloride solution	• Albumin (44 g/liter) • Alpha and beta globulin (6 g/liter) • Sodium (145 mEq/liter) • Chloride (85 mEq/liter) • Potassium (2 mEq/liter) • pH 6.7 to 7.3	Volume replacement in hypovolemic shock, hemorrhagic shock, and hypoproteinemia	• Solution is heat treated to reduce the risk of hepatitis transmission. • It doesn't require crossmatching. • Adverse reactions are unusual. However, patients with heart failure may develop circulatory overload or pulmonary edema. At infusion rates above 10 ml/minute, peripheral vasodilation and hypotension may occur. • Solution doesn't replace lost clotting factors. • Because solution is osmotically equal to plasma, plasma expansion equals the amount of solution infused. • Don't administer cloudy or sedimented solutions.
albumin (normal human serum albumin): albumin protein from human plasma. Supplied in two strengths: 5% albumin (which is osmotically equal to plasma) and 25% albumin (which draws about four times its volume in interstitial fluid into the circulation within 15 minutes of administration).	*5% albumin* • Albumin (50 g/liter) • Sodium (130 mEq/liter) • Potassium (1 mEq/liter) • pH 6.4 to 7.4 *25% albumin* • Albumin (240 g/liter) • Globulins (10 g/liter) • Sodium (130 mEq/liter) • pH 6.4 to 7.4	Volume replacement in hypovolemic shock, hemorrhagic shock, cerebral edema, exchange transfusion, and hypoproteinemia	• Albumin is heat treated to reduce the risk of hepatitis transmission. • It can be given without typing or crossmatching. • Although 25% albumin was once called salt-poor, the term is a misnomer; it contains 130 to 160 mEq/liter of sodium. • Infusion rate depends on the patient's condition and response. For patients in hypovolemic shock, infuse as rapidly as possible to restore vascular volume. For patients with normal vascular volume, infuse 5% solution at 2 to 4 ml/minute, 25% solution at 1 ml/minute. • Monitor the patient for signs and symptoms of allergic reaction: fever, rash, chills. • Don't administer more than 250 g in 48 hours. • Use opened containers immediately; albumin solutions have no preservatives.
dextran (Gentran): Large polysaccharide glucose polymer (combination of simpler molecules) that's water-soluble. Supplied in two strengths: low-molecular-weight dextran (LMD) and high-molecular-weight dextran (HMD). LMD expands vascular volume one to two times more than amount of LMD infused. With HMD, plasma expansion slightly exceeds the volume infused.	*LMD* • 500-ml solution containing 10% dextran (molecular weight 40,000) in 0.9% sodium chloride solution or dextrose 5% in water (D_5W) *HMD* • 500-ml solution containing 6% dextran (molecular weight 70,000) in 0.9% sodium chloride solution or D_5W	Volume replacement in hypovolemic shock, hemorrhagic shock, and thromboembolism prophylaxis (LMD only)	• Dextran solutions may prolong bleeding time. (LMD decreases red blood cell adhesiveness. HMD increases platelet adhesiveness and blood viscosity.) Use cautiously in patients with hemorrhagic or coagulation disorders. • Dextran infusion may interfere with blood typing and crossmatching, so draw blood samples before starting the infusion. • Dextran increases urine specific gravity and osmolality (50% to 70% is excreted unchanged in urine). • Dextran is less expensive than Plasmanate. • Infuse only clear solution. If you see dextran flakes in a stored, unopened I.V. bag, put the bag in warm water until flakes dissolve. • Stop the infusion if the patient develops signs of renal failure—for example, oliguria and increasing levels of blood urea nitrogen or creatinine. • Monitor the patient for an anaphylactic reaction.
hetastarch (Hespan): synthetic starch similar to human glycogen with a side range of molecular weights mixed in 0.9% sodium chloride solution	*In 500 ml* • Sodium (154 mEq/liter) • Chloride (154 mEq/liter) • 6% hetastarch	Volume replacement in hemorrhagic and hypovolemic shock	• Expansion of plasma volume slightly exceeds the amount of hetastarch given. • About 40% of hetastarch dose is excreted in 24 hours. • Use opened containers immediately; hetastarch contains no preservatives. • Monitor the patient for an anaphylactic reaction. • Monitor hematology and coagulation results for prolonged prothrombin, plasma thrombin, and clotting times.

Laboratory tests used to monitor fluid and electrolyte balance

Monitoring certain laboratory tests can help you evaluate your patient's fluid and electrolyte status. This chart presents normal values for relevant blood and urine tests, along with related nursing considerations.

TEST	NORMAL RANGE	NURSING CONSIDERATIONS
BLOOD TESTS		
Serum albumin	3.5 to 4.8 g/dl (35 to 48 g/liter)	• When the albumin level drops, colloidal osmotic pull in the intravascular space decreases; fluid then shifts to the interstitial space, causing edema. • Be sure to consider your patient's albumin level when evaluating total calcium values.
Serum calcium	*Total calcium* 8.9 to 10.3 mg/dl (2.23 to 2.57 mmol/liter)	• Total serum calcium represents the sum of ionized (47%) and nonionized (53%) calcium components. Of the nonionized portion, albumin-bound calcium makes up 40% and the portion chelated to anions (such as phosphate and citrate) accounts for 13%. • Total calcium is the most commonly performed serum calcium test. • To determine the serum calcium level from the serum albumin, first obtain the serum albumin level, then correct total serum calcium for variations in albumin by assuming that each serum albumin change of 1 g/dl (10 g/liter) will alter the total serum calcium level by 0.8 mg/dl (0.2 mmol/liter). However, don't calculate serum calcium this way if your patient has a condition that affects the degree of calcium-albumin binding or the blood pH (which alters the percentage of ionized calcium). Calcium-albumin binding rises with alkalosis and increased free fatty acid levels (common in stressed patients). Increased levels of lactate, bicarbonate, citrate, phosphate, and some substances in radiographic contrast media also may reduce the ionized calcium level.
	Ionized calcium 4.6 to 5.1 mg/dl (1.15 to 1.27 mmol/liter)	• Direct ionized calcium measurement is especially valuable in critically ill patients because ionized calcium is physiologically active. • Be aware that the sampling technique may affect test results. For instance, prolonged tourniquet application or an inappropriate amount of heparin in the collecting syringe may cause misleading results.
Serum chloride	97 to 110 mEq/liter (97 to 110 mmol/liter)	• Below-normal level indicates hypochloremia, as from metabolic alkalosis or hypokalemia. • Above-normal level signifies hyperchloremia, as from excessive administration of isotonic saline solution.
Fasting blood glucose	65 to 110 mg/dl (3.58 to 6.05 mmol/liter)	• Marked serum glucose elevations cause osmotic diuresis, resulting in hypovolemia. • Expect increased levels in patients receiving parenteral glucose therapy.
Serum magnesium	1.3 to 2.1 mEq/liter (0.65 to 1.05 mmol/liter)	• Hemolysis of the sample causes release of magnesium from red blood cells (RBCs) into serum, invalidating test results.
Serum phosphate	2.5 to 4.5 mg/dl (0.81 to 1.45 mmol/liter)	• Evaluate the value in conjunction with serum calcium levels. Keep in mind that phosphate and calcium relate inversely; if the phosphate level increases, the calcium level drops. • Expect a higher serum phosphate level in a child than in an adult. • Infusing I.V. glucose before or during sample collection will cause a decreased value (from carbohydrate metabolism). • Insulin aids entry of extracellular phosphate into cells. • Hemolysis of the sample causes phosphate release from RBCs into serum, invalidating test results.

Laboratory tests used to monitor fluid and electrolyte balance *(continued)*

TEST	NORMAL RANGE	NURSING CONSIDERATIONS
BLOOD TESTS *(continued)*		
Serum potassium	3.5 to 5 mEq/liter (3.5 to 5 mmol/liter)	• Increased value may indicate acidosis, which causes potassium to shift out of cells into blood. • Decreased value may indicate alkalosis, which causes potassium to shift from blood into cells. • Insulin triggers entry of extracellular potassium into cells, causing a transient drop in the serum potassium level. • Serum potassium level may be raised an additional 2.7 mEq/liter by a tight tourniquet around an exercising extremity (as when a patient opens and closes his hand). • Hemolysis of the sample causes movement of potassium from RBCs into serum, invalidating test results.
Serum sodium	135 to 145 mEq/liter (135 to 145 mmol/liter)	• Value relates closely to body water. For adults, each 3-mEq elevation of serum sodium above the normal range represents a deficit of roughly 1 liter of body water. • Expect the value to drop as the serum glucose level rises (from movement of water from cells to extracellular fluid). Every 62-mg/dl increase in the serum glucose level draws enough water from cells to dilute serum sodium concentration by 1 mEq/liter. Thus, if the patient's serum glucose level is 1,000 mg/dl (930 mg/dl above normal), the serum sodium level should decrease 15 mEq/liter.
Blood urea nitrogen (BUN)	8 to 25 mg/dl (2.9 to 8.9 mmol/liter)	• Increased value may result from decreased renal blood flow secondary to fluid volume deficit (which reduces urea clearance). • Conditions that enhance urea production, including excessive protein intake and increased catabolism (as from starvation, trauma, bleeding into the intestines, or catabolic drugs), may elevate BUN levels. • Below-normal value may result from overhydration or low protein intake.
Serum creatinine	0.6 to 1.6 mg/dl (53 to 133 μmol)	• This test evaluates renal disease more sensitively and specifically than BUN because few nonrenal causes of creatinine elevation exist. • Value increases when at least half of the renal nephrons are nonfunctional. • Slight elevations may occur with severe fluid volume depletion (from a reduced glomerular filtration rate).
BUN-creatinine ratio	10:1	• This test helps evaluate hydration status. A ratio above 10:1 suggests hypovolemia, low perfusion pressure to the kidney, or increased protein metabolism. A ratio below 10:1 suggests hepatic insufficiency or low protein intake. • When both BUN and creatinine levels rise but remain in a 10:1 ratio, suspect intrinsic renal disease. (However, this result also may occur when fluid volume depletion causes the glomerular filtration rate to drop.)
Hematocrit	Men: 44% to 52% Women: 39% to 47%	• Hematocrit measures the percentage by volume of packed RBCs in plasma. • Increased value suggests hypovolemia. (RBCs are contained in a relatively smaller plasma fluid volume.) Decreased value suggests hypervolemia. (RBCs are contained in a relatively larger plasma fluid volume.) However, with hemolysis or bleeding, test results don't accurately reflect fluid balance.

(continued)

Laboratory tests used to monitor fluid and electrolyte balance *(continued)*

TEST	NORMAL RANGE	NURSING CONSIDERATIONS
URINE TESTS		
Urine calcium	50 to 300 mg/ 24 hours (depending on dietary intake)	• Value may reach 900 mg/24 hours in patients with hypercalcemia secondary to metastatic tumors. • Subnormal value may indicate hypocalcemia. • Qualitative test is done on a single specimen by observing for precipitate after adding a few drops of calcium oxalate. A heavy white precipitate indicates an above-normal urine calcium level; a clear specimen, a below-normal urine calcium level.
Urine chloride	110 to 250 mEq/liter/24 hours (110 to 250 mmol/24 hours)	• Sodium intake may affect the value. • Value usually approximates urine sodium value in patients with hypovolemia because sodium and chloride are reabsorbed together. • This test helps differentiate the various forms of metabolic alkalosis. A decreased value indicates metabolic alkalosis secondary to vomiting, gastric suctioning, or diuretic therapy. An increased value indicates metabolic alkalosis resulting from profound potassium depletion or mineralocorticoid excess.
Urine potassium	25 to 125 mEq/ liter/24 hours (25 to 125 mmol/24 hours) Random specimen: usually above 40 mEq/liter	• The 24-hour test is used mainly to assess hormonal function and determine if hypokalemia has a renal or nonrenal cause. • Value varies with diet and with serum aldosterone or cortisol level. (Increased amounts of these substances enhance potassium excretion.) • Below-normal value may indicate acute renal failure. In the presence of hypokalemia, however, a below-normal value indicates a nonrenal cause.
Urine sodium	40 to 220 mEq/ liter/24 hours (40 to 220 mmol/24 hours) Random specimen: usually above 40 mEq/liter	• A decreased value indicates hypovolemia characterized by renal sodium conservation to maintain blood volume. • An increased value indicates hypovolemia associated with underlying renal disease, hypoaldosteronism, osmotic diuresis, or diuretic therapy. • Value varies with diet. Be sure to record dietary intake during the test period to permit correct interpretation of test result.
Urine osmolality	Range: 50 to 1,400 mOsm/kg Average: 500 to 800 mOsm/kg	• After an overnight fast of 14 hours, urine osmolality should be triple the serum osmolality. • Value rises with hypovolemia as the kidneys conserve needed fluid, causing greater urine concentration. Value decreases with hypervolemia as the kidneys excrete unneeded fluid, causing more diluted urine. • Simultaneous serum and urine osmolality tests measure renal concentrating ability more accurately than the urine specific gravity test.
Urine pH	4.5 to 8.0	• In pooled daily output, urine pH averages roughly 5.0; in most random specimens, it measures less than 6.6. • Value normally fluctuates throughout the day. • Urine pH reflects serum pH and helps confirm acidosis or alkalosis (except with paradoxical aciduria in hypokalemic alkalosis, or alkaline urine caused by infections or renal tubular acidosis). • Value increases with use of alkalinizing agents (such as sodium bicarbonate and potassium citrate) and decreases with use of acidifying agents (such as ascorbic acid, sodium acid phosphate, and methenamine mandelate). • Specimen should be examined soon after collection to avoid alkalinization from bacteria-induced splitting of urea into ammonia.

Laboratory tests used to monitor fluid and electrolyte balance *(continued)*

TEST	NORMAL RANGE	NURSING CONSIDERATIONS
URINE TESTS *(continued)*		
Urine specific gravity	1.003 to 1.035	• In most random specimens, specific gravity measures 1.012 to 1.025. • In elderly patients, normal range may be lower because of reduced renal concentrating ability. • Value reflects hydration status and varies with urine volume and the solute load to be excreted. • In patients with normal renal function, increased value indicates hypovolemia (the kidneys attempt to retain needed fluid and excrete solutes in a small, concentrated urine volume). • Specific gravity fixed at 1.010 indicates significant renal disease. • Heavy molecules (such as glucose, albumin, and dyes) increase specific gravity disproportionately to the actual concentration. Therefore, urine osmolality is a more accurate test in patients with glycosuria or proteinuria and in those who've recently been injected with radiopaque dyes.

keep firm pressure on the venipuncture site for at least 5 minutes to prevent possible hematoma formation. If a hematoma forms, apply warm soaks.

• If the patient has lingering discomfort or undue bleeding after venipuncture, make sure he lies down. Watch for anxiety or signs of shock, such as hypotension and tachycardia.

• Document the date, time, and site of the venipuncture; the name of the test; the time the sample or specimen was sent to the laboratory; and any adverse reactions the patient experiences, such as hematoma or anxiety.

• Review laboratory test results for indications of fluid or electrolyte imbalance. For accuracy, always consider the patient's history and clinical findings when interpreting results.

Monitoring electrolytes with a vascular intermittent access system

The vascular intermittent access system measures electrolyte levels automatically in patients who have an indwelling arterial or venous line. In just 1 minute, it obtains such critical indices as potassium, calcium, sodium, glucose, hematocrit, and arterial blood gas levels. Then it reinfuses the blood sample into the patient.

By monitoring electrolyte levels almost as they occur, this system allows you to respond quickly to any abnormalities. The arterial or venous line can be accessed as often as every 3 minutes. This avoids the need to draw blood manually for laboratory samples and eliminates problems that an indwelling sensor sometimes causes. Easily transported with the patient from one area to another, it can be used in the operating room, intensive care unit, emergency department, and other special care units.

Equipment

The vascular intermittent access system includes a monitor and a sensor array. It also includes an isotonic I.V. solution with tubing (lactated Ringer's solution) to keep the I.V. line patent. With the appropriate calibrant additives, the solution calibrates the sensors before each measurement. A printer provides a hard copy of test results, and an automatic timer automatically initiates the process at predetermined intervals. (See *Vascular intermittent access system,* page 186.)

Vascular intermittent access system

Used to measure electrolyte levels automatically, the vascular intermittent access system includes a sensor array, an I.V. administration set, I.V. solution with additives for sensor calibration, and a monitor that processes signals from the sensors. A pumping mechanism infuses the solution and withdraws blood samples.

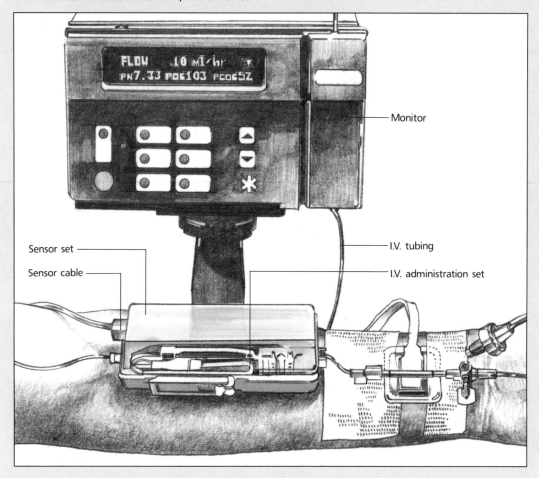

Preparation
Set up the vascular intermittent access system, following the manufacturer's directions. Place the sensor array at the distal end of the I.V. administration set.

Procedure
Perform blood chemistry testing as often as desired by simply pressing the sampling key on the monitor. This triggers a series of automatic steps. First, the sensors are calibrated against known reference values in the I.V. solution. Next, the system reverses its usual pumping action and withdraws a small amount of blood (0.6 ml), which then contacts the sensors. Roughly 30 seconds later, test results appear on the monitor screen. Finally, the system

flushes the blood back into the patient along with the I.V. solution.

Interpretation of findings
Abnormal electrolyte values measured by this system indicate electrolyte imbalances, which can disrupt various body systems and cause serious health problems.

Nursing considerations
• Be aware that the vascular intermittent access system doesn't require long-term compatibility between the sensors and the patient's blood. Except for the few seconds during which the measurement is being made, the sensors are exposed only to the I.V. solution, not the blood.
• Because the system is closed, blood handling by caregivers is avoided and blood loss in the patient is prevented.

Monitoring intra-abdominal pressure

In this procedure, a pressure transducer monitoring system is attached to an indwelling urinary catheter to measure intra-abdominal pressure—pressure within the abdominal cavity. When filled with fluid, the urinary bladder wall acts as a passive diaphragm, allowing transmission of the intra-abdominal pressure into the catheter tubing. The monitoring system converts the signal to a waveform and pressure value, which are displayed on the monitor.

Intra-abdominal pressure monitoring is indicated for patients with conditions that could increase this pressure, such as ascites, abdominal bleeding, intestinal obstruction, or bowel edema or ischemia. Increased intra-abdominal pressure may lead to renal, respiratory, and cardiovascular complications. (See *Dangers of increased intra-abdominal pressure.*)

Equipment
Gather a 16G or 18G needle; an indwelling urinary catheter irrigation tray; sterile 0.9% so-

Dangers of increased intra-abdominal pressure

If your patient has increased intra-abdominal pressure, he may face potential renal, respiratory, and cardiovascular compromise.

Renal complications of increased intra-abdominal pressure ultimately may lead to renal failure. As intra-abdominal pressure rises, the mean glomerular filtration rate and renal blood flow decrease while renal vascular resistance rises. In response, urine output falls. Eventually, renal failure may occur.

Respiratory complications can be equally serious. As intra-abdominal pressure pushes the diaphragm upward, pulmonary compliance diminishes, making the lungs stiffer and harder to ventilate. As a result, peak end-inspiratory pressure rises. The bulging diaphragm also contributes to greater intrathoracic pressure, which compresses the pulmonary alveoli and blood vessels. This may lead to a ventilation-perfusion imbalance and a drop in the partial pressure of arterial oxygen. As blood flow decreases, the arterial pH falls and the lungs and, possibly, some organs may suffer ischemia.

Cardiovascular effects of increased intra-abdominal pressure include reduced cardiac output, increased systemic vascular resistance, elevated right atrial pressure (RAP), and increased pulmonary artery wedge pressure (PAWP). These problems, more common when intra-abdominal pressure exceeds 20 mm Hg, result from various factors. For example, the drop in cardiac output may stem from both rising systemic vascular resistance and reduced venous return caused by increased pressure on the vena cava. RAP and PAWP rise as increased intra-abdominal pressure is transmitted across the diaphragm to the thoracic cavity. However, these hemodynamic elevations may not be true increases but only reflect rising pleural pressures.

dium chloride solution for irrigation; sterile gloves; one or two sterile Kelly clamps; a sterile towel; povidone-iodine swabs; a bedside pressure monitor; a carpenter's level; and a disposable, fluid-filled, pressure transducer monitoring system.

Preparation

Attach the 16G or 18G needle to the pressure transducer tubing. Then flush the transducer tubing with the appropriate flush solution, making sure to remove all air from the tubing. Take all equipment to the patient's bedside.

Explain the purpose of the procedure to the patient. Place him in the supine position, with the head of the bed flat. (If the head remains elevated, thoracic cavity contents will push downward on the abdomen, falsely increasing intra-abdominal pressure.) If the patient can't tolerate a flat position, document the degree of bed elevation and make sure all other staff members use the same elevation when obtaining readings. Although measurements taken with the head slightly elevated will be false-high, you can use them to check for trends in intra-abdominal pressure as long as the elevation remains consistent.

Next, attach the pressure transducer to the monitoring system. Level the transducer with the top of the patient's symphysis pubis by using a carpenter's level or similar device. Then zero and calibrate the transducer, following the directions supplied by the monitor manufacturer. (For details on leveling, zeroing, and calibrating, see Chapter 2.)

Procedure

• Using sterile technique, open the irrigation tray and prepare the irrigation syringe.
• Create a sterile field by placing the sterile towel under the catheter where the catheter tubing connects to the catheter. Place all other sterile supplies on this field.
• Wearing sterile gloves, clamp or cross-clamp the tubing of the urinary drainage bag distal to the aspiration port, using one or two sterile Kelly clamps.
• Disconnect the catheter from the drainage bag. Place the end of the drainage bag tubing on the sterile field.
• With your gloved hand, hold the end of the catheter. Instill 50 to 100 ml of sterile 0.9% sodium chloride solution, using the syringe.
• Pinch the catheter closed to prevent fluid leakage, and remove the irrigating syringe. Reconnect the clamped drainage bag tubing to the catheter.

• Slowly release the Kelly clamp (or clamps) just enough so that air escapes and fluid fills the catheter tubing. Then reclamp the drainage bag tubing distal to the aspiration port. (Air in the tubing may cause a false reading.)
• Prepare the aspiration port with povidone-iodine swabs. Then insert the needle on the pressure tubing into this port.
• Note the intra-abdominal pressure reading on the bedside monitor and watch for the waveform, which should appear as a relatively flat line.
• Remove the needle from the aspiration port.
• Unclamp the Kelly clamp (or clamps). Watch for urinary drainage flow to resume.
• Remove your gloves and discard disposable supplies.
• Document the intra-abdominal pressure reading. Because it may vary with the phase of the respiratory cycle, you should record the reading at end expiration, when the diaphragm rises and intrathoracic pressure has the least effect. This is especially important if the patient is on a mechanical ventilator or is receiving high levels of positive end-expiratory pressure.
• Replace the needle on the pressure tubing with a new sterile needle to prepare for the next intra-abdominal pressure measurement.

Interpretation of findings

Normally, mean intra-abdominal pressure is 0 mm Hg to subatmospheric. It typically increases just after abdominal surgery, possibly rising to 15 mm Hg, or if the patient is wearing a pneumatic antishock garment. At all other times, above-normal intra-abdominal pressure suggests intestinal obstruction, ascites, ruptured abdominal aortic aneurysm, or postoperative bleeding.

Nursing considerations

• Make sure the transducer is leveled, zeroed, and calibrated correctly before each measurement to avoid inaccurate readings.
• If the monitor reveals an abnormal reading, determine the need for interventions to help avert renal, respiratory, and cardiovascular complications. However, be sure to consider other assessment and diagnostic findings in

Benefits of monitoring intra-abdominal pressure

For the patient with abdominal bleeding, monitoring intra-abdominal pressure can be an essential assessment tool. Used with other evaluation techniques, intra-abdominal pressure monitoring can help you detect and correct problems before they become life-threatening.

Suppose, for example, that Jerry Kohler, age 42, was placed in your care.

Initial care
Injured in a motor vehicle accident, Mr. Kohler underwent abdominal surgery to relieve internal bleeding. The surgeon removed his spleen. Surgery was complicated by hemorrhage, with 5,200 ml of blood lost.

Care on your unit
Mr. Kohler was intubated and attached to a mechanical ventilator. On the first postoperative day, you assessed and reported episodes of hypotension and tachycardia. The doctor inserted a pulmonary artery catheter to monitor Mr. Kohler's hemodynamic status. The values obtained—a right atrial pressure (RAP) of 14 mm Hg and a pulmonary artery wedge pressure (PAWP) of 16 mm Hg—suggested that Mr. Kohler was developing cardiovascular complications. Laboratory studies showed a blood urea nitrogen (BUN) level of 17 mg/dl and a serum creatinine level of 1 mg/dl, indicating renal involvement. When Mr. Kohler's urine output dropped to 15 ml/hour, you infused low-dose dopamine at 3 mcg/kg/minute, as ordered.

The doctor ordered intra-abdominal pressure monitoring. You set up the monitoring system and obtained values of 21 to 24 mm Hg, attributing the fluctuation to mechanical ventilation. You started a furosemide drip to help maintain urine output and preserve renal function, as ordered.

On the second postoperative day, Mr. Kohler's urine output was still below normal and his intra-abdominal pressure was rising, though his abdominal girth hadn't increased. Based on low urine output, increasing intra-abdominal pressure, and abnormal BUN and creatinine values, the doctor performed paracentesis, removing 1,700 ml of fluid.

An improving prognosis
After the procedure, Mr. Kohler's intra-abdominal pressure dropped to 6 mm Hg. During the next few hours, his urine output rose to 100 ml/hour and his RAP and PAWP dropped to normal levels.

The next day, Mr. Kohler's intra-abdominal pressure remained stable, his urine output continued to rise, and his BUN and creatinine levels reached normal levels. The doctor determined that Mr. Kohler no longer needed monitoring and mechanical ventilation, and discontinued these interventions.

Conclusion
In Mr. Kohler's case, intra-abdominal pressure measurements helped to detect and monitor worsening renal function and indicated the possible development of cardiovascular complications. With prompt intervention, Mr. Kohler's clinical status improved.

conjunction with intra-abdominal pressure values. Also, analyze successive values for trends rather than focusing solely on isolated values. (See *Benefits of monitoring intra-abdominal pressure.*)
• Make sure you know which laboratory results and clinical findings suggest that your patient's condition is worsening. For instance, increasing BUN and serum creatinine levels may indicate renal dysfunction; if urine output continues to fall, reflecting reduced renal blood flow, the

patient may need I.V. fluids and vasopressor therapy.
• Be aware that each time you measure intra-abdominal pressure, you increase your patient's risk for urinary tract infection and sepsis by interrupting the closed urinary drainage system. To reduce the infection risk, use strict aseptic technique and a new sterile disposable irrigation tray and sterile needle for each measurement. Assess the patient regularly for signs and symptoms of infection by monitoring his tem-

How to monitor intra-abdominal pressure

If your patient has increased intra-abdominal pressure, you may need to monitor it to avert complications. These illustrations show essential steps for setting up the equipment and taking intra-abdominal measurements.

Level the transducer with the top of the patient's symphysis pubis.

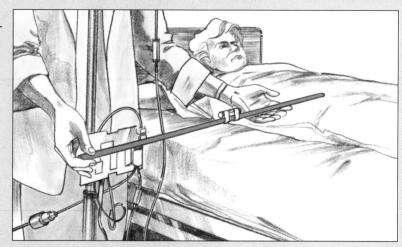

Clamp the catheter distal to the injection port.

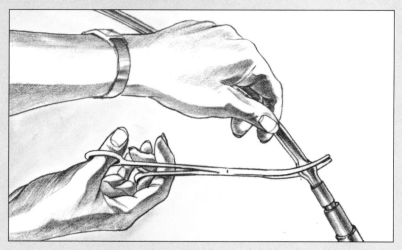

perature and white blood cell count and noting urine color and clarity.
• If the pulmonary artery pressure catheter is in place, monitor the patient's cardiac output, pulmonary artery pressure, right atrial pressure, and mean arterial pressure. Watch for hemodynamic values indicating decreased cardiac output and increased systemic vascular resistance. If cardiac output starts to fall, be prepared to administer inotropic or fluid therapy to support the patient's cardiovascular status and prevent renal failure. (See *How to monitor intra-abdominal pressure.*)
• Monitor the patient's respiratory status continuously. If his intra-abdominal pressure increases, take measures to prevent respiratory complications. For instance, except when taking intra-abdominal pressure readings, always keep the head of the bed elevated (unless contraindicated) to promote maximum lung expansion

Using strict aseptic technique, instill 50 to 100 ml of 0.9% sodium chloride solution.

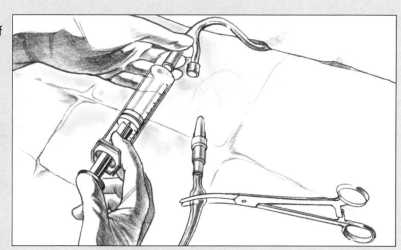

Insert the needle on the pressure tubing into the injection port. Then read the intra-abdominal pressure value on the monitor.

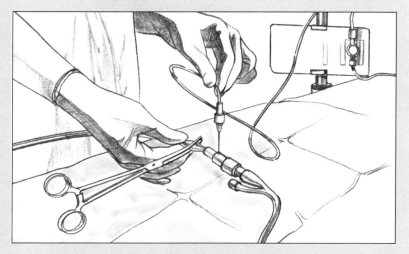

and minimize any ventilation-perfusion imbalance caused by pulmonary alveolar and blood vessel compression. Encourage the patient to cough and deep-breathe to prevent atelectasis, which may worsen the ventilation-perfusion imbalance.
• Discontinue intra-abdominal pressure monitoring, as ordered, when the patient's condition stabilizes. Expect to maintain the indwelling urinary catheter in place even after the monitoring ends.
• Continue to assess the patient's fluid balance by monitoring intake and output, evaluating laboratory studies (especially BUN and serum creatinine levels), and assessing abdominal girth and skin turgor. Changes in abdominal girth usually occur late, after other signs and symptoms appear.

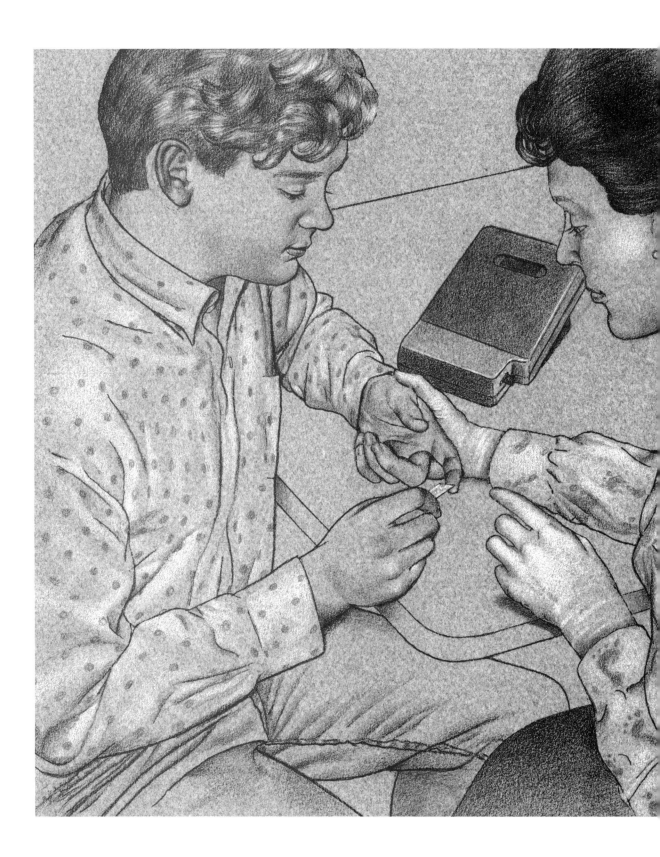

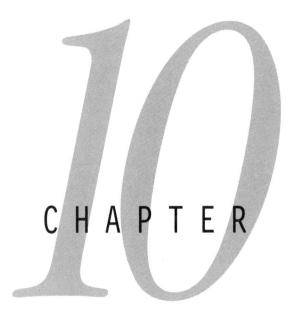

CHAPTER 10

Performing other monitoring techniques

As new monitoring methods and devices have developed, the monitoring of critical functions has become more accurate and efficient. These devices, with their increased automation and use of computers, have eliminated some of the time-consuming, repetitive tasks required by traditional monitoring methods.

Besides the advanced monitoring systems discussed in the previous chapters, you'll encounter others used for various patient needs. This chapter describes how to use intra-aortic balloon counterpulsation (IABC), the automated vital signs monitor, and the pulse amplitude monitor. It also covers bedside monitoring of gastric pH, gastric occult blood, and blood glucose and hemoglobin levels.

For each technique and device discussed, you're responsible for setting up the equipment and preparing the patient. In some cases, you may also be the one who performs the monitoring.

Intra-aortic balloon counterpulsation

Providing temporary support for the heart's left ventricle, IABC mechanically displaces blood within the aorta by means of an intra-aortic balloon attached to an external pump console. It monitors myocardial perfusion and the effects of drugs on myocardial function and perfusion. When used correctly, IABC improves two key aspects of myocardial physiology: It increases the supply of oxygen-rich blood to the myocardium, and it decreases myocardial oxygen demand.

The balloon is usually inserted through the common femoral artery and positioned with its tip just distal to the left subclavian artery. The external pump operates in precise counterpoint to the left ventricle, inflating the balloon with helium early in the diastole phase and deflating it just before systole. As the balloon inflates, it forces blood toward the aortic valve, raising pressure in the aortic root and augmenting diastolic pressure to improve coronary perfusion. It also improves peripheral circulation by forcing blood through the brachiocephalic, common carotid, and subclavian arteries arising from the aortic trunk.

The balloon deflates rapidly at the end of diastole. As a result, aortic volume and pressure decrease. This, in turn, reduces the effort needed by the left ventricle to open the aortic valve. The reduced work load lowers the heart's oxygen needs and, combined with improved myocardial perfusion, helps prevent or minimize myocardial ischemia. (See *How the intra-aortic balloon pump works.*)

IABC is recommended for patients with a wide range of low-cardiac-output disorders or cardiac instability, including refractory anginas, ventricular arrhythmias associated with ischemia, and pump failure caused by cardiogenic shock, intraoperative myocardial infarction (MI), or low cardiac output after bypass surgery. IABC is also indicated for patients with low cardiac output secondary to acute mechanical defects after MI (such as ventricular septal defect, papillary muscle rupture, or left ventricular aneurysm).

Perioperatively, the technique is used to support and stabilize patients with a suspected high-grade lesion who are undergoing such procedures as angioplasty, thrombolytic therapy, cardiac surgery, and cardiac catheterization.

IABC is contraindicated in patients with severe aortic regurgitation, aortic aneurysm, or severe peripheral vascular disease. The procedure may cause numerous complications. The most common, arterial embolism, stems from clot formation on the balloon surface. Other potential complications include extension or rupture of an aortic aneurysm, femoral or iliac artery perforation, femoral artery occlusion, and sepsis. Bleeding at the insertion site may become aggravated by pump-induced thrombocytopenia caused by platelet aggregation around the balloon.

Equipment
The intra-aortic balloon pump control system contains monitor controls and a drive system. The monitor controls allows you to observe and assess the patient's electrocardiogram (ECG), arterial pressure, and balloon pressure waveforms. The drive controls move helium in and out of the catheter by applying pressure to a volume limiter disk inside the console. This ensures adequate inflation and deflation of the balloon. (See *Intra-aortic balloon pump control system,* page 196.)

Preparation
You must prepare both the patient and the equipment for balloon insertion.

Preparing the patient
If time permits, explain to the patient that the doctor will place a special balloon catheter in the aorta to help his heart pump more easily. Briefly explain the insertion procedure, and mention that the catheter will be connected to a large console next to his bed. Tell him that the balloon will temporarily reduce the heart's work load to promote rapid healing of the ventricular muscle. Let him know that it will be removed after his heart can resume an adequate work load.

Make sure the patient or a family member understands and signs a consent form. Verify that the form is attached to his chart.

Next, record the patient's baseline vital signs, including pulmonary artery pressure (PAP). (A pulmonary artery [PA] line should already be in place.) Attach the patient to an ECG device for continuous monitoring. Be sure to apply chest electrodes in a standard lead II position — or in whatever position produces the largest R wave, because the R wave triggers balloon inflation and deflation. Obtain a baseline ECG.

Attach another set of ECG electrodes to the patient unless the ECG pattern is being transmitted from the patient's bedside monitor to the balloon pump monitor through a phone cable. Administer oxygen, as ordered and as necessary.

Make sure that the patient has an arterial line, a PA line, and a peripheral I.V. line in place. The arterial line is used for withdrawing blood samples, monitoring blood pressure, and assessing the timing and effectiveness of the therapy. The PA line allows measurement of PAP, aspiration of blood samples, and cardiac output studies. Increased PAP indicates increased myocardial work load and ineffective balloon pumping. Cardiac output studies are usually performed with and without the balloon to check the patient's progress. The central lumen of the intra-aortic balloon, used to monitor central aortic pressure, produces an augmented pressure waveform that allows you to check for proper timing of the inflation-deflation cycle and demonstrates the effects of counterpulsation, elevated diastolic pressure, and reduced end-diastolic and systolic pressures.

You'll need to insert an indwelling urinary catheter so that you can measure the patient's urine output and assess his fluid balance and renal function. To reduce the risk of infection, shave or clip hair bilaterally from the lower abdomen to the lower thigh, including the pubic area.

Observe and record the patient's peripheral leg pulse and document sensation, movement, color, and temperature of the legs.

How the intra-aortic balloon pump works

Made of polyurethane, the intra-aortic balloon is attached to an external pump console by means of a large-lumen catheter. The illustrations here show the direction of blood flow when the pump inflates and deflates the balloon.

Balloon inflation
The balloon inflates as the aortic valve closes and diastole begins. Diastole increases perfusion to the coronary arteries.

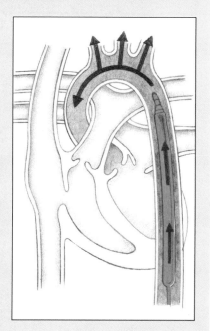

Balloon deflation
The balloon deflates before ventricular ejection, when the aortic valve opens. This permits ejection of blood from the left ventricle against a lowered resistance. As a result, aortic end-diastolic pressure and afterload decrease and cardiac output rises.

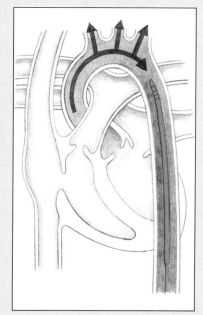

ADVANCED EQUIPMENT

Intra-aortic balloon pump control system

This photograph shows the intra-aortic balloon pump control system, including the control panel. This panel contains the display screen that allows the electrocardiogram and intra-aortic balloon counterpulsation to be monitored. Alarms and triggers can also be controlled from this panel.

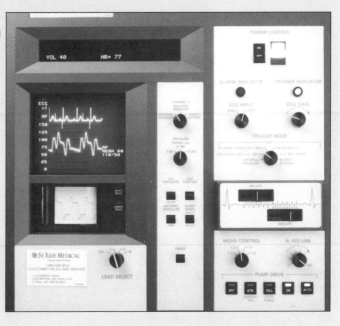

Preparing the equipment

Gather equipment for balloon insertion: balloon catheter and insertion tray, pump control system, 18G angiography needle, #8 French vessel dilator, arterial pressure transducer and flush setup, I.V. infusion set, indwelling urinary catheter, and heparin bolus and heparin infusion solution (unless your hospital uses a substitute). Also obtain sterile drapes, gloves, gown, and mask; suture and dressing materials; a shaving kit; a sterile basin; and povidone-iodine solution. The doctor might request 0.9% sodium chloride solution to lubricate the balloon.

You may also need a defibrillator and emergency drugs, an ECG monitor, a fluoroscope, arterial blood gas (ABG) kits and blood collection tubes for laboratory studies, a PA catheter setup, a temporary pacemaker setup, and an oxygen setup.

Before leaving the manufacturer, an intra-aortic balloon undergoes sophisticated testing

for leaks. It comes prefolded and ready to use and can't be inflated before insertion. The pressure transducer in the external pump console must be balanced and the oscilloscope monitor must be calibrated to ensure accuracy. Depending on your hospital's policy, you or a perfusionist will perform balancing and calibration.

Procedure

The balloon is inserted percutaneously or surgically, in a retrograde or an antegrade direction. The most common insertion method is percutaneous, using a modified Seldinger technique. In this method, the doctor inserts the balloon into the descending thoracic aorta via the femoral artery. In surgical insertion, the femoral artery is usually used. In both percutaneous and surgical insertion, the balloon tip eventually rests 3/8" to 3/4" (1 to 2 cm) distal to the left subclavian artery. The balloon's position must be confirmed by fluoroscope or X-ray.

Percutaneous insertion
• The doctor accesses the vessel with an 18G angiography needle and removes the inner stylet. Then he passes the guide wire through the needle and removes the needle.
• After passing a #8 French vessel dilator over the guide wire into the vessel, the doctor removes the vessel dilator, leaving the guide wire in place.
• Next, the doctor passes an introducer (dilator and sheath assembly) over the guide wire into the vessel until 1″ (2.5 cm) remains above the insertion site. He then removes the inner dilator, leaving the introducer sheath and guide wire in place.
• After passing the balloon over the guide wire into the introducer sheath, the doctor advances the catheter into position, ³⁄₈″ to ³⁄₄″ distal to the left subclavian artery.
• The doctor attaches the balloon to the control system to initiate counterpulsation. The balloon catheter then unfurls.

Surgical insertion
• After making an incision and isolating the femoral artery, the doctor attaches a Dacron graft to a small opening in the arterial wall.
• He then passes the catheter through this graft. With fluoroscopic guidance as needed, he advances the catheter up the descending thoracic aorta and positions the catheter tip between the left subclavian artery and the renal arteries.
• The doctor sews the Dacron graft around the catheter at the insertion point and connects the other end of the catheter to the pump console. (See *Surgical insertion sites for the intra-aortic balloon.*)
• If the balloon can't be inserted through the femoral artery, the doctor inserts it in an antegrade direction through the anterior wall of the ascending aorta. He positions it ³⁄₈″ to ³⁄₄″ beyond the left subclavian artery and brings the catheter out through the chest wall.

Interpretation of findings
Normally, balloon inflation immediately follows aortic valve closure and deflation occurs during isovolumetric contraction, just before the aortic valve opens. The normal waveform will display

Surgical insertion sites for the intra-aortic balloon

If an intra-aortic balloon can't be inserted percutaneously, the doctor will insert it surgically using a femoral or transthoracic approach.

Femoral approach
Insertion through the femoral artery requires a cutdown and an arteriotomy. The doctor passes the balloon through a Dacron graft that has been sewn to the artery.

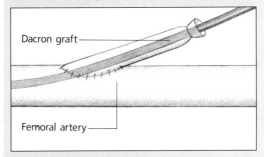

Dacron graft

Femoral artery

Transthoracic approach
If femoral insertion is unsuccessful, the doctor may use a transthoracic approach. He inserts the balloon in an antegrade direction through the subclavian artery and then positions it in the descending thoracic aorta.

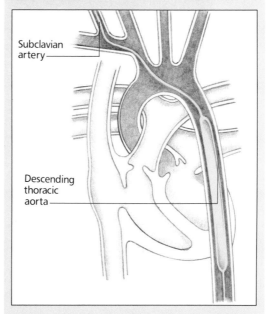

Subclavian artery

Descending thoracic aorta

Interpreting intra-aortic balloon waveforms

During intra-aortic balloon counterpulsation (IABC), you can use electrocardiogram and arterial pressure waveforms to determine whether the balloon pump is functioning properly.

Normal inflation-deflation timing

Balloon inflation usually occurs after aortic valve closure; deflation, during isovolumetric contraction, just before the aortic valve opens. In a properly timed waveform, like the one shown at right, the inflation point lies at or slightly above the dicrotic notch. Both inflation and deflation cause a sharp V. Peak diastolic pressure exceeds peak systolic pressure, peak systolic pressure exceeds assisted peak systolic pressure, and patient aortic end-diastolic pressure is 5 to 15 mm Hg higher than balloon aortic end-diastolic pressure.

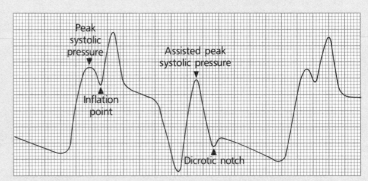

Early inflation

With *early inflation,* the inflation point lies before the dicrotic notch. Early inflation dangerously increases myocardial stress and decreases cardiac output.

Early deflation

With *early deflation,* a U shape appears and peak systolic pressure is less than or equal to assisted peak systolic pressure. This will not decrease afterload or myocardial oxygen consumption.

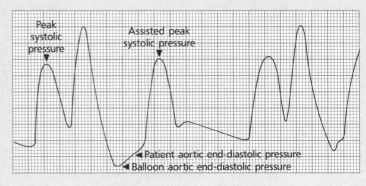

a rise in peak diastolic pressure, which indicates an increase in coronary perfusion pressure and a reduction in patient aortic end-diastolic pressure. The balloon aortic end-diastolic pressure should be less than the patient's normal aortic end-diastolic pressure. This reflects a reduction

in myocardial oxygen consumption and afterload. (See *Interpreting intra-aortic balloon waveforms.*)

Early inflation occurs when the balloon inflates before the aortic valve closes. On the waveform, the inflation point will precede the

Late inflation

With *late inflation,* the dicrotic notch precedes the inflation point, and the notch and the inflation point create a W shape. This can lead to a reduction in peak diastolic pressure, coronary and systemic perfusion augmentation time, and augmented coronary perfusion pressure.

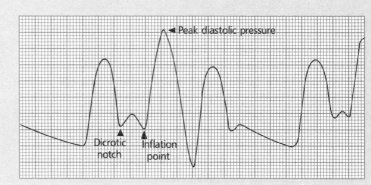

Late deflation

With *late deflation,* peak systolic pressure exceeds assisted peak systolic pressure. This threatens the patient by increasing afterload, myocardial oxygen consumption, cardiac work load, and preload. It occurs when the balloon has been inflated for too long.

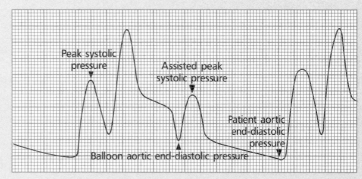

Proper timing with reduced augmentation

Sometimes, inflation and deflation are properly timed but the balloon doesn't inflate enough. When this happens, peak diastolic pressure equals or drops below peak systolic pressure. You'll need to evaluate the patient's condition to determine the cause of reduced augmentation.

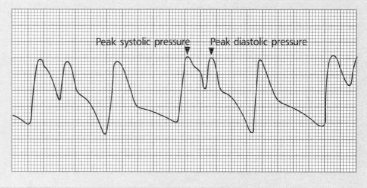

dicrotic notch. Early inflation is dangerous because it increases myocardial stress and decreases cardiac output. You can see these effects in premature aortic valve closure, incomplete ventricular emptying, decreased stroke volume, and increased preload and myocardial oxygen consumption.

Early deflation occurs when the balloon deflates before isovolumetric contraction occurs, allowing aortic refilling before ventricular ejection. The waveform will show aortic refilling and balloon aortic end-diastolic pressure will return to the normal patient aortic end-diastolic pressure reading, which may appear as a notch or shelflike area. Systolic unloading won't occur as the heart is pumping against the same resistance it encountered without IABC support, and peak systolic pressure will be less than or equal to assisted peak systolic pressure. Early deflation doesn't reduce after-load or myocardial oxygen consumption.

Late inflation occurs when the balloon inflates after the aortic valve closes, shortening the period of diastolic augmentation. On the waveform, the dicrotic notch precedes the inflation point and a characteristic W shape appears. Late inflation may cause reductions in coronary and systemic perfusion augmentation time, augmented coronary perfusion pressure and, possibly, peak diastolic pressure.

Late deflation occurs when the balloon remains inflated too long and impedes ejection. The waveform will show a balloon aortic end-diastolic pressure equal to or higher than the patient aortic end-diastolic pressure and will indicate depressed systolic ejection (signified by peak systolic pressure exceeding assisted peak systolic pressure). Late deflation poses a threat to the patient because it increases afterload, myocardial oxygen consumption, cardiac work load, and preload. It also reduces stroke volume and cardiac output, prolongs isovolumetric contraction, delays aortic valve opening, and depresses systolic ejection. If the patient has mechanical defects, such as a ventricular aneurysm, mitral regurgitation, or a septal defect, serious consequences may result.

If peak systolic pressure equals or exceeds peak diastolic pressure, suspect *reduced augmentation* (balloon inflation). If this occurs, first recheck balloon inflation-deflation timing. If timing is normal, evaluate the entire clinical picture to determine the cause of reduced augmentation. For instance, the balloon may be too low in the aorta or it may be too small for the patient. Reduced augmentation also may occur if stroke volume exceeds IABC effects, if the patient has hypertension or hypovolemia, or if the patient has received large amounts of drugs that reduce systemic vascular resistance. Also check to see if the controls are set to deliver a reduced volume.

Nursing considerations
• Before using the IABC control system, make sure you know what the alarms and messages mean and how to respond to them. *Caution:* You must respond immediately to alarms and messages. (See *Responding to control system alarms,* pages 202 and 203.)
• If the control system malfunctions or becomes inoperable, don't let the balloon catheter remain dormant for more than 30 minutes. Get another control system and attach it to the balloon; then resume pumping. In the meantime, inflate the balloon manually, using a 60-cc syringe and room air a minimum of once every five minutes, to prevent thrombus formation in the catheter.
• Obtain a chest X-ray to determine correct balloon placement.
• Assess and record pedal and posterior tibial pulses as well as color, sensation, and temperature in the affected limb every 15 minutes for 1 hour, then hourly. Notify the doctor immediately if you detect circulatory changes; the balloon may need to be removed.
• Observe and record the patient's baseline arm pulses, arm sensation and movement, and arm color and temperature every 15 minutes for 1 hour after balloon insertion, then every 2 hours while the balloon is in place. Loss of left arm pulses may indicate upward balloon displacement. Notify the doctor of any changes.
• Monitor the patient's urine output every hour. Note baseline blood urea nitrogen (BUN) and serum creatinine levels, and monitor these levels daily. Changes in urine output, BUN, and serum creatinine levels may signal reduced renal perfusion from downward balloon displacement.
• Auscultate and record bowel sounds every 4 hours. Check for abdominal distention and tenderness as well as changes in the patient's elimination patterns.
• Measure the patient's temperature every 1 to 4 hours. If it's elevated, obtain blood samples for a culture, send them to the laboratory immediately, and notify the doctor. Culture any drainage at the insertion site.
• Monitor the patient's hematologic status. Ob-

serve for bleeding gums, blood in the urine or stools, petechiae, and bleeding at the insertion site. Monitor his platelet count, hemoglobin levels, and hematocrit daily. Expect to administer blood products to maintain hematocrit at 30%. If the platelet count drops, expect to administer platelets.

• Monitor partial thromboplastin time every 6 hours while the heparin dose is adjusted to maintain the partial thromboplastin time at 1½ to 2 times the normal value, then every 12 to 24 hours while the balloon remains in place.

• Measure PAP and pulmonary artery wedge pressure (PAWP) every 1 to 2 hours, as ordered. A rising PAWP reflects preload, signaling increased ventricular pressure and work load; notify the doctor if this occurs. Some patients require I.V. nitroprusside during IABC to reduce preload and afterload.

• Obtain samples for ABG analysis, as ordered.

• Monitor serum electrolyte levels — especially sodium and potassium — to assess the patient's fluid and electrolyte balance and help prevent arrhythmias.

• Wash your hands carefully before patient contact, and use sterile technique during balloon insertion and dressing changes. Pay special attention to hygiene when caring for the indwelling urinary catheter and peripheral line.

• Change the dressing at the balloon insertion site every 24 hours or as needed, using strict sterile technique. Don't let povidone-iodine solution come in contact with the catheter.

• Make sure that the head of the bed is elevated no more than 30 degrees. If necessary, restrain the affected leg below the insertion site to prevent hip flexion, which could kink the catheter and disrupt the helium flow. A knee immobilizer works best because it doesn't restrict blood flow to the leg.

• Check for gas leaks from the catheter or balloon, which may be signaled by an alarm on the pump console. If the balloon ruptures, blood will appear in the catheter. If blood appears in the connecting tubing of the catheter, discontinue pumping and notify the doctor immediately.

• Watch for pump interruptions, which may result from loose ECG electrodes or leadwires,

static or 60-cycle interference, catheter kinking, or improper body alignment.

• Turn and reposition the patient every 2 hours, keeping the affected leg straight.

• Provide oral hygiene at least every 4 hours.

• Give pain medication, as ordered, to relieve discomfort at the insertion site.

• If angina occurs, notify the doctor.

• Watch for signs and symptoms of a dissecting aortic aneurysm: a blood pressure differential between the left and right arms; elevated blood pressure; pain in the chest, abdomen, or back; syncope; pallor; diaphoresis; dyspnea; a throbbing abdominal mass; and a reduced red blood cell count with an elevated white blood cell count. Notify the doctor immediately if you note any of these findings.

• The balloon may be removed if limb circulation is seriously compromised or if the patient's condition is considered inoperable or beyond recovery, at the doctor's discretion.

• Document all aspects of patient assessment and care, including the patient's response to therapy. If you're responsible for the IABC device, document all routine checks, problems, and troubleshooting measures. If a technician is responsible for the device, record only when and why the technician was notified and how his actions affected the patient. Also document any teaching you've provided to the patient or his family.

Weaning the patient from the balloon

• Assess the cardiac index, systemic blood pressure, and PAWP to help the doctor evaluate the patient's readiness for weaning — usually about 24 hours after balloon insertion.

• To begin weaning, gradually decrease the frequency of balloon augmentation to 1:2, 1:4, and 1:8, as ordered. Although your hospital has its own weaning protocol, be aware that assist frequency is usually maintained for an hour or longer. If the patient's hemodynamic indices remain stable during this time, weaning may continue.

• Avoid leaving the patient on a low augmentation setting for more than 2 hours to prevent embolus formation.

• Assess his tolerance of weaning. Signs and

(Text continues on page 204.)

TROUBLESHOOTING

Responding to control system alarms

When your patient undergoes intra-aortic balloon counterpulsation (IABC), you must respond immediately to any equipment problems. This chart describes the problems most often encountered in the Model 700 IABP Control System, a popular device.

PROBLEM	POSSIBLE CAUSES	NURSING INTERVENTIONS
High gas leakage (automatic mode only)	Balloon leakage or abrasion	Check for blood in tubing. Stop pumping. Contact the doctor to remove the balloon as soon as possible.
	Condensation in extension tubing, volume limiter disk, or both	Remove condensate from tubing and volume limiter disk. Refill, autopurge, and resume pumping.
	Kink in balloon catheter or tubing	Check catheter and tubing for kinks and loose connections. Refill and resume pumping.
	Tachycardia (rapid flow of helium causing insufficient fill pressure)	Change wean control to 1:2 or operate in ON (manual) mode. *Note:* Gas alarms are off in manual mode. Autopurge balloon every 1 to 2 hours, and monitor balloon pressure waveform closely.
	Malfunctioning or loose volume limiter disk	Replace or tighten volume limiter disk. Refill, autopurge, and resume pumping.
	System leak	Perform leak test.
Balloon line block (automatic mode only)	Kink in balloon catheter or tubing	Check catheter and tubing for kinks. Refill and resume pumping.
	Balloon catheter not unfurled, sheath positioned too high, or balloon positioned too high	Contact doctor to verify placement; balloon may have to be repositioned or inflated manually.
	Condensation in tubing, volume limiter disk, or both	Remove condensate from tubing and volume limiter disk. Refill, autopurge, and resume pumping.
	Balloon too large for aorta	Decrease volume control percentage by one notch.
	Malfunctioning volume limiter disk or incorrect volume limiter disk size	Replace volume limiter disk, refill, autopurge, and resume pumping.
No electrocardiogram (ECG) trigger	Inadequate signal	Adjust ECG gain, and change lead or trigger mode.
	Lead disconnected	Replace lead.
	Improper ECG input mode (skin or monitor) selected	Adjust ECG input to appropriate mode (skin or monitor).

TROUBLESHOOTING

Responding to control system alarms *(continued)*

PROBLEM	POSSIBLE CAUSES	NURSING INTERVENTIONS
No arterial pressure trigger	Arterial line damped	Flush line.
	Arterial line open to atmosphere	Check connections on arterial pressure line.
Trigger mode change	Trigger mode changed while pumping	Resume pumping.
Irregular heart rhythm	Patient in irregular rhythm (such as atrial fibrillation or ectopic beats)	Change to R or QRS sense (if necessary) to accommodate irregular rhythm.
Erratic atrioventricular (AV) pacing	Demand for paced rhythm occurs while in AV sequential trigger mode	Change to pacer reject trigger or QRS sense.
Noisy ECG signal	Malfunctioning leads	Replace leads; check ECG cable.
	Electrocautery in use	Switch to AP trigger.
Internal trigger	Trigger mode set on internal 80 beats/minute	Select alternative trigger if patient has a heartbeat or rhythm. *Caution:* Internal trigger should be used only during cardiopulmonary bypass surgery or cardiac arrest.
Purge incomplete	OFF button pressed during autopurge, interrupting purge cycle	Initiate autopurge again or initiate pumping.
High fill pressure	Malfunctioning volume limiter disk	Replace volume limiter disk, refill, autopurge, and resume pumping.
	Occluded vent line or valve	Attempt to resume pumping. If this fails to correct problem, contact manufacturer.
No balloon drive	No volume limiter disk	Insert volume limiter disk, and lock it securely in place.
	Tubing disconnected	Reconnect tubing, refill, autopurge, and resume pumping.
Incorrect timing	Inflate and deflate controls improperly set	Place inflate and deflate controls at set midpoints. Reassess timing and adjust as necessary.
Low volume percentage	Volume control percentage not on 100%	Assess cause of decreased volume and reset if necessary.

symptoms of poor tolerance include confusion and disorientation, urine output below 30 ml/hour, cold and clammy skin, chest pain, arrhythmias, ischemic ECG changes, and elevated PAP. If the patient develops any of these problems, notify the doctor at once.

Removing the balloon
• The balloon is removed when the patient can tolerate counterpulsation in 1:4 or 1:8 and no longer needs augmentation. The control system is turned off and the connective tubing is disconnected from the catheter to ensure balloon deflation.
• The doctor withdraws the balloon until the proximal end of the catheter contacts the distal end of the introducer sheath.
• The doctor then applies pressure below the puncture site and removes the balloon and introducer sheath as a unit, allowing a few seconds of free bleeding to prevent thrombus formation.
• To promote distal bleedback, the doctor applies pressure above the puncture site.
• Apply direct pressure to the site for 30 minutes or until bleeding stops. (In some hospitals, this is the doctor's responsibility.)
• If the balloon was inserted surgically, the doctor will close the Dacron graft and suture the insertion site. The cardiologist usually removes a percutaneous catheter.
• After balloon removal, provide wound care according to hospital policy. Record the patient's pedal and posterior tibial pulses, and the color, temperature, and sensation of the affected limb. Enforce bed rest as appropriate (usually for 24 hours).

Automated vital signs monitoring

An automated vital signs monitor measures a patient's vital signs independently, freeing you to carry out other patient care activities. A noninvasive device, the monitor measures pulse rate, systolic and diastolic blood pressures, and mean arterial pressure at preset intervals.

Some models also monitor the patient's temperature.

Because the monitor works automatically, many patients who would otherwise need the closer observation of an intensive care unit can stay in a medical-surgical unit. Such patients include those with chronic renal failure or chronic congestive heart failure; those receiving such I.V. drugs as low-dose dobutamine, dopamine, or nitroglycerin; and those who've recently undergone surgery, certain diagnostic tests, or short procedures (such as cardiac catheterization).

Equipment
Many types of automated vital signs monitors are available. Find out the manufacturer of the monitor you're using, and obtain an instruction manual for the correct model. (See *Automated vital signs monitor.*) Besides the monitor itself, you'll need an I.V. pole.

Preparation
To prepare the monitor for use, place it securely on the I.V. pole and plug it into an electrical outlet to help preserve the batteries. Turn on the monitor and allow it to warm up.

Explain to the patient what the monitor is and how it works. Tell him that the monitor will automatically measure his blood pressure at preset intervals, so he shouldn't be alarmed when the cuff inflates. Warn him that the first few cuff inflations may be uncomfortable until the monitor determines his blood pressure range.

Procedure
• Before using the monitor, assess its accuracy. Determine the patient's pulse rate and blood pressure manually, using the same arm you'll place in the monitor cuff. Compare your results with initial monitor readings; if they differ, suspect monitor malfunction. Get a new monitor, and notify the appropriate department so that someone can arrange for repair of the old one.
• Place the monitor cuff on the patient's arm, making sure that the ARTERY arrow is over the palpated brachial artery. Secure the cuff for a snug fit.

Automated vital signs monitor

Various automated vital signs monitors are available. As this photograph of the Dinamap monitor shows, the monitor is compact and lightweight enough to be placed on an I.V. pole for use at the patient's bedside. The monitor will display heart rate; systolic, diastolic, and mean blood pressures; and the time interval when the machine will measure the patient's vital signs.

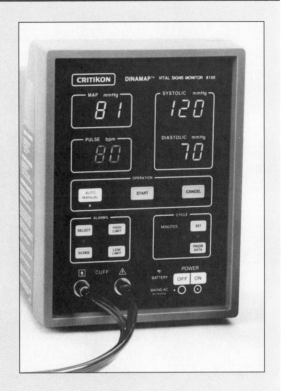

• Select the automatic mode, which lets you program how often the monitor should take vital signs. With most models, a manual mode lets you take the patient's vital signs at any time without interfering with preset time intervals.
• Set the high and low alarms according to the manufacturer's directions.
• After you start the monitor, stay with the patient until the monitor completes its first vital signs measurement.

Interpretation of findings
The monitor displays the patient's vital signs on the appropriate screens. If the displayed results seem unusual (for example, extremely high or low blood pressure values), reactivate the monitor to reassess vital signs or take the patient's vital signs manually. Consult the manu-

facturer's instructions to make sure you're using the monitor correctly. (See *Correcting problems with an automated vital signs monitor,* page 206.)

If you note a significant change in vital signs from one reading to the next, check the patient's clinical status and notify the doctor.

Nursing considerations
• Assess the color, temperature, and capillary refill time of the arm or leg with the blood pressure cuff. Remove the cuff every 4 hours and assess the skin under it to make sure that it's dry and not being pinched by the cuff.
• To ease the patient's anxiety, explain to him and his family the meaning of the numbers displayed on the screen.
• Take the patient's vital signs manually once every shift to assess the accuracy of monitor

Correcting problems with an automated vital signs monitor

PROBLEM	POSSIBLE CAUSES	NURSING INTERVENTIONS
No value or error message displayed	Cardiac arrhythmia	Check patient's clinical status (for example, blood pressure, pulses, and mental status) and take measures to stabilize him.
	Kinked or occluded tubing	Unkink tubing; if patient is leaning against tubing, reposition him.
	Leak in tubing or cuff	Replace cuff set.
	Patient movement, shivering, or seizures	Remind patient that he shouldn't move his arm. Increase his body temperature with blankets and give medication, as ordered, to decrease seizures.
	Heart rate too low (for example, below 40 beats/minute)	Use alternative method to determine blood pressure, such as Doppler ultrasound stethoscope.
Extremely high blood pressure value displayed	Cuff too small	Use correct size cuff. (Check measurements inside cuff or in operating manual.)
	Cuff positioned below heart level	Place cuffed limb at heart level.
Extremely low blood pressure value displayed	Cuff too large	Use correct size cuff. (Check measurements inside cuff or in operating manual.)
	Cuff positioned above heart level	Place cuffed limb at heart level.
	Faulty internal calibration	Replace monitor and call for service.
Only mean blood pressure value displayed or no value displayed (00/00/00)	Rapid blood pressure fluctuation caused by cardiac arrhythmia or vasoactive drugs	Use alternative method to determine blood pressure, such as Doppler ultrasound stethoscope.
	Patient movement, shivering, or seizures	Use alternative method to determine blood pressure, such as Doppler ultrasound stethoscope.
	Heart rate too low	Use alternative method to determine blood pressure, such as Doppler ultrasound stethoscope.
	Patient weight under 20 lb (9 kg)	Use appropriate pediatric or neonatal cuff and tubing. Or use alternative device to determine blood pressure, such as Doppler ultrasound stethoscope.
No heart rate or blood pressure display on a clinically stable patient	Inadequate circulation to limb	Change limb being used to monitor vital signs.
	Faulty cuff or sensor	Try another cuff. If that doesn't help, change entire unit.

values. Be sure to use the same arm or leg that the monitor is using.
• Document the results of your assessment checks and manual checks.
• When the patient no longer needs the automated vital signs monitor, turn it off and remove the cuff from his arm or leg. Clean the monitor and cuff according to the manufacturer's instructions.

Pulse amplitude monitoring

Determining the presence and strength of peripheral pulses, an essential part of cardiovascular assessment, helps you to evaluate the adequacy of peripheral perfusion. A pulse amplitude monitor simplifies this procedure. A sensor taped to the patient's skin over a pulse point sends signals to a monitor, which measures the amplitude of the pulse and displays it as a waveform on a screen. The system continuously monitors the patient's peripheral pulse so that you can perform other patient care duties.

The pulse amplitude monitor can be used after peripheral vascular reconstruction on the upper or lower extremities or after percutaneous transluminal peripheral or coronary angioplasty (either with the sheaths in place or after they've been removed).

Because the sensor monitors only relatively flat pulse points, it can't be used for the posterior tibial pulse point. Also, movement will distort the waveform, so the patient must stay as still as possible during monitoring. The patient shouldn't have lesions on the skin where the pulse will be monitored because the sensor must be placed directly on this site. The sensor and tape could irritate the lesion, or the lesion could impair transmission of the pulse amplitude.

Equipment
You'll need a pulse amplitude display monitor and a sensor. This is a fairly new piece of equipment and may not be available in many hospitals. (See *Pulse amplitude monitor and sensor,* page 208.)

Preparation
To prepare the patient, explain how the pulse amplitude monitor works. Next, locate the pulse that you want to monitor. Mention that you'll tape the sensor to the site you've selected, usually the foot.

Plug the monitor into a grounded outlet. Although the monitor has battery power for up to 24 hours, it should be plugged in when the battery isn't needed.

Turn on the monitor and allow it to warm up, which may take up to 10 seconds. Plug the sensor cable into the monitor; then tap the sensor gently. If tapping causes interference on the display screen, you can assume the sensor-monitor connection is functioning properly.

Procedure
• Place the sensor over the strongest point of the pulse you're going to monitor. While observing the display screen, move the sensor until you see a strong upright waveform.
• Without moving the sensor from this site, peel off the adhesive strips and affix the sensor securely to the patient's foot. The sensor must maintain proper skin contact, so be sure to tape it firmly.
• Adjust the height of the pulse wave signal to half the height of the display screen. This will give the waveform room to fluctuate as the pulse amplitude increases and decreases.
• Set the low and high waveform amplitude alarms so that you'll be alerted to any waveform changes.

Interpretation of findings
If the patient has a strong peripheral pulse, you'll see an adequate waveform. (See *Identifying a normal pulse amplitude waveform,* page 209.)

If the sensor doesn't pick up an adequate signal, suspect a weak pulse or significant vessel calcification.

ADVANCED EQUIPMENT

Pulse amplitude monitor and sensor

The pulse amplitude monitor helps you assess peripheral perfusion by noninvasively checking the presence and strength of a patient's peripheral pulse. A sensor placed on the pulse point of an extremity measures the amplitude of the peripheral pulse, and the monitor screen continuously displays a pulse amplitude waveform.

This illustration shows a sensor taped to the patient's foot and connected to the pulse amplitude monitor.

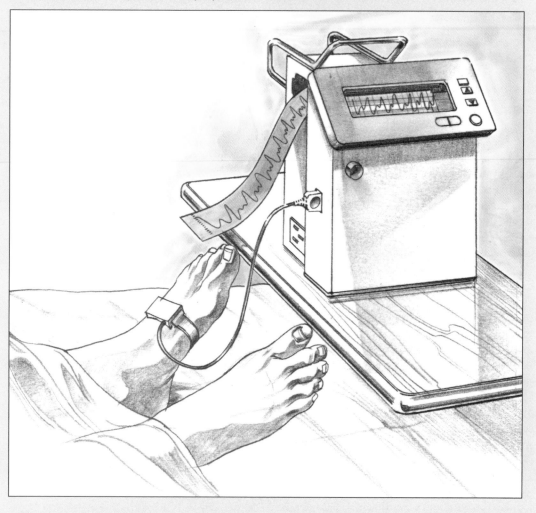

Nursing considerations

• Be aware that although the waveform displayed by a pulse amplitude monitor may resemble an ECG or blood pressure waveform, it's not the same.

• Don't apply much pressure on the pulse sensor film or press on it with a sharp object because such stress may warp or destroy the sensor.

Identifying a normal pulse amplitude waveform

If your patient has adequate peripheral perfusion, the pulse amplitude
monitor will usually display a normal
waveform, like the one shown here.
This waveform resembles the waveform seen when a patient has an arterial line.

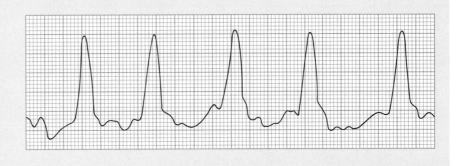

• Never place the sensor over an open wound
or ulcerated skin.
• Print out a strip of the patient's waveform,
and place the strip in the patient's chart during
every shift and whenever you note a change in
the waveform or the patient's condition. Along
the left side of the strip, you'll see a reference
scale used to measure pulse amplitude height.
This scale should be included in your documentation.
• If waveform amplitude decreases, assess the
patient's leg for capillary refill time, temperature, color, and sensation. The amplitude
change may stem from a malfunction in the
monitor itself (such as a low battery) or from
a thrombus, a hematoma, or a significant
change in the patient's hemodynamic status.
• If the display screen is blank when you turn
on the machine, check whether the monitor is
plugged in. If it's plugged in but the screen remains blank, the screen may need repair.
• If the screen is functioning but no waveform
appears on it, first check the sensor-monitor
connection. Then check the sensor by gently
tapping it to see if interference appears on the
screen. If the sensor is working properly, relo-
cate the peripheral pulse on the patient's foot
and reapply the sensor. If your interventions
don't work, the screen may need servicing.
• To discontinue monitor use, peel the sensor

tapes from the patient's skin. Turn the machine
off but keep it plugged in. Discard the sensor
and, if necessary, wipe the monitor with a
mild soap solution.

Bedside gastric pH and occult blood monitoring

Bedside testing kits, such as Gastroccult, help
you assess your patient's gastric pH level and
determine whether he's experiencing occult
gastric bleeding. This information helps guide
drug therapy for gastric bleeding, which typically involves antacids or H_2-receptor antago-
nists. GI tonometry, another means of indirect
gastric pH measurement, is also gaining wider
use. (See *Using GI tonometry,* page 210.)
    Gastric bleeding is a particular risk for pa-
tients with such conditions as cardiac disease,
sepsis, multiple trauma, liver failure, hypotension, respiratory failure, or renal failure. Patients
who've recently undergone major surgery are
also at higher risk for GI bleeding. The physiologic stress may interfere with the body's normal mechanism for protecting the gastric mucosa; without such protection, the mucosa may
ulcerate and bleed.

ADVANCED EQUIPMENT

Using GI tonometry

An alternative to bedside testing kits, GI tonometry measures the partial pressure of carbon dioxide (P_{CO_2}) in the gastric mucosa. By using the gastric P_{CO_2} value in a special equation along with the patient's arterial bicarbonate (HCO_3^-) level, you can estimate gastric pH.

Because GI tonometry indirectly measures systemic oxygenation, it's especially useful for detecting hypoxia early in critically ill patients. Hypoxia typically decreases gastric pH.

How the method works

Measurements are obtained by using a standard nasogastric (NG) sump tube incorporated into a silicone balloon system. The doctor inserts the sump tube as he would an NG tube. Once the balloon enters the patient's stomach, he fills it with 0.9%

sodium chloride solution. The balloon, permeable to carbon dioxide (CO_2), lies close to the gastric mucosa; CO_2 diffuses through the balloon into the 0.9% sodium chloride solution (as shown below). After 60 to 90 minutes, the P_{CO_2} of the 0.9% sodium chloride solution is tested; the result correctly reflects gastric mucosal P_{CO_2}.

The test also requires an arterial sample for blood gas analysis. To determine gastric pH, you'll need the results of these tests: the P_{CO_2} of the 0.9% sodium chloride solution and HCO_3^- level of the arterial sample. They're used in the Henderson-Hasselbalch equation, as shown here:

$$pH = \frac{6.1 + \log 10 \text{ (arterial } HCO_3^-)}{0.03 \times P_{CO_2} \text{ of 0.9\% sodium chloride}}$$

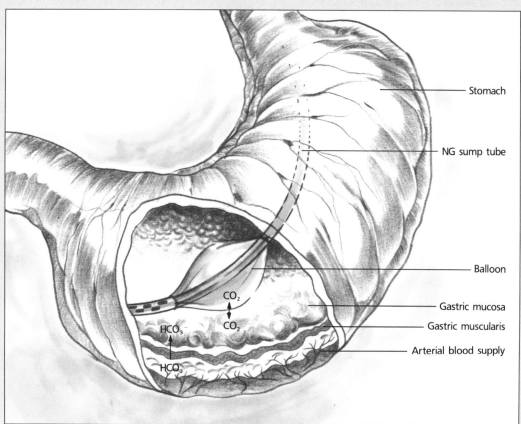

Equipment

You'll need the testing kit and the appropriate developing solution, two piston irrigating syringes, and 0.9% sodium chloride solution (or sterile water) to irrigate the nasogastric (NG) tube.

Preparation

To prepare the patient, make sure that the NG tube is in place. If the tube is connected to suction, disconnect the suction and plug the tube before aspirating stomach contents for testing. Have the patient lie on his left side to promote pooling of gastric contents.

Procedure

• Using a piston syringe, withdraw 10 to 15 ml of the patient's gastric secretions from the NG tube. As you aspirate secretions, you also remove any fluid or other elements that may alter pH and occult blood test results, so discard this sample.
• With the second piston syringe, withdraw a small amount (1 to 5 ml) of secretions for testing.
• Place a small portion of the secretions on the testing card, in the areas designated for pH testing and occult blood testing. Close the flap on the card.
• Turn the testing card over and raise the flap. Apply the developer to the affected areas, wait the recommended time, and then read the results.

Interpretation of findings

To determine if your patient's pH level is normal, compare it to the normal indicators on the test card.

If the patient's secretions contain occult blood, the testing area will turn blue; the more occult blood in the secretions, the more intense the blue reaction. If blue doesn't appear, the test result is negative.

Nursing considerations

• Don't aspirate secretions with a syringe that you've used to administer drugs.
• If you've administered medication through the NG tube, wait 30 minutes before measuring gastric pH or testing for occult blood. This is especially important for gastric pH testing; if you test prematurely, the results may reflect the pH of the medication rather than that of the patient's secretions. If possible, test the pH of drugs you're giving by NG tube to help prevent test interference. (Be aware that such drugs as ranitidine and cimetidine won't interfere with occult blood testing or distort pH values.)
• If the doctor orders NG tube irrigation, test the pH of the irrigating fluid for the same reason (0.9% sodium chloride solution, for instance, has a pH of 5 to 5.5).
• Read the testing cards in adequate light to ensure accurate color interpretations.
• Take the test sample directly from the NG tube, not from the drainage collection container.
• Wash the syringes carefully after testing, using a solution with a pH that you've tested or already know.

Bedside blood glucose and hemoglobin monitoring

Increasingly, nurses are monitoring blood glucose and hemoglobin levels at the patient's bedside. The fast, accurate results obtained this way allow immediate intervention, if necessary. In contrast, with traditional monitoring methods, blood samples must be sent to the laboratory for interpretation. A blood sample that sits at room temperature for an hour may undergo glycolysis, which reduces glucose concentration by 3% to 30%, leading to inaccurate test results.

Numerous testing systems are available for bedside monitoring. Bedside systems are also convenient for the patient's home use. HemoCue, a widely used system, gives accurate results without having to dispense, pipette, or mix blood and reagents to obtain readings. Thus, it eliminates the risk of leakage, broken tubes, and splattered blood.

How to use a bedside blood glucose and hemoglobin monitor

Monitoring blood glucose and hemoglobin levels at the patient's bedside is a straightforward procedure. Follow the three steps shown below to use the HemoCue system to obtain a blood sample and place it in the photometer for a reading.

After you pierce the skin, the microcuvette draws blood automatically.

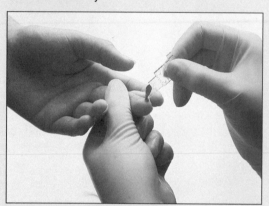

Next, place the microcuvette into the photometer.

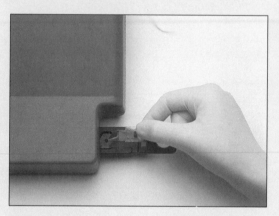

Equipment

To use the HemoCue system, you'll need a microcuvette, a photometer, sterile gloves, alcohol sponges, and gauze pads. The plastic, disposable microcuvette functions as a combination pipette, test tube, and measuring vessel. It contains a reagent that produces a precise chemical reaction as soon as it contacts blood.

The photometer is powered by a battery or an AC adapter. One model is calibrated at the factory and rarely needs to be recalibrated, returning to zero between tests. Use the control cuvette included with each system to test photometer function. (See *How to use a bedside blood glucose and hemoglobin monitor.*)

Preparation

Explain the test purpose to the patient. Tell him he'll feel a pinprick in his finger during blood sampling.

Turn the photometer on. If it hasn't been used recently, insert the control cuvette to make sure that it's working properly.

Procedure

• Select a puncture site—usually the fingertip or earlobe for an adult, or the heel or great toe for an infant.
• Wash your hands and put on sterile gloves.
• Wipe the puncture site with an alcohol sponge, and dry it thoroughly with a gauze pad.
• Pierce the skin quickly and sharply with the microcuvette, which automatically draws a precise amount of blood (approximately 5 μl).
• Place the microcuvette into the photometer. Results appear on the photometer screen within 40 seconds to 4 minutes.
• Place a gauze pad over the area until the bleeding stops.

Interpretation of findings

Normal glucose values range from 70 to 100 mg/dl; normal hemoglobin values range from 12.5 to 15 g/dl.

An above-normal glucose level (hyperglycemia) may indicate diabetes mellitus or the use of steroid drugs. A below-normal glucose level

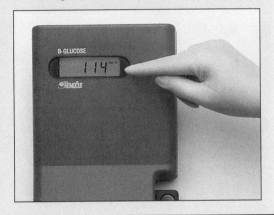

The photometer screen displays the blood glucose and hemoglobin levels.

may indicate overly rapid glucose use, which may occur with strenuous exercise or infection, resulting in tissues receiving insufficient glucose.

A below-normal hemoglobin value may indicate anemia, recent hemorrhage, or fluid retention, causing hemodilution. An elevated hemoglobin value suggests hemoconcentration from polycythemia or dehydration.

Nursing considerations
• Before using a microcuvette, note its expiration date. Microcuvettes can be stored for up to 2 years. However, after the microcuvette vial is opened, the shelf life is 90 days.
• Before taking a blood sample, operate the photometer with the control cuvette to check for proper function.
• To ensure an adequate blood sample, don't use a cold, cyanotic, or swollen area as the puncture site.
• Document the values obtained from the photometer as well as any interventions.

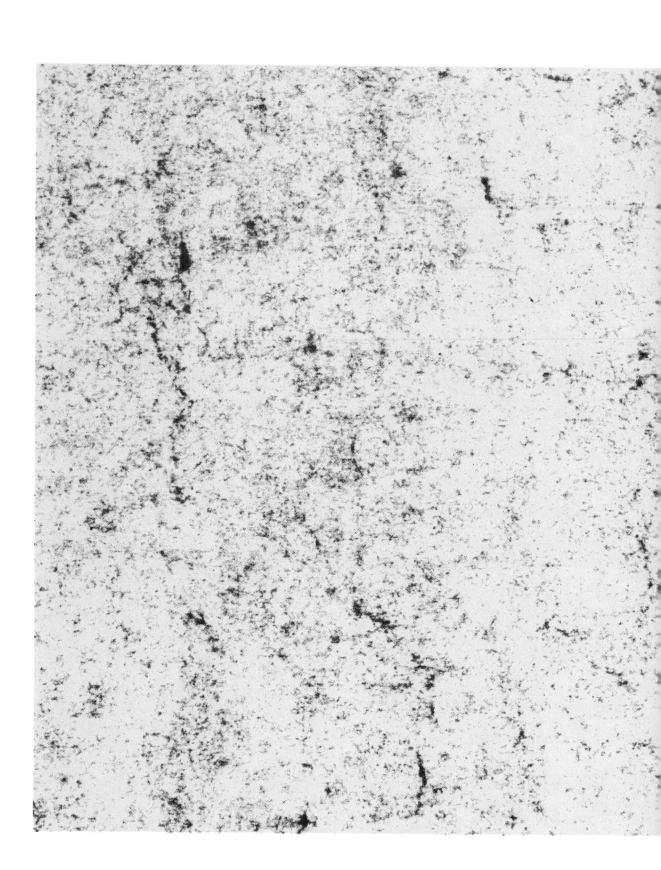

Suggested readings and acknowledgments

Alspach, G. *Core Curriculum for Critical Care Nursing,* 2nd ed. Philadelphia: W.B. Saunders Co., 1991.

Andrus, C. "Intracranial Pressure: Dynamics and Nursing Management," *Journal of Neuroscience Nursing* 23(2):85-92, April 1991.

Bavin, T.K. "Nursing Considerations for Patients Requiring Cardiopulmonary Support," *AACN Clinical Issues in Critical Care Nursing* 2(3):500-514, August 1991.

Bobak, I., et al. *Maternity and Gynecologic Care, the Nurse and the Family,* 4th ed. St. Louis: Mosby Publishing, Inc., 1989.

Campbell, M.L., and Greenberg, C.A. "Reading Pulmonary Artery Wedge Pressures at End-Expiration," *Focus on Critical Care* 15(2):60-63, April 1988.

Carnevali, D.L., and Patrick, M. *Nursing Management of the Elderly,* 3rd ed. Philadelphia: J. B. Lippincott Co., 1992.

Carroll, G.C. "Blood Pressure Monitoring," *Critical Care Clinics* 4(3):411-34, July 1988.

Chenevey, B. "Overview of Fluids and Electrolytes," *Nursing Clinics of North America* 22(4):749-59, December 1987.

Daily, E.K. "Hemodynamic Monitoring." In *Critical Care Nursing: Clinical Management through the Nursing Process.* Edited by Dolan, J. Philadelphia: F.A. Davis, 1991.

Dennison, R.D., "Understanding the Four Determinants of Cardiac Output," *Nursing90* 20(7):35-41, July 1990.

Dickman, C., et al. "Continuous Regional Cerebral Blood Flow Monitoring in Acute Craniocerebral Trauma," *Neurosurgery* 28(3):467-72, March 1991.

Gardner, P.E. "Cardiac Output: Theory, Technique, and Troubleshooting," *Critical Care Nursing Clinics of North America* 1(3):577-87, September 1989.

Hickey, J. *Clinical Practice of Neurological and Neurosurgical Nursing,* 3rd ed. Philadelphia: J.B. Lippincott Co., 1992.

Holder, C., and Alexander, J. "A New and Improved Guide to I.V. Therapy," *AJN* 90(2):43-47, February 1990.

Holmes, J., and Magiera, L. *Maternity Nursing.* New York: Macmillan Publishing Co., 1987.

Jansen, J.R.C., et al. "Reliability of Cardiac Output Measurements by the Thermodilution Method." In *Update in Intensive Care and Emergency Medicine.* Edited by Vincent, J.R. Berlin: Springer-Verlag, 408-41, 1989.

Methany, N. *Fluid and Electrolyte Balance: Nursing Considerations,* 2nd ed. Philadelphia: J.B. Lippincott Co., 1992.

Nursing Procedures. Springhouse, Pa.: Springhouse Corp., 1992.

Paolella, L.P., et al. "Topographic Location of the Left Atrium by Computed Tomography: Reducing Pulmonary Artery Catheter Calibration Error," *Critical Care Medicine* 16(11):1154-156, November 1988.

Poyss, A. "Assessment and Nursing Diagnosis in Fluid and Electrolyte Disorders," *Nursing Clinics of North America* 22(4):773-83, December 1987.

Scott, J.R. *Obstetrics and Gynecology,* 6th ed. Philadelphia: J.B. Lippincott Co., 1989.

Smith, R.G., and Cleavinger, M. "Current Perspectives on the Use of Circulatory Assist Devices," *AACN Clinical Issues in Critical Care Nursing* 2(3):488-99, August 1991.

Sommers, M. "Rapid Fluid Resuscitation: How to Correct Dangerous Deficits," *Nursing90* 20(1):52-59, January 1990.

Tucker, S. *Pocket Guide to Fetal Monitoring,* 2nd ed. St. Louis: Mosby Publishing, Inc., 1992.

Tuman, K.J., et al. "Pitfalls in Interpretation of Pulmonary Artery Catheter Data," *Journal of Cardiothoracic Anesthesia* 3(5):625-41, October 1989.

Yipintsoi, T., and Wood, E.H. "The History of Circulatory Indicator Dilution." In *Dye Curves: The Theory and Practice of Indicator Dilution.* Edited by Bloomfield, D. Baltimore, MD: University Park Press, 1-19. Reprinted by Books in Demand, UMI, 1974.

Acknowledgments

Abbott Critical Care Systems, Abbott Laboratories
Mountain View, Calif.

Edwards Critical-Care Division, Baxter Healthcare Corporation
Irvine, Calif.

Camino Laboratories
San Diego, Calif.

Clinical Neuro Systems Inc.
Exton, Pa.

Codman & Shurtleff, Inc.
Randolf, Mass.

Cordis Corp.
Miami Lakes, Calif.

Pudenz-Schultz Medical Corp.
Goleta, Calif.

Viggo-Spectramed
Oxnard, Calif.

Advanced skilltest

You can test your knowledge of monitoring critical functions by answering the following multiple-choice questions. The answers, along with rationales, appear on pages 221 to 223.

1. Indications for cardiac monitoring include all of the following *except:*

    a. monitoring the heart rate.

    b. detecting ST-segment changes.

    c. alerting caregivers to pain and discomfort.

    d. identifying arrhythmias.

2. Electrodes placed on the skin detect the electrical current traveling through the heart. Another name for this current is:

    a. a vector.

    b. energy.

    c. a bipolar system.

    d. a positive complex.

3. To set up a cardiac monitoring system, you do all of the following *except:*

    a. set the heart rate and the high- and low-limit alarms.

    b. activate the pacemaker channel to avoid double-sensing of pacer artifacts and QRS complexes (if the patient has a pacemaker).

    c. turn the bedside monitor on.

    d. start a peripheral I.V. line.

4. With a five-electrode electrocardiograph (ECG) monitoring system, you must place each limb electrode at the point where the limb joins the trunk. Where would you place the chest electrode of the V lead?

    a. At the fifth intercostal space in the left midaxillary line

    b. At the fourth intercostal space along the right sternal border

    c. At the fourth intercostal space along the left sternal border

    d. At the third intercostal space in the left midaxillary line

5. Which ECG leads are most reliable for detecting a new bundle-branch block in a patient with a recent myocardial infarction?

    a. V_1 or MCL_1 or V_3 or MCL_3

    b. V_1 or MCL_1 or V_6 or MCL_6

    c. V_3 or MCL_3 or V_5 or MCL_5

    d. V_3 or MCL_3 or V_6 or MCL_6

6. The ST segment of the ECG waveform, which represents early myocardial repolarization, typically deviates from the baseline if myocardial ischemia occurs. When is such a deviation considered significant?

    a. When it exceeds 2 mm

    b. When it exceeds 3 mm

    c. When it exceeds 0.5 mm

    d. When it exceeds 1 mm

7. A pressure monitoring system must accurately reproduce and display physiologic vibrations or frequencies. This capacity is called:

    a. resonant frequency.

    b. hydrostatic pressure.

    c. frequency response.

    d. dynamic pressure.

8. Optimally, the signals reproduced by a pressure monitoring system are critically damped, or diminished. In an overdamped system, the signals are excessively diminished. Overdamping does *not* result from:

    a. noncompliant tubing.

    b. compliant tubing.

    c. air bubbles.

    d. additional stopcocks.

9. To obtain accurate values from a pressure monitoring system, you must zero the transducer to offset the effect of atmospheric pressure. Zeroing is adversely affected by all of the following *except:*

    a. insufficient transducer warm-up time.

    b. opening the stopcock to air.

    c. atmospheric pressure changes in the patient's room.

    d. moving the transducer after zeroing it.

10. Once you've evaluated the dynamic response of the pressure monitoring system, the only way to verify transducer accuracy is by applying a known value to it. Which procedure is *not* appropriate when doing this?

    a. Perform the square wave test.

    b. Detach a sphygmomanometer cuff; then attach the end of sterile, fluid-filled pressure extension tubing to the zero port of the stopcock. Pump the hand bulb to 200 mm Hg; the monitor display should read 200 mm Hg.

    c. Apply a water column to the transducer; then apply a hydrostatic pressure of approximately 22 mm Hg. The monitor display should read 22 mm Hg.

    d. Use a calibration device attached to the back of the disposable transducer, and apply a negative pressure (which is converted to a positive pressure on the monitor).

11. Direct arterial pressure monitoring is more accurate in patients with low cardiac output and high systemic vascular resistance. Direct monitoring is *not* preferred for patients with:

    a. obesity.

    b. severe edema.

    c. diabetes mellitus.

    d. hypovolemia and vasoconstriction.

12. Which artery is rarely used for direct arterial pressure monitoring in adults?

    a. Radial artery

    b. Axillary artery

    c. Brachial artery

    d. Femoral artery

13. Which of the following does *not* cause erroneous direct arterial pressure readings?

    a. Lack of air in the catheter

    b. A positional catheter

    c. Improper zeroing of the transducer

    d. Additional stopcocks or extension tubing

14. After your patient's arterial line is discontinued:

    a. check the catheter insertion site for bleeding.

    b. assess circulation in the extremity distal to the insertion site.

    c. apply a pressure dressing (for a femoral insertion site).

    d. do all of the above.

15. Cardiac output — the volume of blood pumped by the ventricle in 1 minute — is influenced by the heart rate and the amount of blood ejected during each heartbeat. Another term for the amount of blood ejected during each heartbeat is:

    a. cardiac reserve function.

    b. afterload.

    c. contractility.

    d. stroke volume.

16. Pulmonary artery perforation can occur in any patient with a pulmonary artery catheter. However, this complication is most common in patients with:

    a. obesity.

    b. pulmonary hypotension.

    c. advanced age and pulmonary hypertension.

    d. hypovolemia.

17. Which nursing measure would *not* reduce anxiety and promote safety in a patient with a pulmonary artery catheter?

    a. Explain to the patient that the catheter is monitoring pressures in his heart and lungs.

    b. Inform the patient that he can move about normally as long as he stays in bed.

    c. Administer mild analgesics to relieve tenderness at the insertion site.

    d. Reassure the patient that the catheter poses little danger to his health.

18. Central venous pressure (CVP) monitoring helps the health care team evaluate venous return to the heart and indirectly reflects how well the patient's heart is pumping. Normal CVP ranges from:

    a. 4 to 10 mm Hg.

    b. 10 to 15 mm Hg.

    c. 1 to 7 mm Hg.

    d. 1 to 4 mm Hg.

19. Cardiac output may diminish from any condition that weakens myocardial contraction, including myocardial infarction, cardiomyopathy, cardiac tamponade, acidosis, hypoxia, and cardiac depressant drug therapy. Which condition may *increase* cardiac output?

    a. Systemic inflammatory response syndrome

    b. Arteriosclerosis

    c. Valvular disease

    d. Hypertension

20. Which of the following does *not* determine stroke volume?

    a. Heart rate

    b. Contractility

    c. Afterload

    d. Preload

21. To obtain accurate cardiac output measurements using the thermodilution technique, you must make sure that:

    a. the indicator has been measured accurately.

    b. the indicator has been thoroughly mixed with blood.

    c. the indicator hasn't been recirculated or lost.

    d. all of the above.

22. Cerebral perfusion pressure (CPP) is an estimate of cerebral blood flow. For adults, CPP normally ranges from:

    a. 120 to 150 mm Hg.

    b. 50 to 70 mm Hg.

    c. 70 to 100 mm Hg.

    d. 25 to 50 mm Hg.

23. For continuous intracranial pressure (ICP) monitoring, the surgeon may place the sensor anywhere in the brain *except* the:

    a. arterioles.

    b. ventricles.

    c. subarachnoid space.

    d. parenchyma.

24. ICP monitoring is recommended for any patient who's at risk for intracranial hypertension. ICP monitoring is *not* indicated for patients with:

    a. subarachnoid hemorrhage.

    b. a tumor that obstructs the ventricular system.

    c. cerebral aneurysm.

    d. headache.

25. When caring for a patient who's undergoing ICP monitoring, you should:

    a. avoid stimulating him before obtaining ICP readings, and make sure his head is in the same position for all readings.

    b. correlate ICP increases with any activity taking place around the patient.

    c. identify baseline ICP before starting a care activity and then monitor for ICP changes during the activity; ensure that ICP returns to baseline within 5 minutes after the activity ends.

    d. do all of the above.

26. The most serious complication of ICP monitoring and cortical blood flow monitoring is:

    a. hemorrhage.

    b. cerebrospinal fluid leakage.

    c. infection.

    d. an inaccurate monitor value.

27. Which statement about pulse oximetry is true?

    a. Pulse oximetry reliably detects hypoxemia in a patient with carbon monoxide poisoning.

    b. Pulse oximetry readings aren't affected by ambient light.

    c. Pulse oximetry provides continuous data about the amount of oxygen dissolved in plasma.

    d. Pulse oximetry may yield false-low values in a patient with venous pulsations.

28. During end-tidal carbon dioxide ($ETCO_2$) monitoring, a rounded alveolar plateau on the waveform represents:

    a. normal carbon dioxide concentration in exhaled gas.

    b. reduced pulmonary blood flow.

    c. esophageal intubation.

    d. incomplete exhalation.

29. If your patient's mixed venous oxygen saturation ($S\bar{v}O_2$) value rises from 68% to 80%, what would you suspect?

    a. His oxygen delivery has decreased.

    b. His oxygen consumption has increased.

    c. His oxygen delivery has increased.

    d. His oxygen delivery has decreased and his oxygen consumption has increased.

30. Which condition does *not* cause hypoxia in the fetus?

    a. Hydramnios

    b. Cord compression

    c. Maternal hypertension

    d. Dorsal recumbent position of the mother

31. If variable decelerations appear on your patient's fetal heart rate monitor, which measure should you take first?

    a. Discontinue oxytocin.

    b. Notify the doctor.

    c. Change the patient's position.

    d. Increase the I.V. infusion rate.

32. Fetal scalp blood sampling provides information about fetal pH and the partial pressures of arterial oxygen and carbon dioxide. What is the normal pH of fetal blood?

    a. 7.20

    b. 7.25 to 7.35

    c. 7.20 to 7.24

    d. 7.40 to 7.50

33. The most abundant electrolytes in intracellular fluid (ICF) are:

    a. potassium and sodium.

    b. potassium and chloride.

    c. potassium and phosphate.

    d. sodium and chloride.

34. Using the vascular intermittent access system, you can measure your patient's:

    a. blood gases.

    b. serum electrolytes.

    c. hematocrit.

    d. all of the above.

35. Intra-aortic balloon (IAB) counterpulsation temporarily supports the left ventricle through controlled mechanical displacement of blood in the aorta. This procedure is indicated for patients with:

    a. aortic aneurysms.

    b. ventricular arrhythmias.

    c. severe clotting disorders.

    d. severe aorto-iliac disease.

36. The IAB is usually inserted into the:

    a. radial artery, with the balloon tip just lateral to the left subclavian artery.

    b. left subclavian vein.

    c. right anterior jugular vein.

    d. common femoral artery, with the balloon tip just distal to the left subclavian artery.

37. Pulse amplitude monitoring is *not* used:

    a. after peripheral vascular reconstruction surgery.

    b. if the patient has Alzheimer's disease.

    c. if the patient has undergone coronary angioplasty.

    d. after percutaneous transluminal peripheral angioplasty.

38. The automated vital signs monitor allows a patient who needs continuous vital signs monitoring to remain on the medical-surgical unit, avoiding transfer to an intensive care unit (ICU). However, transfer to the ICU is required if the patient:

    a. has chronic renal failure.

    b. has chronic congestive heart failure.

    c. is receiving I.V. nitroglycerin.

    d. has ventricular arrhythmias.

Answers and rationales

1. c. Cardiac monitoring is used to monitor the heart rate, detect ST-segment changes, and identify arrhythmias. It doesn't tell the nurse when the patient is experiencing pain, shortness of breath, or other symptoms.

2. a. The electrical current that travels through the heart is called a vector. A bipolar ECG monitoring system uses two electrodes placed at opposite poles of the heart's electrical field. When electrical current travels toward the positive electrode, the ECG records a positive complex.

3. d. Cardiac monitoring doesn't require insertion of an I.V. line or infusion of an I.V. solution (except during a thallium stress test).

4. b. With a five-electrode ECG monitoring system, you'd place the chest electrode of the V lead at the fourth intercostal space along the right sternal border. The V_6 lead belongs at the fifth intercostal space in the left midaxillary line.

5. b. V_1 or MCL_1 or V_6 or MCL_6 is the best lead for detecting a new bundle-branch block in a patient with a recent myocardial infarction.

6. d. An ST-segment deviation of more than 1 mm from the baseline is considered significant.

7. c. Frequency response is the ability to accurately reproduce and display the vibrations or frequencies applied to the pressure monitoring system. To ensure adequate frequency response, the pressure monitoring system must have good reproducibility or fidelity. Resonant frequency refers to the vibrations sensed in the pressure tubing during systole. Hydrostatic (head-height) pressure depends on the vertical height and density of fluid in a vessel. Dynamic pressure refers to dynamic flow changes occurring within a vessel or cardiac chamber when blood travels through it.

8. a. The ideal tubing for a pressure system is noncompliant. With compliant (soft) tubing, some vibrations are lost, causing overdamping. Air bubbles and additional stopcocks that interrupt the fluid-filled path also can diminish vibrations excessively and cause overdamping.

9. b. Opening the stopcock to air is one of the steps in the procedure you perform when zeroing the transducer. Insufficient transducer warm-up time, atmospheric pressure changes in the patient's room, and transducer movement after zeroing can adversely affect zeroing.

10. a. You perform the square wave test to verify the accuracy and dynamic response of the monitoring system. Then, to verify transducer accuracy, you perform one of the other three procedures described here.

11. c. Unlike the other patients listed here, diabetic patients don't necessarily require direct arterial pressure monitoring.

12. b. In adults, the radial, brachial, and femoral arteries are most commonly used for arterial pressure monitoring. The axillary artery and dorsalis pedis are rarely used.

13. a. Air in the catheter—not lack of it—can cause erroneous arterial pressure readings, as can the other factors listed here.

14. d. After arterial line removal, you should check the catheter insertion site for bleeding, assess circulation in the extremity distal to the insertion site, and apply a pressure dressing if the femoral artery was used.

15. d. Stroke volume is the amount of blood ejected during each heartbeat. Cardiac output equals heart rate multiplied by stroke volume. Stroke volume is determined by preload, afterload, and contractility. These three components are interrelated and play an important role in maintaining oxygen

delivery to the tissues. Cardiac reserve function is the heart's ability to store energy or increase blood flow when it's overtaxed—for example, when the heart rate increases.

16. c. Pulmonary artery perforation is most likely to occur in elderly patients with pulmonary hypertension.

17. b. To help prevent catheter dislodgment, you should advise the patient to use caution when moving about in bed.

18. c. Normal CVP ranges from 1 to 7 mm Hg (as reflected by the mean value).

19. a. Systemic inflammatory response syndrome (sepsis) increases both cardiac output and myocardial oxygen demand. Arteriosclerosis, valvular disease, and hypertension reduce cardiac output.

20. a. Heart rate affects—but doesn't determine—stroke volume. Contractility, afterload, and preload determine stroke volume. Contractility refers to the intensity of myofibril contraction. Afterload is the resistance the ventricles must overcome to eject blood. Preload is ventricular wall tension at end diastole, which is affected mainly by venous return to the heart.

21. d. All of these conditions are required to ensure accurate cardiac output measurements using the thermodilution technique.

22. c. In adults, normal CPP measures 70 to 100 mm Hg.

23. a. An ICP sensor can be placed in the ventricles, subarachnoid or epidural space, or brain parenchyma. It can't be placed in an arteriole.

24. d. ICP monitoring isn't indicated for patients with headache unless diagnostic tests suggest the need. It is indicated for patients with trauma, subarachnoid hemorrhage, tumors that obstruct the ventricular space, intracranial hemorrhage, cerebral aneurysm, or Reye's syndrome.

25. d. All of these nursing measures help ensure accurate ICP values.

26. c. Infection is the most serious complication of both ICP monitoring and cortical blood flow monitoring.

27. d. Venous pulsations may cause false-low arterial oxygen saturation measurements. In a patient with carbon monoxide poisoning, more complete assessment of oxygenation is warranted because pulse oximetry reflects only functional hemoglobin saturation. Ambient light may cause unreliable pulse oximetry readings; the sensor should be covered to protect the optical elements from light. Pulse oximetry continuously measures the amount of oxygen combined with hemoglobin, not the amount dissolved in plasma.

28. d. Incomplete exhalation may cause a rounded plateau, representing impaired alveolar emptying, and the monitor value won't accurately estimate $ETCO_2$. With reduced pulmonary blood flow or esophageal intubation, the monitor won't detect exhaled carbon dioxide and won't display a waveform.

29. c. $S\bar{v}O_2$ rises when oxygen delivery increases or when sepsis occurs (because tissues can't extract enough oxygen for their needs). Decreased oxygen delivery and increased oxygen consumption — separately or in combination — may reduce $S\bar{v}O_2$.

30. a. Hydramnios does not cause fetal hypoxia, while cord compression, maternal hypertension, or a maternal dorsal recumbent position can.

31. c. A change in maternal position, especially the left lateral decubitus position, will remove pressure on the umbilical cord and correct maternal hypotension or hypertension.

32. b. The normal pH of fetal blood ranges from 7.25 to 7.35.

33. c. Potassium and phosphate are the most abundant electrolytes in ICF. Potassium affects resting membrane potentials and is important in muscle contraction and myocardial membrane responsiveness. Phosphate is essential for energy metabolism and combines with calcium to form a key component for bones and teeth.

34. d. The vascular intermittent access system allows measurement of blood gases, serum electrolytes, and hematocrit.

35. b. IAB counterpulsation is indicated in patients with ventricular arrhythmias associated with ischemia. It's contraindicated in patients with aortic aneurysm, severe clotting disorders, aorto-iliac disease, or aortic regurgitation.

36. d. The IAB is usually inserted through the common femoral artery and positioned with the balloon tip just distal to the left subclavian artery.

37. b. Pulse amplitude monitoring is ineffective if the patient moves continuously (for example, from shivering or uncooperativeness) because these movements will distort the waveforms. A patient with Alzheimer's disease may not remember instructions to stay as still as possible. Pulse amplitude monitoring can be used after vascular reconstruction or angioplasty.

38. d. The patient with ventricular arrhythmias requires ECG monitoring, which isn't available on a medical-surgical unit.

Index

i refers to illustration; t refers to a table

i refers to illustration; t refers to a table